Equine Gait Analysis: Translating Science into Practice

Equine Gait Analysis: Translating Science into Practice

Guest Editors

Hilary M. Clayton
Lindsay St. George

MDPI

Basel • Beijing • Wuhan • Barcelona • Belgrade • Novi Sad • Cluj • Manchester

Guest Editors
Hilary M. Clayton
Large Animal Clinical Sciences
Michigan State University
East Lansing
USA

Lindsay St. George
School of Health, Social Work and Sport
University of Central Lancashire
Preston
United Kingdom

Editorial Office
MDPI AG
Grossp eteranlage 5
4052 Basel, Switzerland

This is a reprint of the Special Issue, published open access by the journal *Animals* (ISSN 2076-2615), freely accessible at: https://www.mdpi.com/journal/animals/special_issues/GQ9P0LSAQX.

For citation purposes, cite each article independently as indicated on the article page online and as indicated below:

Lastname, A.A.; Lastname, B.B. Article Title. *Journal Name* **Year**, *Volume Number*, Page Range.

ISBN 978-3-7258-4131-8 (Hbk)
ISBN 978-3-7258-4132-5 (PDF)
https://doi.org/10.3390/books978-3-7258-4132-5

Cover image courtesy of Hilary M. Clayton

Contents

About the Editors

Hilary M. Clayton

Hilary M. Clayton is a veterinarian, researcher, and horsewoman. For more than 45 years, she has performed innovative research in the areas of equine locomotor biomechanics, lameness, rehabilitation, conditioning programs for equine athletes, and the interaction between rider, tack, and horse. She has published 8 books and more than 250 peer-reviewed papers on these topics. Clayton served as the Mary Anne McPhail Dressage Chair in Equine Sports Medicine at Michigan State University's College of Veterinary Medicine from 1997 until she retired from academia in 2014. She continues to conduct collaborative research with colleagues in universities around the world. Dr. Clayton was awarded a Fellowship from the Royal College of Veterinary Surgeons in 2018. She is a charter diplomate and past president of the American College of Veterinary Sports Medicine and Rehabilitation. She is an Honorary Fellow of the International Society for Equitation Science and has been inducted into the Roemer Foundation/USDF Hall of Fame, the International Equine Veterinarians Hall of Fame, the Midwest Dressage Association Hall of Fame, and the Saskatoon Sports Hall of Fame. She is a lifelong rider and has competed in many equestrian sports, most recently focusing on dressage in which she trains through the Grand Prix level.

Lindsay St. George

Lindsay is a Research Fellow at the University of Central Lancashire, where she completed her PhD in 2017. She is research-active in equine and human biomechanics, with a special interest in using surface electromyography (sEMG) to investigate athletic performance in horses and how muscles facilitate normal and abnormal gait. Her current research also involves the development of best practice and the standardization of methods for acquiring, processing, and analyzing equine sEMG signals. She has also been involved in conducting research for the Fédération Équestre Internationale (FEI), the international governing body for equestrian sport. Lindsay's research on equine biomechanics and the use of sEMG within this field have been published widely in the *Equine Veterinary Journal*, the *American Journal of Veterinary Research, Frontiers in Veterinary Science, PLOS One*, and the *Journal of Electromyography and Kinesiology*. She is the recipient of competitive research awards, including a 2021 Morris Animal Foundation Fellowship to evaluate the impact of equine lameness on movement and muscle activity with colleagues at Utrecht University and Delsys/Altec Inc. and the 2018 British Society of Animal Science Steve Bishop Early Career Award. Lindsay is an accredited Animal Scientist (Associate) (R.Anim.Sci) through the Royal Society of Biology and the British Society of Animal Science Register of Accredited Animal Scientists and Animal Technologists. Currently, Lindsay is involved in several national and international equine research collaborations, as well as supervising postgraduate student research. She acts as a reviewer for several scientific journals and disseminates her knowledge and expertise outside of academia through podcasts, layperson articles, book chapters, webinars, and workshops.

Preface

From ancient cave paintings to modern research labs, equine locomotion remains a source of fascination. The past half-century has seen what Professor René van Weeren describes as the "Second Golden age of equine locomotion research". Recent developments have been made possible through advances in computerization, micro-electronics, artificial intelligence, and the development of lightweight, wireless sensors that have allowed equine gait analysis to migrate from the sophisticated research laboratory to the field. Researchers, veterinarians, and equestrians can now acquire high-quality data from horses in motion during clinical evaluations or athletic pursuits. This Special Issue is dedicated to showcasing applications for existing and new techniques in equine gait analysis and to demonstrating their value in analyzing a broad spectrum of equestrian activities. The plethora of topics covered in this Special Issue include clinical diagnostic and surveillance applications for lameness and field studies to evaluate and monitor equine gait and athletic performance. The novel areas of investigation covered in this reprint include characterizations of gait type and quality of movement; the harnessing of artificial intelligence for lameness detection; the electromyographic evaluation of muscle function during canter; the evaluation of limb–arena surface interactions during jumping, thresholds for upper body asymmetry parameters during straight and circular motion, a comparison of axial and limb movement asymmetries of high-level dressage horses during fitness-to-compete (in-hand) and ridden conditions at trot; and the effect of tack design on performance. Some of the studies are based on well-established techniques, such as videography, used with or without dedicated software to aid in data reduction. Other studies make use of novel, emerging techniques, made possible through the development of body-mounted motion and electromyography sensors, as well as cell phone apps that take advantage of the smartphone's built-in camera and artificial intelligence to quantify asymmetries in equine gait. Applications of artificial intelligence, markerless motion capture, and wearable electromyography and motion sensors are undoubtedly only the tip of an emerging iceberg in the transference of science into the hands of practitioners and equestrians via field-deployable and user-friendly applications for analyzing equine gait. The future in this arena of research is promising.

Hilary M. Clayton and Lindsay St. George
Guest Editors

animals

MDPI

Article

Is Markerless More or Less? Comparing a Smartphone Computer Vision Method for Equine Lameness Assessment to Multi-Camera Motion Capture

Felix Järemo Lawin [1], Anna Byström [2], Christoffer Roepstorff [1], Marie Rhodin [2], Mattias Almlöf [1], Mudith Silva [1], Pia Haubro Andersen [2], Hedvig Kjellström [3] and Elin Hernlund [1,2,*]

1 Sleip AI, Birger Jarlsgatan 58, 11426 Stockholm, Sweden
2 Department of Anatomy, Physiology and Biochemistry, Swedish University of Agricultural Sciences, 75007 Uppsala, Sweden
3 KTH Royal Institute of Technology, Division of Robotics, Perception and Learning, 10044 Stockholm, Sweden
* Correspondence: elin.hernlund@slu.se; Tel.: +46-18-672142

Simple Summary: Lameness, an alteration of the gait due to pain or dysfunction of the locomotor system, is the most common disease symptom in horses. Yet, it is difficult for veterinarians to correctly assess by visual inspection. Objective tools that can aid clinical decision making and provide early disease detection through sensitive lameness measurements are needed. In this study, we describe how an AI-powered measurement tool on a smartphone can detect lameness in horses without the need to mount equipment on the horse. We compare it to a state-of-the-art multi-camera motion capture system by simultaneous, synchronised recordings from both systems. The mean difference between the systems' output of lameness metrics was below 2.2 mm. Therefore, we conclude that the smartphone measurement tool can detect lameness at relevant levels with easy-of-use for the veterinarian.

Abstract: Computer vision is a subcategory of artificial intelligence focused on extraction of information from images and video. It provides a compelling new means for objective orthopaedic gait assessment in horses using accessible hardware, such as a smartphone, for markerless motion analysis. This study aimed to explore the lameness assessment capacity of a smartphone single camera (SC) markerless computer vision application by comparing measurements of the vertical motion of the head and pelvis to an optical motion capture multi-camera (MC) system using skin attached reflective markers. Twenty-five horses were recorded with a smartphone (60 Hz) and a 13 camera MC-system (200 Hz) while trotting two times back and forth on a 30 m runway. The smartphone video was processed using artificial neural networks detecting the horse's direction, action and motion of body segments. After filtering, the vertical displacement curves from the head and pelvis were synchronised between systems using cross-correlation. This rendered 655 and 404 matching stride segmented curves for the head and pelvis respectively. From the stride segmented vertical displacement signals, differences between the two minima (MinDiff) and the two maxima (MaxDiff) respectively per stride were compared between the systems. Trial mean difference between systems was 2.2 mm (range 0.0–8.7 mm) for head and 2.2 mm (range 0.0–6.5 mm) for pelvis. Within-trial standard deviations ranged between 3.1–28.1 mm for MC and between 3.6–26.2 mm for SC. The ease of use and good agreement with MC indicate that the SC application is a promising tool for detecting clinically relevant levels of asymmetry in horses, enabling frequent and convenient gait monitoring over time.

Keywords: monocular motion analysis; objective lameness assessment; equine orthopaedics; animal pose estimation; optical motion capture

1. Introduction

Objective measurement of a horse's motion at the trot has become an important part of the diagnostic procedures performed during clinical lameness investigation. These measurements, which have been used in clinical practice for more than a decade, trace the vertical displacement of axial body segments: the head, the pelvis and sometimes the withers. Using reflective markers or inertial sensors attached to a point on each body segment, a time series signal is generated. In trot, the vertical displacement signal takes the shape of a sinusoidal double wave from each stride and it is the position of the two peaks and valleys of this signal which are used for lameness analysis.

The degree of asymmetry in the vertical displacement signal i.e., the difference between the two peaks and valleys respectively is known to indicate asymmetric loading of the left versus right limb during the midstance and the push-off phases of the stride [1–3]. Measurements of these asymmetries provide the veterinarian with high-resolution data that help overcome the limited time resolution of the human visual system [4,5]. These objective data seem crucial for quality control of the clinical procedure, since subjective lameness assessment has been shown to have moderate to low agreement between veterinarians [6,7] and is affected by expectation bias [8]. The metrics derived from objective motion analysis show high sensitivity for single-limb lameness, acting as early indicators to detect asymmetric loading of the limbs [9]. However, the specificity for lameness on a population level is less clear. Motion asymmetries are commonly observed in cross-sectional studies of different horse populations, such as Warmblood riding horses [10,11], Thoroughbred race horses [12], working Polo horses [13], elite eventing horses [14], endurance horses [15] and young Standardbred trotters [16], with a prevalence ranging between 50–90 percent. Although these asymmetries are of the same magnitude as in horses investigated for lameness in a clinical setting [17], it is currently unknown if these asymmetry levels indicate that a large proportion of horses in training are lame or if the asymmetries can be explained by other factors, such as laterality. A key approach to the further investigation of this issue is to perform longitudinal monitoring of individual horses over time. For this to be possible, a reliable, ease of use and low-cost measuring system is required.

Several motion analysis systems have been developed for clinical use based on inertial measurement units (IMUs) [18–20]. Also available is a multi-camera marker-based motion capture (MC) system [21]. This MC-system, is considered to be the gold standard for measuring body segment movement for kinematic gait analysis [22]. It relies on reflective markers attached to a horse's body. These markers are detected and tracked by a set of cameras that are geometrically calibrated and temporally synchronized. By using the synchronized tracks of the marker positions in the camera images, MC-systems reconstruct the 3D coordinates using multi-view triangulation. It has been shown that under favourable conditions, the accuracy of the computed estimates of the 3D positions over time is less than a millimetre for the MC-systems [23]. However, placing markers on the horse are resource and time-consuming in a clinical situation, and the equipment is a substantial financial investment for a veterinary practice. This impedes the system's large-scale clinical and scientific use.

During the previous decade, the field of computer vision was revolutionized by methods based on deep neural networks [24–26]. These networks are computer algorithms that consist of multi-layered (referred to as deep) compositions of parametric functions that can be trained on large datasets to perform classification and regression tasks. Deep learning has demonstrated increased robustness to differing scenarios, light conditions, and noise levels compared to traditional computer vision methods. Estimation of poses of the human body from images has been enabled by deep learning and as a result of this development, it has become possible to perform motion analysis from video, e.g., from a smartphone camera [27]. Recent works on horse lameness classification [28,29] have demonstrated a progressive movement towards the application of computer vision and deep learning within objective motion analysis. However, a binary disease classifier of "lame" versus "not lame" is a difficult approach for clinical use, given that lameness is often not a binary state and that the deep learning algorithms act in a black box manner, rendering distrust from medical professionals [30]. Instead, providing a clinician with computer vision derived metrics to support medical decision making is a more implementable approach. But until now, the methodological accuracy of deep neural networks for quantification of clinically used lameness metrics has not been investigated.

In this work, we validate a new single-camera markerless (SC) system designed for equine lameness assessment which uses images from a smartphone camera video stream. To achieve robust detection and tracking, the system employs a series of neural networks. These networks were trained to detect and track the pelvis, head and hooves in video streams of trotting horses. The system also detects the trotting direction of the horse, away from or towards the camera, to determine which parts of the horse are visible for measuring. The network designs were inspired by previously proposed methods for object detection [28,31] and segmentation [32,33]. Unlike the MC-system, the deep neural networks of the SC-system do not require that markers are placed on the horse. Instead, the networks learn to detect the points of interest on the horse's body visible in the images through training on large datasets.

The specific aim of the study was to compare this new markerless smartphone system to a state-of-the-art multi-camera marker-based system with respect to waveform similarity of the derived vertical displacement signals and the limits of agreement for their extracted lameness metrics.

2. Materials and Methods

2.1. Study Protocol

Twenty-five horses were recorded as they underwent motion analysis at the orthopedic gait laboratory situated in the Equine Clinic of the University Animal Hospital in Uppsala, Sweden. The recordings were performed simultaneously with a multi-camera marker-based motion capture system and a single smartphone camera markerless system. The experimental setup is illustrated in Figure 1. The study subjects were a convenience sample selected from the horses visiting the clinic during the 10-day data collection period, without any exclusion criteria. The horses were of different breeds, sizes (range 128 to 180 cm to the withers) and colours (black, bay, chestnut, grey). All owners gave their written informed consent to participate. The study did not in any way alter the clinical procedures or add physical manipulation of the animals. Hence, no ethical approval was required according to the national animal ethics legislation.

2.2. Data Collection

During data collection, each horse was guided by a handler (the owner, or a researcher running at the horse's left side) to trot at least two times back and forth on a 30 m concrete runway in a corridor. The horses were jogged at the handler's preferred speed.

We employed a MC-system with 13 cameras (Qualisys AB, Motion Capture Systems). The MC cameras were placed $\approx$ 4 m over the ground and in a manner such that the union of the field of view of each camera covered as much of the runway as possible while still maintaining sufficient overlap between neighboring cameras to perform tracking and triangulation of the marker positions. The recording rate was set to 200 Hz. We attached spherical reflective markers in the median plane over the poll on the horse's head and between the tubera sacrale of the pelvis, allowing the MC-system to detect and track the markers over time. Additional markers were placed, but not used in this study (see Figure 2).

The smartphone (iPhone12 Pro Max) was placed $\approx$ 1.6 m above the ground on a tripod facing the direction of the horse trot recording 4k video (2160 $\times$ 3840 pixels) at 60 Hz. The video streams recorded were input to the SC-system. Example frames from the smartphone camera recordings are shown in Figure 2.

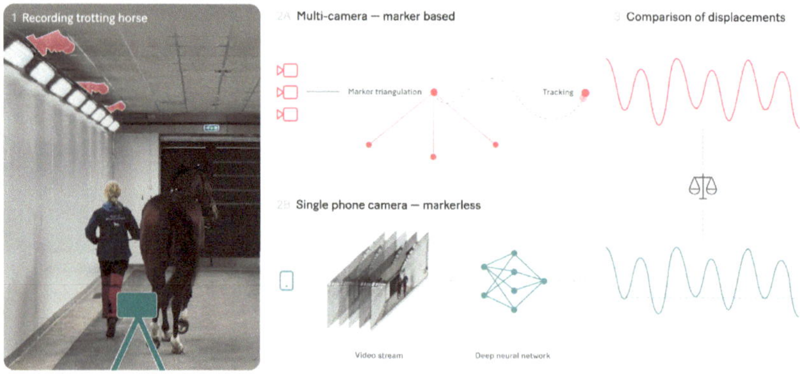

Figure 1. Illustration of the experimental setup. We recorded horses trotting back and forth in a corridor with a multi-camera system and a single smartphone camera. The multi-camera system detected and tracked reflective markers attached to the horse. Marker positions were triangulated into 3D coordinates from which vertical displacement curves were extracted. The single-camera system used deep neural networks to predict the vertical displacement curves of the head and pelvis from the images in the smartphone video stream. We then compared the displacement curves from the two systems using normalised peak and valley differences.

For each recording, the MC-system and the smartphone camera were triggered at approximately the same time such that the data streams from both systems would cover the same sequence of events.

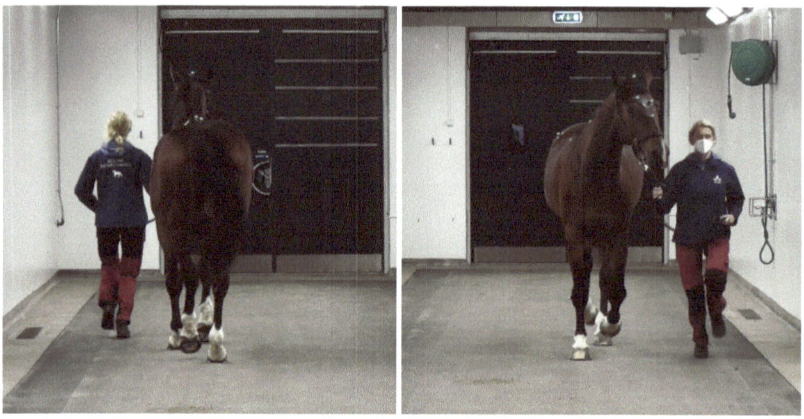

Figure 2. Example images from data set (horse 21) taken from the video recorded by the markerless single-camera system (SC). Attached to the horse's skin by double adhesive tape are the spherical reflective markers used by the multi-camera marker-based system (MC) for tracking head and pelvic motion. The markers on the poll and between the tubera sacrale were used.

2.3. Signal Extraction

The MC-system software (Qualisys Track Manager—QTM, Qualisys AB) automatically tracked the reflective markers and generated 3D coordinates corresponding to the positions of the markers in each frame. The 3D marker coordinates from QTM were exported to .mat files (MATLAB). From these coordinates, vertical displacements were extracted for each frame, one for the head marker and one for the pelvis marker. This resulted in two vertical displacement signals (VDS), $y_{mc}^{head}(t)$ and $y_{mc}^{pelvis}(t)$ for head and pelvis respectively, where t is time in seconds.

For the SC-system, deep neural networks were applied (software of Sleip AI AB) on the input video stream from the smartphone camera. The deep neural networks were trained to output the pixel coordinates of horse body parts for each frame of the video. The training material for the deep neural networks contained horses of many different coat colours and varying conformation, but none had physical markers attached to the skin. Head ($y_{sc}^{head}(t)$) and pelvis ($y_{sc}^{pelvis}(t)$) VDS was calculated from the pixel coordinates. Additionally, the VDS of all four hooves were extracted from the SC-system for stride splitting purposes (see Section 2.4). Both the MC-system and the SC-system data were further processed using custom written python scripts.

Note that the pelvis was visible to the SC-system only when the horse was trotting away from the camera, while the head was mostly visible in both directions. Consequently, SC generally produced data from a higher number of strides with head tracking than strides with pelvic tracking. The following analyses only included strides with data matched from both systems for the body segment in question (head and pelvis). Horses were removed from the dataset where less than 10 matching strides were available for either head or pelvis since we deemed that insufficient for statistical relevance.

2.4. Stride Split and Signal Filtering

The recorded data contained noise, due to measurement errors and because the horses seldom trot in a consistent manner throughout a trot-up. This noise was present for both the MC-system and the SC-system data. Thus, the VDS had to be band-pass filtered in order to remove the noise without affecting the frequency content of the signal that related to movement asymmetries and lameness [34].

In order to perform the VDS filtering described in [34], the within horse mean stride frequency of a measurement was needed. This was estimated by extracting strides from the hoof VDS of the SC-system. Firstly, we performed a pre band-pass filtering of the hoof VDS to remove trends and high-frequency noise. Specifically, a 7th order Butterworth digital filter with a lower bound cut-off frequency of 0.6 Hz and an upper bound cut-off frequency of 2.2 Hz. This allowed us to determine in which time intervals the left hoof was above the right hoof and vice versa, ultimately enabling the classification of left and right strides.

Next, the lengths of the intervals were used to compute the stride frequency, which in turn was used to set the bounds of the 10th order Butterworth band-pass filter applied to the VDS of the pelvis and head. Specifically, we set the lower bound to 0.75 times the stride frequency, to not alter frequency content related to the movement asymmetry [34]. Similarly, the upper bound was set to 2.42 times the stride frequency to not attenuate the frequency content related to the symmetric movement, while omitting higher frequency content and noise.

2.5. Signal Synchronization

Since the MC and SC recordings were triggered manually, the extracted signals were not adequately synchronized in time. To synchronize the vertical displacement signals we computed cross-correlations to find the relative time shift t_{shift} that solved the following maximization problem:

$$t_{shift} = \arg\max_{t}\left((y_{mc}^{pelvis} \star y_{sc}^{pelvis})(t) + (y_{mc}^{head} \star y_{sc}^{head})(t) \right). \quad (1)$$

Here $\star$ denotes the correlation operator. The signals were band-pass filtered according to Section 2.4 before synchronization.

2.6. Asymmetry Quantification

In this section, we introduce a number of definitions that we use in the remaining parts of the paper. First, we define a stride segment as a section of the VDS corresponding to a time interval of a full stride. To extract the stride segment we utilize the extreme values (see the illustration in Figure 3). Tracing of the vertical displacement of the horse's head or pelvis while it trots yields a sine-shaped signal as depicted in Figure 3. The valleys (local minima) and peaks (local maxima) of the signal are associated with the vertical forces generated during impact (the more force, the lower the valley position) and the relative timing of horizontal and vertical forces during the propulsive phase of the stride respectively (less push-off rendering a lower peak position). Differences between consecutive peaks or valleys can be quantified into an asymmetry index [22], which can be used as an indicator of lameness severity. Depending on the measurement technique and due to variation in horse size, these values may need to be normalised to be comparable [35,36]. Therefore, normalisation of these values to the range of motion (R) is used in the SC-system to obtain values that are more independent of horse size.

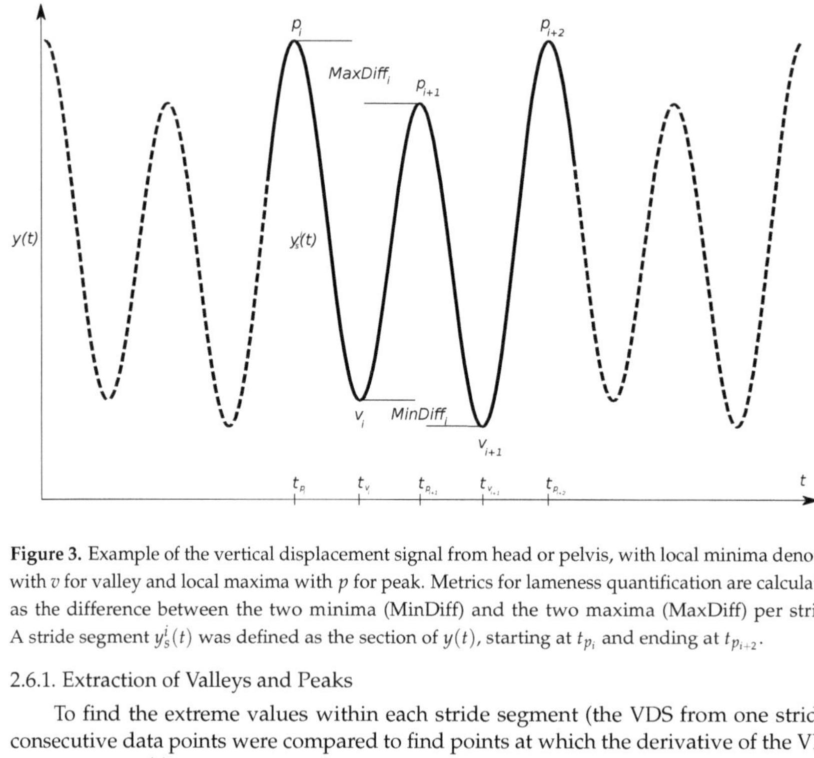

Figure 3. Example of the vertical displacement signal from head or pelvis, with local minima denoted with v for valley and local maxima with p for peak. Metrics for lameness quantification are calculated as the difference between the two minima (MinDiff) and the two maxima (MaxDiff) per stride. A stride segment $y_s^i(t)$ was defined as the section of $y(t)$, starting at t_{p_i} and ending at $t_{p_{i+2}}$.

2.6.1. Extraction of Valleys and Peaks

To find the extreme values within each stride segment (the VDS from one stride), consecutive data points were compared to find points at which the derivative of the VDS was zero. Let $y(t)$ be the VDS value at time t. We defined the peaks $p_i = y(t_{p_i}), i = 1, 2, \ldots,$ as the local maximum values and the valleys $v_j = y(t_{v_j}), j = 1, 2, \ldots,$ as the local minimum values. Further, we assumed that $t_{p_i} < t_{p_{i+1}}$ and $t_{v_j} < t_{v_{j+1}}$. We extracted a sequence of consecutive peaks and valleys $p_i, p_{i+1}, v_j, v_{j+1}$ such that $t_{p_i} < t_{v_j} < t_{p_{i+1}} < t_{v_{j+1}} < t_{p_{i+2}}$.

In horses showing moderate to severe lameness, the changes in motion asymmetry can cause extreme asymmetries in $y(t)$. In these cases, local extreme values might be canceled out, interrupting the assumed stride pattern of two peaks and two valleys in sequence. Instead, a single peak or valley signal pattern occurs. To handle this, we implemented a robust extreme value extraction method. The reasoning behind this method is that $y(t)$ contains two dominant harmonics [1]. The first harmonic corresponds to the stride frequency, thus contributing to the asymmetry of the signal. The second harmonic corresponds to twice the stride frequency and should dominate $y(t)$ if the horse is healthy. In our approach, we extracted extreme values based on the curve shape of the second harmonic. We first removed the asymmetric component of $y(t)$ by performing high-pass filtering with a frequency bound higher than the first harmonic. Next, we employed local extreme value extraction on the high-pass filtered signal. Finally, we refined the selection by selecting the extreme values from the original $y(t)$ within 50 ms of the estimated value. As a result, we were able to estimate normalised peak/valley differences at any degree of lameness.

2.6.2. Normalised Differences for Valleys and Peaks

From the extracted stride peaks we computed local extreme value differences per stride i, consisting of the following scalars,

$$\mathrm{MinDiff}_i = v_{i+1} - v_i \tag{2}$$

$$\mathrm{MaxDiff}_i = p_i - p_{i+1}\,. \tag{3}$$

These values provide information about the asymmetries between the right and left leg impact and push-off. However, since different horses have different amplitudes in their vertical displacement trajectories, these values are not comparable. In this work, we instead use the normalised extreme value differences (NEVd), which show more independence from the scale of the vertical displacement. The NEVd-values were computed using the following operations,

$$V_i = \frac{\mathrm{MinDiff}_i}{R_i} \tag{4}$$

$$P_i = \frac{\mathrm{MaxDiff}_i}{R_i} \tag{5}$$

$$\text{where } R_i = \max(p_i, p_{i+1}) - \min(v_i, v_{i+1})\,.$$

Here, normalization was performed by division by the range-of-motion R_i. Thus, the NEVd-values measures asymmetry as a rate of R_i.

2.6.3. Outlier Removal

To remove occasional strides with erroneous measurements from the analysis, we performed a series of outlier removal steps.

While the noise in the vertical displacement signals is partly suppressed by band-pass filtering, the signal quality becomes inadequate for asymmetry analysis when the noise is too prevalent. Therefore, we first removed strides where the stride segments contained a substantial amount of high-frequency noise. A stride segment was deemed to contain too much high frequency noise when the majority of the frequency content amplitudes were found above 10 Hz in at least a quarter of a stride interval.

As a second step, we performed a linear discriminant analysis (LDA). In addition to $\mathrm{MinDiff}_i$ and $\mathrm{MaxDiff}_i$ from Equation (4), we used the peak valley differences $p_i - v_i$ and $p_{i+1} - v_{i+1}$ to represent each stride as features. We then removed NEVd-values from the analysis that corresponded to strides that were considered outliers in the LDA.

2.7. System Comparisons

We compared the MC and SC systems on the data set of trotting horses described in Section 2.2. For each recorded sample, we used MC and SC to generate vertical displacement signals. From these, we extracted and compared stride segments and NEVd-values between the two systems. The following sections detail the implementation and setup of the comparison.

2.7.1. Comparison Metrics

To compare the extracted asymmetry indices between the MC and SC systems the following deviations were calculated from the synchronized NEVd-vales,

$$\Delta V^i = \text{MinDiff}_i^{sc} - \text{MinDiff}_i^{mc} \tag{6}$$

$$\Delta P^i = \text{MaxDiff}_i^{sc} - \text{MaxDiff}_i^{mc} \ . \tag{7}$$

To recover an estimate of geometric deviation, we multiplied ΔV^i and ΔP^i with the range of motion $R_{i,mc}$ computed from the NEVd-values of the MC signal.

In practice, lameness indication is deduced from the trial mean of the NEVd-values $\bar{V} = 1/N \sum_i^N \text{MinDiff}_i$ and $\bar{P} = 1/N \sum_i^N \text{MaxDiff}_i$, where N is the number of strides in the trial after the outlier removal in Section 2.6.3. We computed the trial mean deviations as,

$$\Delta \bar{V} = \bar{V}^{sc} - \bar{V}^{mc} \tag{8}$$

$$\Delta \bar{P} = \bar{P}^{sc} - \bar{P}^{mc} \ . \tag{9}$$

We further scaled $\Delta \bar{V}$ and $\Delta \bar{P}$ with the mean range of motion $\bar{R}_{mc} = 1/N \sum_i^N R_{i,mc}$ to estimate the geometric deviation.

2.7.2. Statistical Analysis

Bland-Altman analysis [37] was used to evaluate the statistical agreement between the MC and SC-systems for head and pelvis NEVd-values. The Bland-Altman analysis was subdivided into deviations for MinDiff and MaxDiff and was performed both on trial and stride level.

In addition to the comparison of the NEVd-values, we compared the shapes of the band pass filtered vertical displacement signals using the root mean square deviations (RMSD),

$$RMSD = \sqrt{\frac{\sum_{m=1}^{M_i} \left(R_{i,sc}^{mc} \cdot y_{sc}(t_{m,sc}^i) - y_{mc}(t_{m,mc}^i) \right)^2}{M_i}} \tag{10}$$

$$\text{where } R_{i,sc}^{mc} = \frac{R_{i,mc}}{R_{i,sc}} \ .$$

Here, M = 23 is the number of trials, i.e number of horses in the dataset. $t_{m,sc}^i$ and $t_{m,mc}^i$ are equally spaced points in time for sampling the vertical displacement signals corresponding to the ith synchronized stride, i.e $t_{1,sc}^i = p_{i,sc}$, $t_{M,sc}^i = p_{i+2,sc}$, $t_{1,mc}^i = p_{i,mc}$ and $t_{M_i,mc}^i = p_{i+2,mc}$. Note that we scaled the y_{sc} samples to the geometric scale of y_{mc}. Further, since y_{sc} and y_{mc} have different frame rates, we aligned and re-sampled the signals with linear interpolation before applying (10).

3. Results

In this section, we outline the results from the experiments described in Section 2.7. In total, the results below were generated from 23 of the 25 horses in the initial data set, after the exclusion of two horses with less than 10 synchronized strides. From the included horses we extracted a total of 655 stride observations of the head motion and 404 stride observations of the pelvic motion. Descriptive statistics of the head measurements from the 23 trials can be found in Table 1 and the pelvis measurement in Table 2.

Table 1. Descriptive statistics for head measurements from the 23 included horses showing number of matched strides per trial (N) and the mean trial deviations between the two systems for the valley values $\Delta\bar{V}$ (MinDiff) and peak values $\Delta\bar{P}$ (MaxDiff). Also, the actual trial means for the $\bar{V}$ (MinDiff) and the $\bar{P}$ are presented per trial for the multi-camera marker-based (*mc*) and the single-camera markerless (*sc*) systems, followed by their within trial standard deviation (σV and σP). From the *mc*, the trial mean range of motion of the vertical displacement signal is presented.

Horse	N	$\Delta\bar{V}$	$\Delta\bar{P}$	$\bar{V}^{sc}$	$\bar{V}^{mc}$	$\bar{P}^{sc}$	$\bar{P}^{mc}$	σV^{sc}	σV^{mc}	σP^{sc}	σP^{mc}	$\bar{R}_{mc}$
1	16	−0.4	−4.8	−1.5	−1.1	13.1	17.9	15.2	15.4	18.1	16.5	66.6
2	23	−2.1	8.7	−9.4	−7.3	43.0	34.3	12.3	10.4	19.7	20.8	82.2
3	29	2.3	−1.9	−1.6	−3.9	9.5	11.4	17.7	15.0	13.6	14.1	70.4
4	38	4.1	3.4	−39.8	−44.0	−0.8	−4.2	14.3	15.7	14.8	16.8	71.2
5	28	−0.3	2.2	70.0	70.3	−17.5	−19.8	17.4	15.2	17.2	14.5	109.6
6	26	4.4	5.7	−39.2	−43.6	−3.9	−9.6	16.8	19.1	15.8	15.8	68.5
7	19	3.3	−3.1	5.4	2.1	3.3	6.3	13.5	14.2	19.9	21.1	77.5
8	22	−0.6	−3.7	7.1	7.7	8.8	12.5	15.7	11.9	11.0	10.4	73.6
9	29	1.0	−5.0	−39.7	−40.7	15.7	20.6	9.1	10.6	9.5	10.0	70.8
10	36	−0.6	0.6	1.8	2.4	−19.1	−19.8	22.3	22.0	20.7	21.4	95.2
11	27	0.0	0.4	−57.8	−57.9	13.0	12.5	11.5	13.1	16.4	15.2	90.1
12	28	−2.5	1.9	−11.7	−9.2	−18.5	−20.4	14.3	13.5	17.5	14.9	71.0
13	22	−0.0	1.6	62.8	62.8	−3.7	−5.3	8.9	8.2	10.8	10.3	79.8
14	22	0.3	−0.9	−1.6	−1.9	8.7	9.6	9.7	13.8	6.1	10.6	39.0
15	29	1.5	−1.8	27.0	25.5	−14.1	−12.4	13.8	13.1	11.2	11.6	75.2
16	19	−6.8	0.2	22.8	29.6	10.9	10.7	19.1	26.2	18.6	28.1	75.5
17	34	−0.2	−3.7	3.7	3.9	−4.2	−0.5	18.9	17.5	19.6	18.7	95.0
18	24	1.8	−3.1	14.9	13.1	−13.1	−10.1	8.3	7.9	13.6	11.4	57.9
19	35	−0.4	−2.1	0.2	0.6	24.2	26.3	6.9	6.4	8.6	6.0	51.0
20	41	−0.5	1.7	−21.6	−21.0	7.0	5.3	11.9	12.6	9.1	8.5	71.4
21	16	−0.4	1.2	−23.5	−23.0	5.8	4.6	8.4	7.7	6.7	7.4	43.0
22	36	2.2	−1.8	−13.0	−15.2	−1.5	0.3	8.5	8.2	12.3	10.5	50.9
23	56	−4.2	−0.1	−18.2	−14.0	−16.3	−16.2	18.7	17.6	18.8	18.9	74.7
mean	28.5	1.7	2.6	21.5	21.8	12.0	12.6	13.6	13.7	14.3	14.5	72.2

Table 2. Descriptive statistics for pelvic measurements from the 23 included horses showing the number of matched strides per trial (N) and the mean trial deviations between the two systems for the valley values $\Delta\bar{V}$ (MinDiff) and peak values $\Delta\bar{P}$ (MaxDiff). Also, the actual trial means for the $\bar{V}$ (MinDiff) and the $\bar{P}$ are presented per trial for the multi camera marker based (*mc*) and the single camera markerless system (*sc*), followed by their within trial standard deviation (σV and σP). From the *mc*, the trial mean range of motion of the vertical displacement signal is presented.

Horse	N	$\Delta\bar{V}$	$\Delta\bar{P}$	$\bar{V}^{sc}$	$\bar{V}^{mc}$	$\bar{P}^{sc}$	$\bar{P}^{mc}$	σV^{sc}	σV^{mc}	σP^{sc}	σP^{mc}	$\bar{R}_{mc}$
1	13	1.0	−0.1	−0.1	−1.1	6.6	6.6	8.4	6.1	8.2	8.3	83.4
2	15	1.7	4.3	−0.4	−2.1	0.6	−3.8	11.0	8.6	10.0	8.6	82.3
3	16	−1.8	2.1	−0.6	1.2	−2.7	−4.8	6.5	4.0	8.9	5.6	82.6
4	24	4.3	6.5	−15.8	−20.1	21.0	14.5	9.3	7.9	9.6	8.1	92.5
5	17	5.5	−0.5	5.7	0.2	4.3	4.8	5.1	4.3	10.3	11.3	79.3
6	15	4.8	5.9	−12.8	−17.6	27.2	21.3	11.0	7.5	8.9	6.3	92.8
7	17	1.5	0.0	−0.1	−1.5	−5.2	−5.2	6.8	6.9	10.5	8.5	74.8
8	13	1.1	3.1	2.1	1.0	−8.6	−11.6	8.0	8.1	9.2	4.7	76.7
9	15	−0.8	2.2	−13.0	−12.2	−4.3	−6.5	7.1	4.6	6.0	6.0	67.5
10	22	4.6	2.1	9.0	4.4	2.2	0.1	6.5	7.7	15.8	16.0	77.7
11	15	−1.7	0.7	−7.0	−5.3	−11.9	−12.6	6.4	8.3	10.2	9.6	88.0
12	14	−0.9	1.1	−4.5	−3.6	2.6	1.5	6.4	4.8	7.3	7.9	64.7

Table 2. *Cont.*

Horse	N	$\Delta\bar{V}$	$\Delta\bar{P}$	$\bar{V}^{sc}$	$\bar{V}^{mc}$	$\bar{P}^{sc}$	$\bar{P}^{mc}$	σV^{sc}	σV^{mc}	σP^{sc}	σP^{mc}	$\bar{R}_{mc}$
13	11	3.9	2.4	−12.6	−16.5	9.0	6.6	9.7	6.9	8.1	8.5	70.8
14	14	1.3	0.9	−5.1	−6.4	13.0	12.0	5.8	6.7	9.0	8.6	74.8
15	14	−2.3	−3.0	5.8	8.1	−16.9	−13.9	5.7	3.1	6.0	3.3	75.3
16	13	4.2	−1.1	11.8	7.7	−25.8	−24.7	10.5	13.0	13.8	8.7	75.7
17	18	−1.4	−0.8	−10.6	−9.3	−1.4	−0.6	12.2	11.2	11.4	11.5	103.7
18	15	−3.2	−0.3	−2.8	0.4	−13.1	−12.8	5.6	4.6	7.1	3.3	85.5
19	26	1.2	−1.2	−9.6	−10.8	4.4	5.6	3.6	3.4	4.3	4.6	39.6
20	21	−4.9	1.3	−7.2	−2.3	0.1	−1.2	6.5	6.6	11.6	9.0	87.8
21	21	0.8	2.6	−38.0	−38.9	48.5	46.0	7.1	6.8	12.7	8.6	97.7
22	25	−1.5	2.8	−10.2	−8.7	−1.4	−4.2	6.6	5.1	5.5	6.1	67.0
23	30	1.0	0.4	−21.5	−22.6	12.5	12.1	8.9	9.8	8.8	8.0	72.6
mean	17.6	2.4	2.0	9.0	8.8	10.6	10.1	7.6	6.8	9.3	7.9	78.8

We split the comparisons into per-stride and per-trial comparisons. In the per-stride comparisons, we treated each stride as a sample and performed statistical analysis on the stride-based deviations ΔV_i and ΔP_i. In the per-trial comparison, we treated each horse as a sample and performed statistical analysis on deviations computed from the mean NEVd values $\Delta\bar{V}_i$ and $\Delta\bar{P}_i$.

3.1. Per-Stride Comparisons

An example of the time-domain curves from the MC and SC for all strides in a recorded trial (horse 11) are displayed in Figure 4. The displayed stride segments of the two systems show high resemblance, resulting in similar conclusions on lameness diagnosis. We provide more examples from the experiment in Appendix A.

The Bland-Altman analysis for head and pelvis lameness metrics is illustrated in Figures 5 and 6 respectively. The deviations are similar for both valley and peak differences and generally higher for head than for pelvis signals. Moreover, the correlations between the NEVd-values are high and the deviations are generally small, rarely exceeding 21 mm for the head signals and 14 mm for pelvis.

We further provide histograms over the deviations for head and pelvis in Figure 7. The histograms include both V and P-values. In addition, these plots show the empirical estimates of normal distributions computed from the stride samples. The distributions of the absolute values for stride mean residuals are presented in Figure 8.

Finally, we provide mean RMSD values in Table 3 to give an estimate of curve similarity. Note that RMSD, as computed in Table 3, is sensitive to small time shifts. As the synchronization between signals $y_{sc}(t)$ and $y_{mc}(t)$ is approximate, the RMSD does not only reflect curve similarity but also errors in the synchronization.

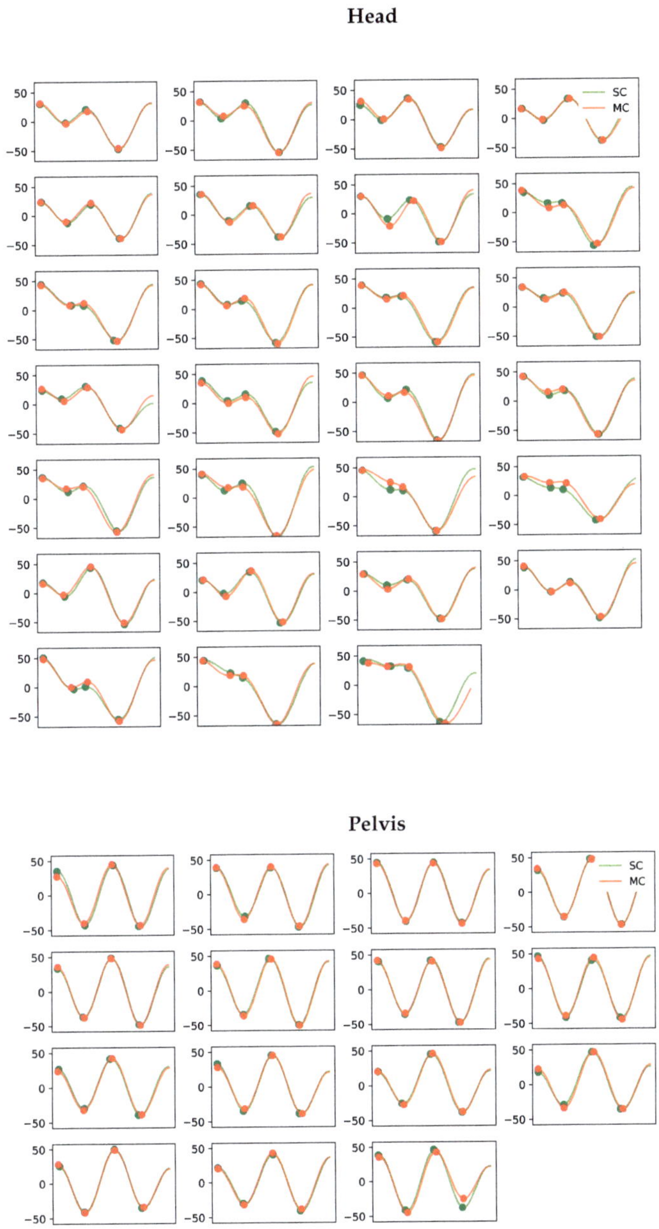

Figure 4. Example of the vertical displacement signal per stride for the head and pelvis for horse 11. Each subplot contains the matched stride segments for the markerless single-camera system (SC) in green and the multi-camera marker-based motion capture system (MC) in red. The y-axis shows the vertical displacement in millimetres. The four dots on each curve indicate the positions of the two peaks and two valleys extracted using the approach in Section 2.6.2. We observe that despite the high variability in curve shape between strides, there is a notable resemblance between the two systems.

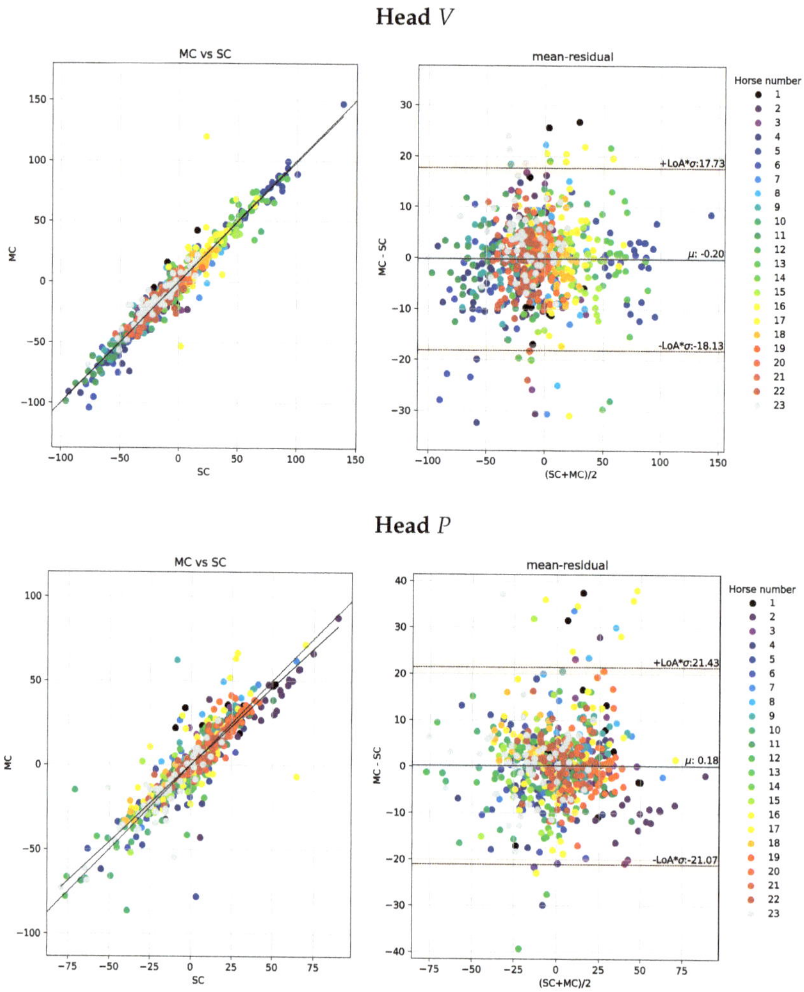

Figure 5. Scatter plots of the head metrics obtained per stride (n = 655) observed by the multi-camera marker-based motion capture system (MC) plotted against the observation by the single-camera markerless system (SC) are shown in the left sub-panels. Agreements between the systems, with limits of agreement (LoA) displayed as orange horizontal lines, are presented in the Bland-Altman plots in the right sub-panels. In the top row, we show the ΔV (MinDiff) and in the bottom row, we show ΔP (MaxDiff) defined in Section 2.7.1. For the purpose of visibility, we have fixed the range of the y-axis, causing a few samples with large residuals to be out of range. In the left plot, we have out of range residuals at 97.0 and −55.2, and in the right plot out of range residuals are at −48.9, −81.5, 70.9, 56.0, −47.1 −71.5, −44.4. While these samples have large errors they have little impact on the overall statistics.

Pelvis V

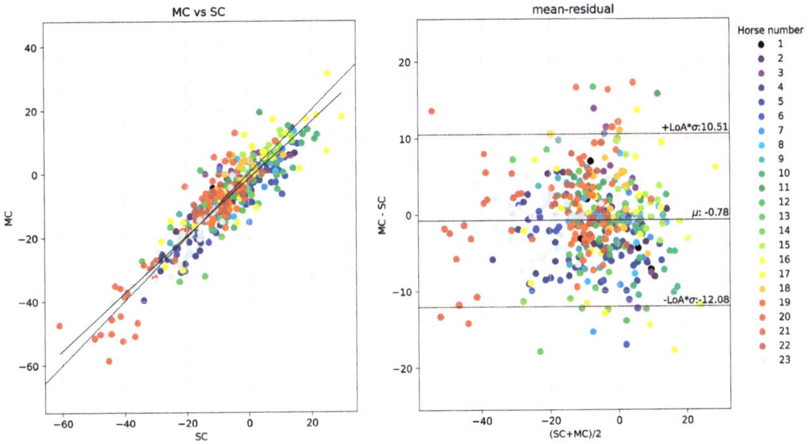

Pelvis P

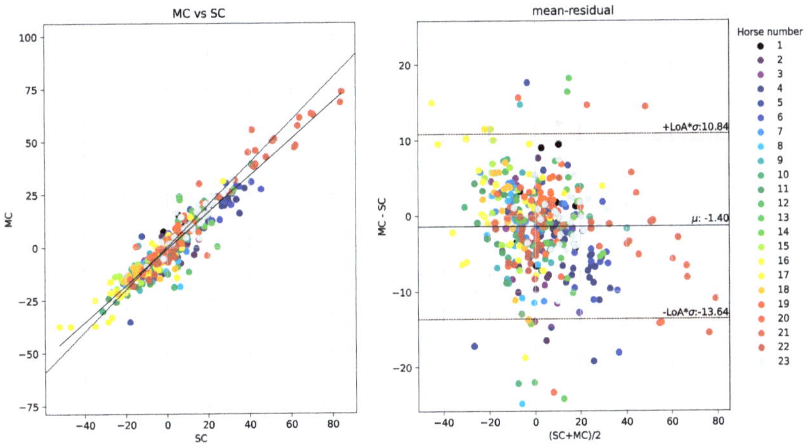

Figure 6. Scatter plots of the pelvic metrics obtained per stride (n = 404) observed by the multi-camera marker-based motion capture system (MC) plotted against the observation by the single-camera markerless system (SC) are shown in the left sub-panels. Agreements between the systems with limits of agreement (LoA) displayed as orange horizontal lines are presented in the Bland-Altman plots (right sub-panels). In the top row, we show the ΔV (MinDiff) and the bottom row we show ΔP (MaxDiff) defined in Section 2.7.1.

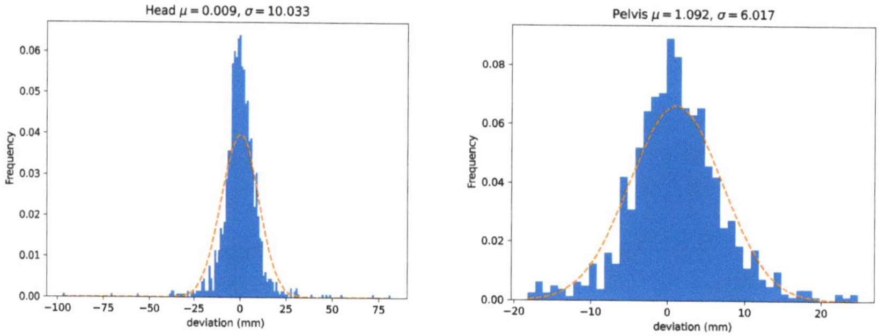

Figure 7. Distributions of the per-stride deviations for head (**left**) and pelvis (**right**). Here we have combined both peak and valley deviations defined in Section 2.7.1 (ΔV and ΔP). The dashed line displays the normal distribution estimated from the means and standard deviations of the between-systems deviations.

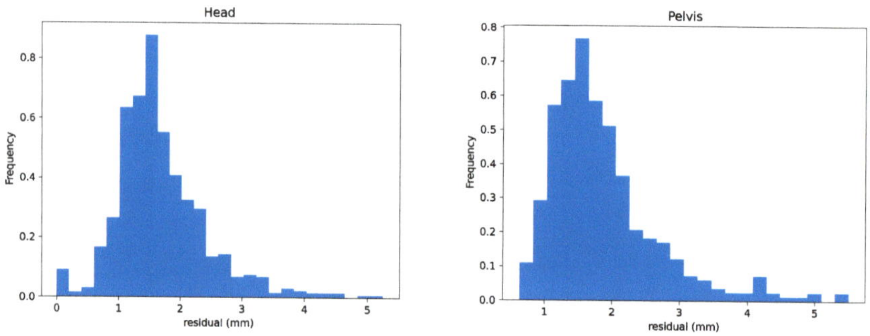

Figure 8. Distributions of the absolute values for stride mean residuals for head (**left**) and pelvis (**right**).

Table 3. Results summary for the measurement deviations between the systems over the entire dataset. In the top 6 rows we provide combined per-trial deviations ($\bar{D}$) using both deviations for the normalised MinDiff ($\Delta\bar{V}$) and MaxDiff ($\Delta\bar{P}$). For both head and pelvis, we compute the overall absolute mean, maximum and minimum deviations. In the bottom two rows we provide mean root mean square deviations (RMSD) as a comparison of the shape of the vertical displacement signals.

Per Trial	
head $\bar{D}$	2.2 mm
pelvis $\bar{D}$	2.2 mm
head max D	8.7 mm
pelvis max D	6.5 mm
head min D	0.0 mm
pelvis min D	0.0 mm
Per Stride	
head mean RMSD	5.0 mm
pelvis mean RMSD	3.5 mm

3.2. Per-Trial Comparisons

In this section, we provide the results from the per-trial comparison between MC and SC. In Table 3 we present statistics over the entire dataset from the per-trial mean NEVd-values. In this case, we combine $\bar{V}$ and $\bar{P}$. Thus, each stride contributes with two deviation values. For these, we compute the overall absolute mean, maximum and minimum absolute deviations as,

$$\bar{D} = \frac{\sum_{m=1}^{M} |\Delta \bar{V}_m| + \sum_{m=1}^{M} |\Delta \bar{P}_m|}{2M} \tag{11}$$

$$\max D = \max(\{|\Delta \bar{V}_m|\}_{m=1}^{M} \cup \{|\Delta \bar{P}_m|\}_{m=1}^{M}) \tag{12}$$

$$\min D = \min(\{|\Delta \bar{V}_m|\}_{m=1}^{M} \cup \{|\Delta \bar{P}_m|\}_{m=1}^{M}), \tag{13}$$

where $M = 23$ is the number of trials, i.e number of horses in the dataset, and $\cup$ denotes the union of the sets of $\{|\Delta \bar{V}_m|\}_{m=1}^{M}$ and $\{|\Delta \bar{P}_m|\}_{m=1}^{M}$.

Similar to the per-stride comparison in Section 3.1, we use Bland-Altman plots [37] to inspect the statistical agreements. The plots for head and pelvis are shown in Figures 9 and 10, respectively. Not unexpectedly, the deviations between systems are smaller for the per-trial mean NEVd-values than for the per-stride comparison in Section 3.1, rarely exceeding 6.4 ms. Similar to the per-stride comparison, the differences between $\bar{V}$ and $\bar{P}$ are small. However, the per-trial deviations show similar values for pelvis and head, which could be due to the fact that the two systems jointly observed more strides for the head signal than the pelvis.

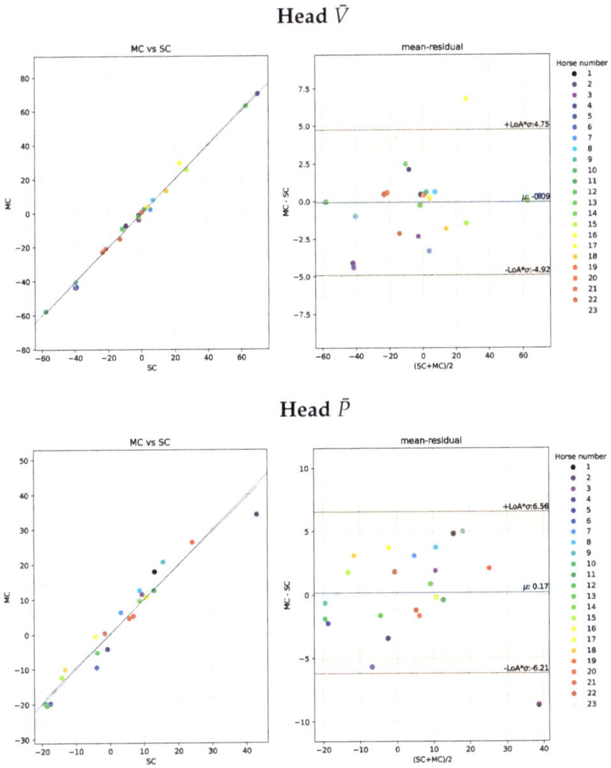

Figure 9. Trial-level scatter plots of the head metrics from the 23 included horses measured by the marker-based motion capture system (MC) versus the single-camera markerless system (SC) are presented in the left panel. Agreements between the systems, with limits of agreement (LoA) displayed as orange horizontal lines, are presented in the Bland-Altman plots in the right sub-panels. In the top row, we show $\Delta\bar{V}$ (trial mean MinDiff) and in the bottom row, we show $\Delta\bar{P}$ (trial mean MaxDiff) defined in Section 2.7.1.

In addition, we provide histograms over all the deviations (both $\bar{V}$ and $\bar{P}$) for head and pelvis in Figure 11. These plots also show the empirical estimates of normal distributions computed from the stride samples.

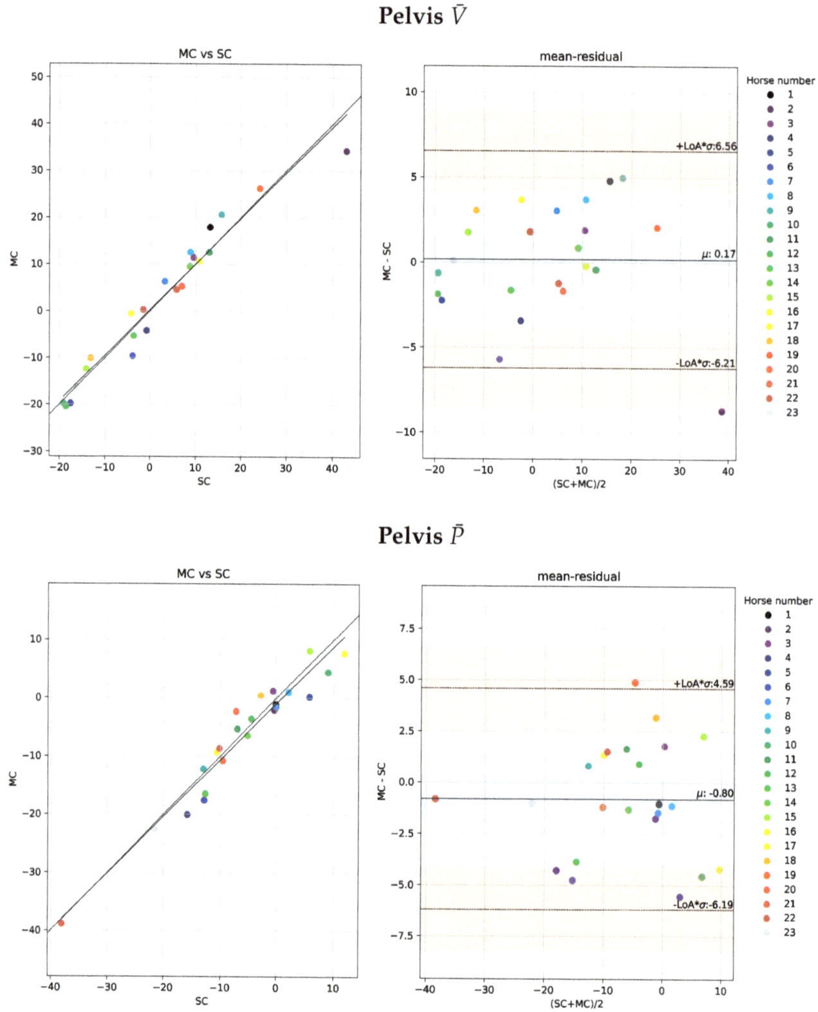

Figure 10. Trial-level scatter plots of the pelvic metrics from the 23 included horses measured by the marker-based motion capture system (MC) versus the single-camera markerless system (SC) are presented in the left panel. Agreements between the systems, with limits of agreement (LoA) displayed as orange horizontal lines, are presented in the Bland-Altman plots in the right sub-panels.In the top, we show $\Delta\bar{V}$ (trial mean MinDiff) and in the bottom row, we show $\Delta\bar{P}$ (trial mean MaxDiff) defined in Section 2.7.1.

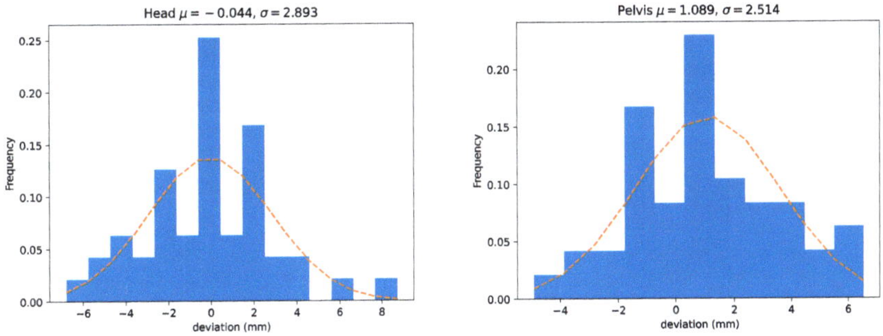

Figure 11. Distributions of the per-trial deviations for head (**left**) and pelvis (**right**). Here we have combined both peak and valley deviations defined in Section 2.7.1 ($\Delta\bar{V}$ and $\Delta\bar{P}$). The dashed line shows the normal distribution estimated from the means and standard deviations of the deviations.

4. Discussion

In this work, we demonstrated that deep neural networks and computer vision can be applied to reliably perform orthopaedic gait analysis for horses when trotted in hand on the straight during lameness assessment. The recorded average per-trial errors of 2.17 mm (head) and 2.19 mm (pelvis) are well below the previously recorded between-measurement-variation, of 18 mm (head) and 6 mm (pelvis) of horses trotting in a MC-system with several repetitions over two consecutive days and a one-month follow-up [21]. The results thus indicate that the average per-trial errors of the SC-extracted variables compared to the MC-extracted variables were small enough to not be a major hindrance when used for objective lameness assessment.

From a clinical perspective, the ease-of-use of the SC-system studied has a clear benefit since it allows affordable, repeated observations of equine patients, which can help to understand the considerable between trial variations observed in gait asymmetry [21].

When comparing the results of this study to another validation study performed on an IMU-based system (compared to a MC-system), it was found that stride-by-stride limits of agreement for the pelvic variables were approximately twice the magnitude for the SC-system described in this work [20]. It has to be acknowledged that comparing results from different samples can be a confounding factor in this case, but it still presents a general indication of how a computer vision based solution may compare to an IMU-based solution. Unfortunately, limits of agreement for the IMU-system in the Bosch et al. study [20] versus our SC-system can not be compared for the head variables since these were not presented in the IMU-system validation study.

The reported accuracy of the SC-system could also be compared to a previous test-retest repeatability study of an IMU-system, where the 95% confidence interval was reported as approximately 6 mm for head asymmetries and 3 mm for pelvic asymmetries [38]. However, a later study comparing that IMU-system to a different IMU-system, also developed for detecting equine lameness, found that the limits of agreement between the two systems were in this same range [36]. Further, it was found that the system used by [38] consistently underestimated the amount of movement asymmetry compared to the other IMU-system, which had previously been shown to give values comparable to optical motion capture. It has been suggested that the confidence intervals reported by Keegan et al [38] should be adjusted to 8 and 4 mm [13] for the other IMU-system, and this is likely a suitable adjustment also for an MC-system.

There were two outlier trials with a recorded per-trial mean deviation of 8.71 mm (head) and 6.54 mm (pelvis). Notably, these outliers occurred for horses with large asymmetries (see horse 2 in Table 1 and horse 4 in Table 2), and did not change the sign of the calculated variables or the clinical interpretation of the gait data. Hence, these deviations would not confuse which limb was affected by the asymmetry. We hypothesized that these errors might be due to difficulties in detecting and tracking the head and pelvis when they were occluded e.g., the horse lowering its head and hiding it behind the trunk, or lifting the tail obscuring the pelvic region.

Another SC-system utilizing deep neural networks to detect and track trotting horses for the purpose of lameness assessment has been previously described [39]. Although their approach was similar to the method presented in this study, the authors did not quantify movement symmetry metrics directly. Instead, they focused on lame limb classification. It is also worthwhile noting that a SC-system has been developed and shown to be able to perform reliable gait analysis of human subjects [27]. The level of precision described is said to open up for several potential applications in human medicine.

Is markerless more or less? A dichotomous answer cannot be given here. There are technical drawbacks related to using computer vision techniques implemented in a SC-system aimed towards objective equine lameness assessment, lower accuracy and lack of 3D motion to name two. However, these drawbacks have to be weighed against the benefit of having a lightweight, portable and low-cost system available for data collection, that allows repeatable observations of the horse. Other systems, such as IMUs and MC are typically more expensive, are sometimes limited to laboratory environments and require more interaction in terms of placing markers and sensors on the horse. Inevitably, this leads to fewer measurements being done and it is well known that low sample sizes of horses are the standard in many equine biomechanics studies. This study has shown that a simple application on a smartphone can be a tool for flexible and reliable collection of kinematic asymmetry data from horses. By extension, this opens up opportunities for larger-scale biomechanics research studies in non-laboratory environments. Coupling this with current advances in machine learning, where computers efficiently learn from data to perform predictions, we suggest that SC can be used to accelerate our understanding of horse locomotion and horse welfare.

Limitations

In the current study, all measurements were performed in the same clinical indoor environment on a limited number of horses (n = 23). The SC-system would likely be more challenged if there was a severe lack of light or if for example heavy rain obscured the visibility of the horse in the video. However, testing under such conditions was not within the scope of this study and would have been impossible to perform given that the state-of-the-art MC-system is a permanent indoor installation. The smartphone was placed on a tripod during the data collection, as handheld recordings would demand a stabilisation algorithm to be applied to the video. As such, further research is required to evaluate the SC-system under handheld conditions. Also, the length of the runway was 30 m, hence a greater distance between the camera and the horse has not been investigated. We did, however, analyse the error per stride index and did not find increasing deviations of the lameness metrics studied.

There are today several iPhone models with different camera specifications, such as image resolution and sampling rate. This study was limited to the use of an iPhone12 Pro Max where the resolution was set to 2160 × 3840 pixels and the frame rate to 60 Hz. Newer iPhone models come with even better camera specifications. Further research should investigate whether these models would improve the output from the SC-system even further.

The neural networks used in the SC-system were trained on image data of horses that did not have markers attached to the skin. Therefore, the skin-attached reflective markers used in this validation study could be suspected to partly obscure the anatomical region of interest and potentially present a problem to the SC-system. Visual inspection of the tracking from the SC-system, did however show very stable detection of the anatomical segments. This is confirmed by the comparison to the output of the MC-system.

This study only investigated vertical movement asymmetry of head and pelvis in a straight line. 3D motion comparisons would be of interest in the future, in order to provide a more detailed analysis of horse locomotion e.g., limb retraction and protraction angles studied from lateral view or on a circle. However, 3D lifting from a 2D image is an inherently complicated computer vision task where more advanced methods would be required, and so these kinematic variables were not investigated in this preliminary study.

5. Conclusions

We conclude that objective gait analysis for lameness assessment in horses can be reliably performed using a smartphone and computer vision analysis built on deep neural networks. The measurement deviation, when compared to a state-of-the-art motion capture system, is larger compared to IMU-based systems [20], but the error is clearly lower than observed levels of "between trial variation" from earlier studies [21]. The ease-of-use of the system makes repeated observations of a horse's lameness more feasible, which can provide more objective data points for treatment evaluation.

Author Contributions: Conceptualisation, E.H., M.R., P.H.A. and H.K.; methodology, E.H., F.J.L., A.B. and C.R.; software, F.J.L., C.R., M.S., M.A. and A.B.; validation, F.J.L., E.H., C.R. and A.B.; formal analysis, F.J.L.; investigation, F.J.L., E.H.; resources, E.H., M.R.; data curation, F.J.L.; writing—original draft preparation, F.J.L., E.H. and C.R.; writing—review and editing, all authors; visualisation, F.J.L.; supervision, E.H. and H.K.; project administration, E.H.; funding acquisition, E.H., P.H.A. and M.R. All authors have read and agreed to the published version of the manuscript.

Funding: This research was funded by the Swedish Research Council FORMAS grant number 2018-00737, Marie-Claire Cronstedts Stiftelse grant number 2018.4.2-2084 and CareNet grant number SLU ua 2020.4.1-4651.

Institutional Review Board Statement: Animal ethical approval was not applicable for this study according to Swedish legislation since it involves privately owned horses which were not subjected to any invasive procedures or alterations to the clinical decisions due to entering the study.

Informed Consent Statement: Written informed consent has been obtained from the the animal owners to publish this paper.

Data Availability Statement: Raw stride-level data from all included horses (and all strides) are presented as Appendix A to the manuscript.

Acknowledgments: Thanks to the staff at Equine Orthopaedic Clinic of the University Animal Hospital in Uppsala for support with recordings.

Conflicts of Interest: The funder had no role in the design of the study; in the collection, analyses, or interpretation of data; in the writing of the manuscript; or in the decision to publish the results. Authors affiliated to the company Sleip AI (F.J.L., C.R., M.A., M.S. and E.H.) declare a conflict of interest since the company provides a commercially available diagnostic tool for detecting lameness in horses from a smartphone. The developed computer vision technique is validated in the current paper.

Abbreviations

The following abbreviations are used in this manuscript:

SC	Single-camera markerless system
MC	Multi-camera marker-based system
VDS	Vertical displacement signal
NEVd	Normalised extreme value differences
MaxDiff	Difference between local maxima values within a stride
MinDiff	Difference between local minima within a stride
P	Normalised difference between local maxima values of the VDS per stride
V	Normalised difference between local minima values of the VDS per stride
$\bar{P}$	Trial mean P
$\bar{V}$	Trial mean V
σP	Trial standard deviation of P
σV	Trial standard deviation of V

ΔP	Deviation between two corresponding P's from different systems
ΔV	Deviation between two corresponding V's from different systems
$\Delta\bar{P}$	Deviation between two corresponding $\bar{P}$'s from different systems
$\Delta\bar{V}$	Deviation between two corresponding $\bar{V}$'s from different systems
$\bar{D}$	Mean absolute deviation over dataset
$\max D$	Maximum absolute deviation over dataset
$\min D$	Minimum absolute deviation over dataset
R	Range of motion of the VDS per stride
LDA	Linear Discriminant Analysis
LoA	Limit of Agreement

Appendix A. All Stride Curves

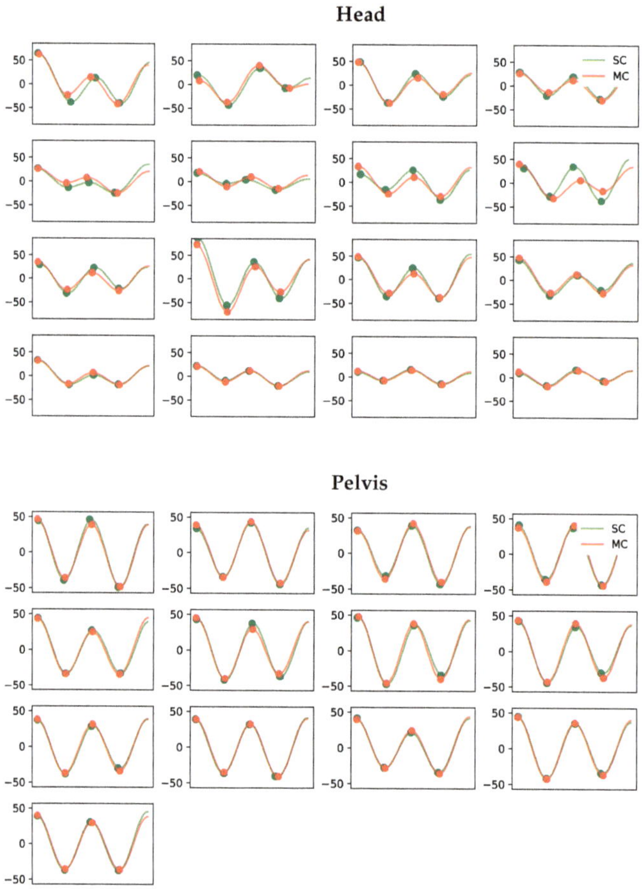

Figure A1. Vertical displacement signals per stride for the head and pelvis for horse 1. Each subplot contains the matched stride segments for the single-camera markerless system (SC) in green and the multi-camera marker-based system (MC) in red. The y-axis shows the vertical displacement in millimeters. The four dots on each curve indicate the positions of the two peaks and two valleys extracted using the approach in Section 2.6.2.

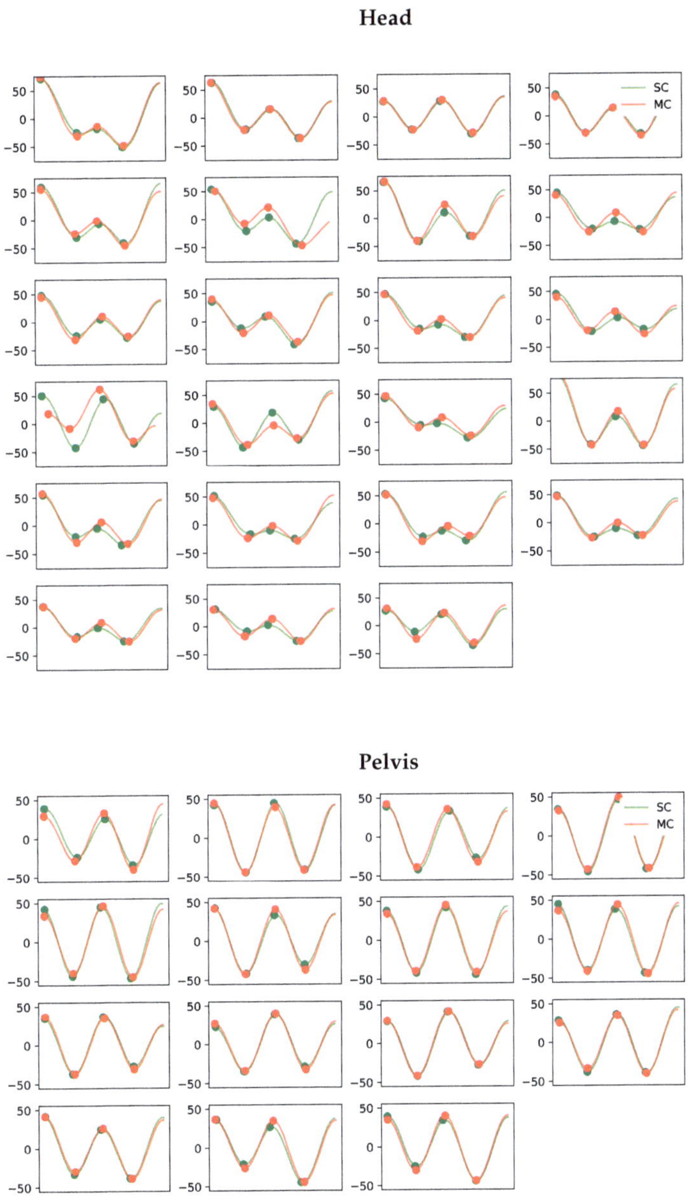

Figure A2. Vertical displacement signals per stride for the head and pelvis for horse 2. Each subplot contains the matched stride segments the single-camera markerless system (SC) in green and the multi-camera marker-based system (MC) in red. The y-axis shows the vertical displacement in millimeters. The four dots on each curve indicate the positions of the two peaks and two valleys extracted using the approach in Section 2.6.2.

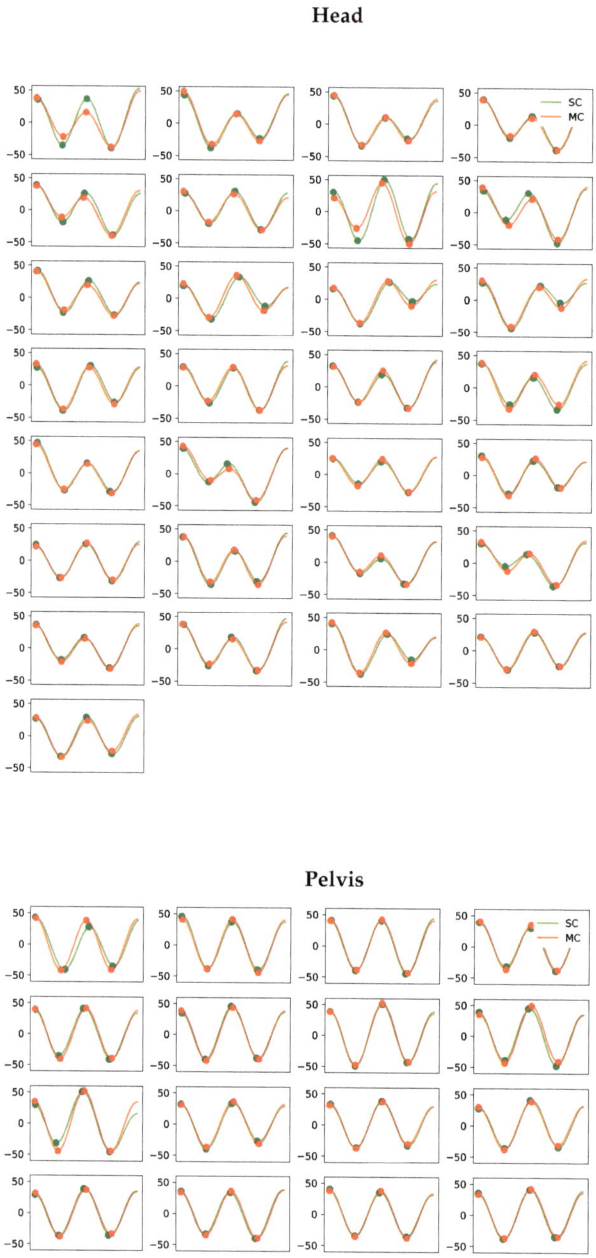

Figure A3. Vertical displacement signals per stride for the head and pelvis for horse 3. Each subplot contains the matched stride segments for the single-camera markerless system (SC) in green and the multi-camera marker-based system (MC) in red. The y-axis shows the vertical displacement in millimeters. The four dots on each curve indicate the positions of the two peaks and two valleys extracted using the approach in Section 2.6.2.

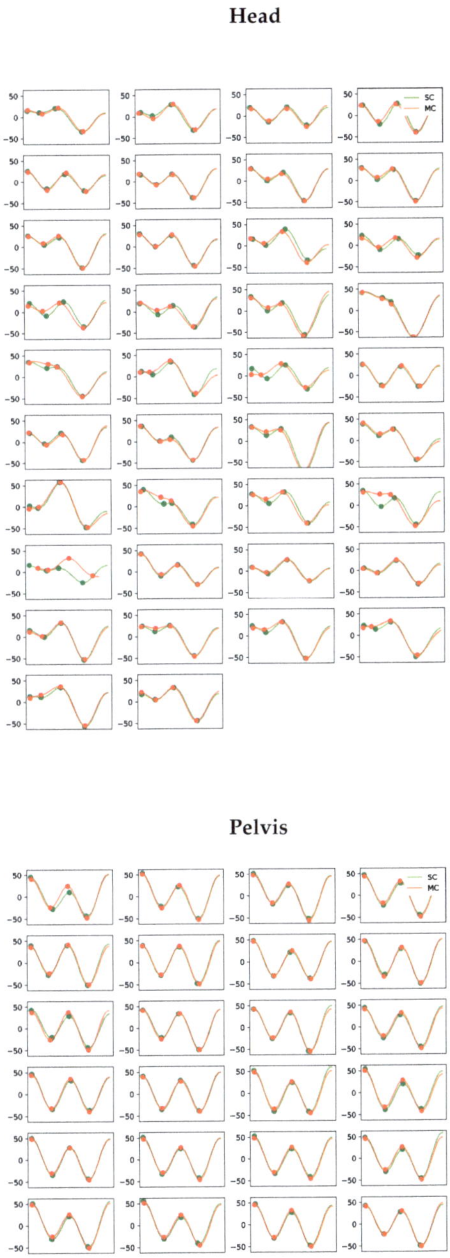

Figure A4. Vertical displacement signals per stride for the head and pelvis for horse 4. Each subplot contains the matched stride segments forthe single-camera markerless system (SC) in green and the multi-camera marker-based system (MC) in red. The y-axis shows the vertical displacement in millimeters. The four dots on each curve indicate the positions of the two peaks and two valleys extracted using the approach in Section 2.6.2.

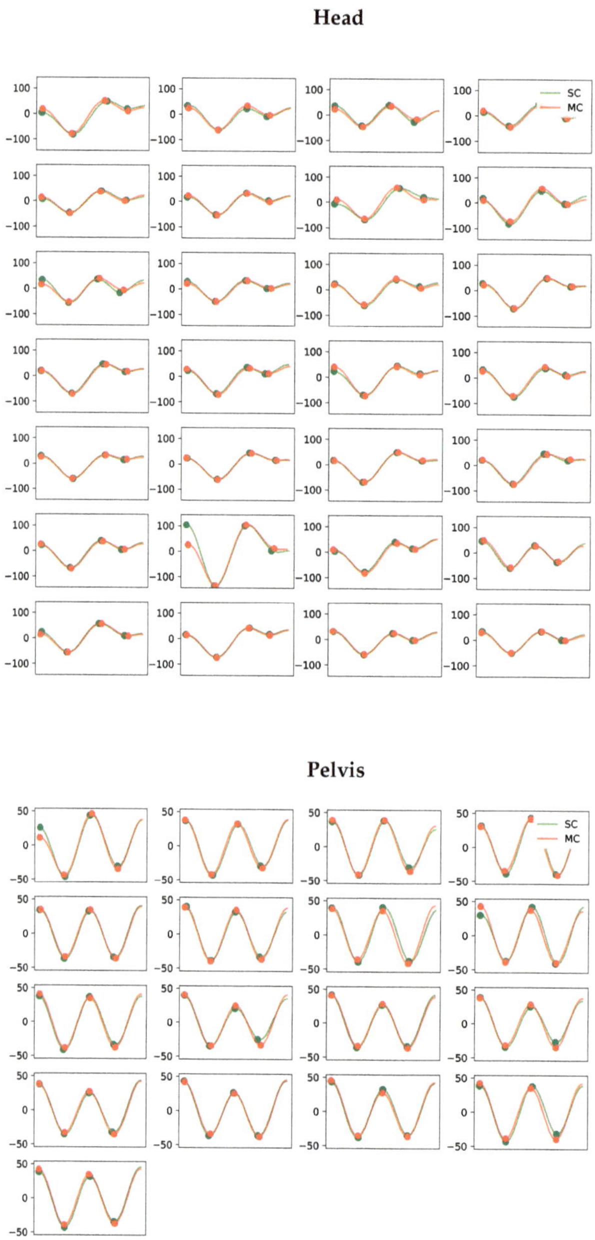

Figure A5. Vertical displacement signals per stride for the head and pelvis for horse 5. Each subplot contains the matched stride segments for the single-camera markerless system (SC) in green and the multi-camera marker-based system (MC) in red. The y-axis shows the vertical displacement in millimeters. The four dots on each curve indicate the positions of the two peaks and two valleys extracted using the approach in Section 2.6.2.

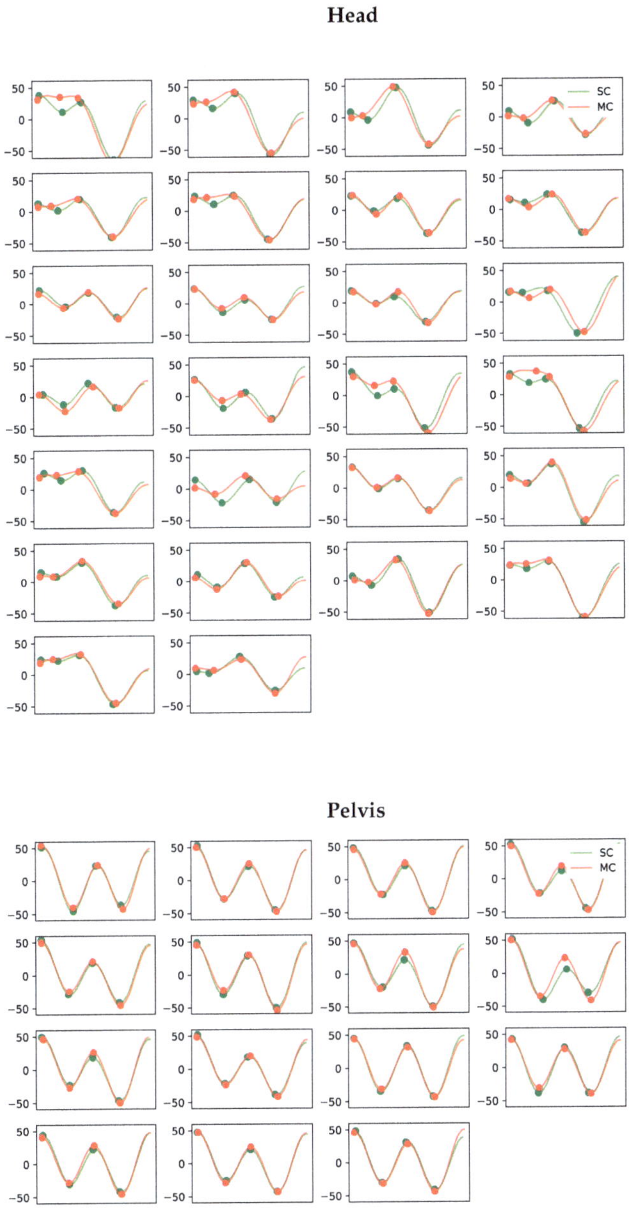

Figure A6. Vertical displacement signals per stride for the head and pelvis for horse 6. Each subplot contains the matched stride segments for the single-camera markerless system (SC) in green and the multi-camera marker-based system (MC) in red. The y-axis shows the vertical displacement in millimeters. The four dots on each curve indicate the positions of the two peaks and two valleys extracted using the approach in Section 2.6.2.

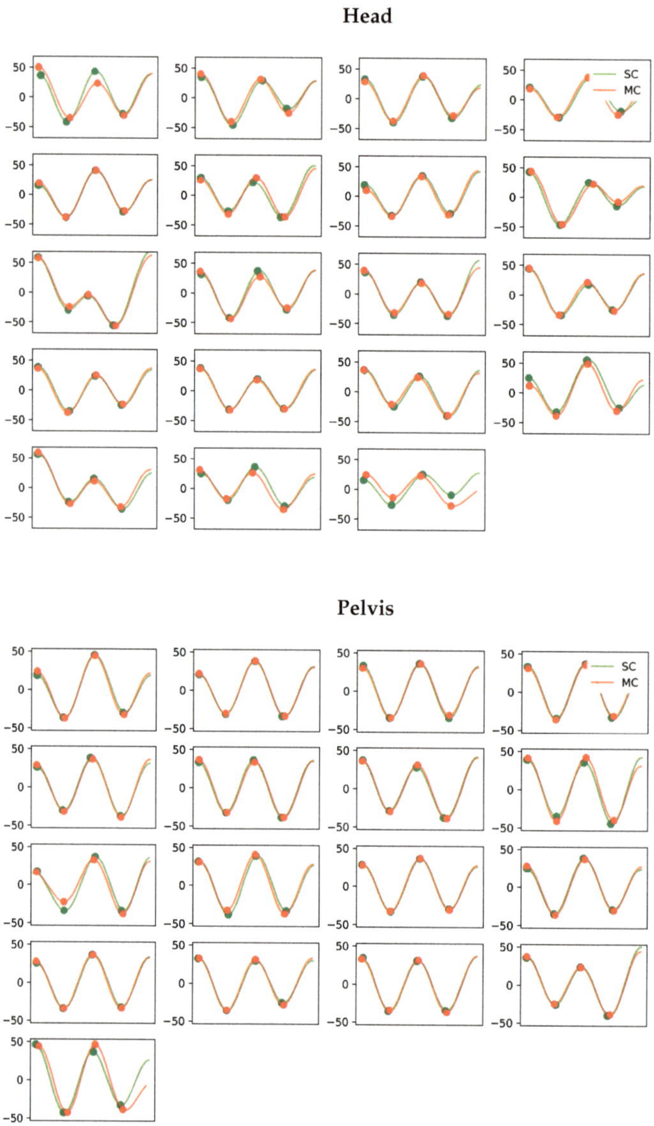

Figure A7. Vertical displacement signals per stride for the head and pelvis for horse 7. Each subplot contains the matched stride segments for the single-camera markerless system (SC) in green and the multi-camera marker-based system (MC) in red. The y-axis shows the vertical displacement in millimeters. The four dots on each curve indicate the positions of the two peaks and two valleys extracted using the approach in Section 2.6.2.

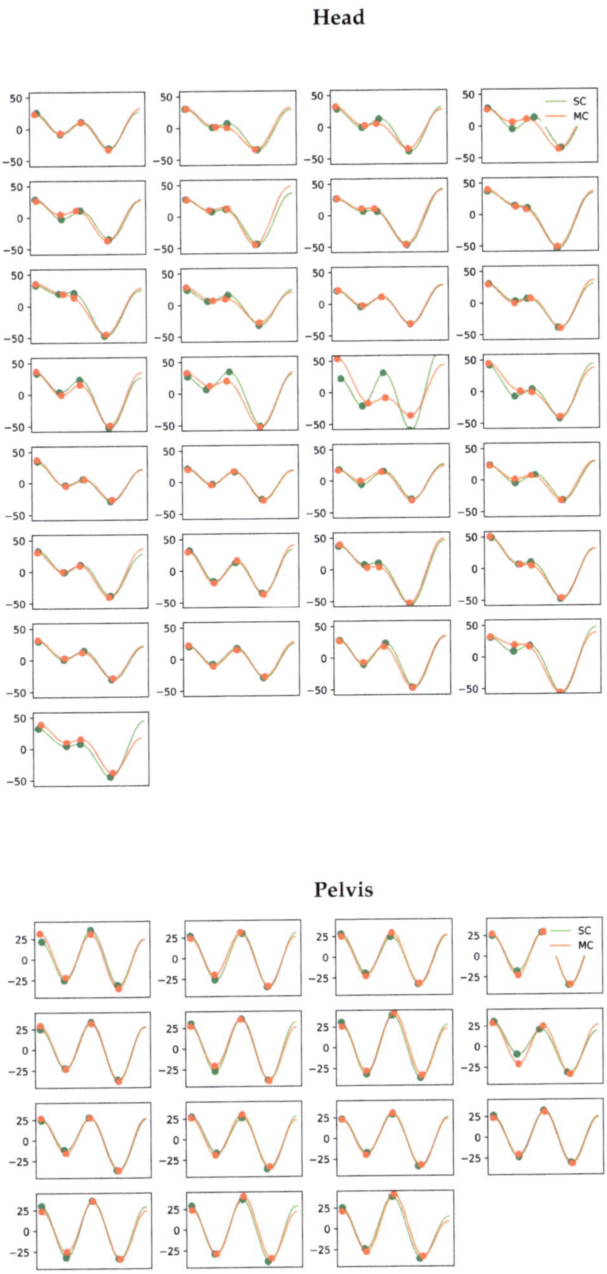

Figure A8. Vertical displacement signals per stride for the head and pelvis for horse 9. Each subplot contains the matched stride segments for the single-camera markerless system (SC) in green and the multi-camera marker-based system (MC) in red. The y-axis shows the vertical displacement in millimeters. The four dots on each curve indicate the positions of the two peaks and two valleys extracted using the approach in Section 2.6.2.

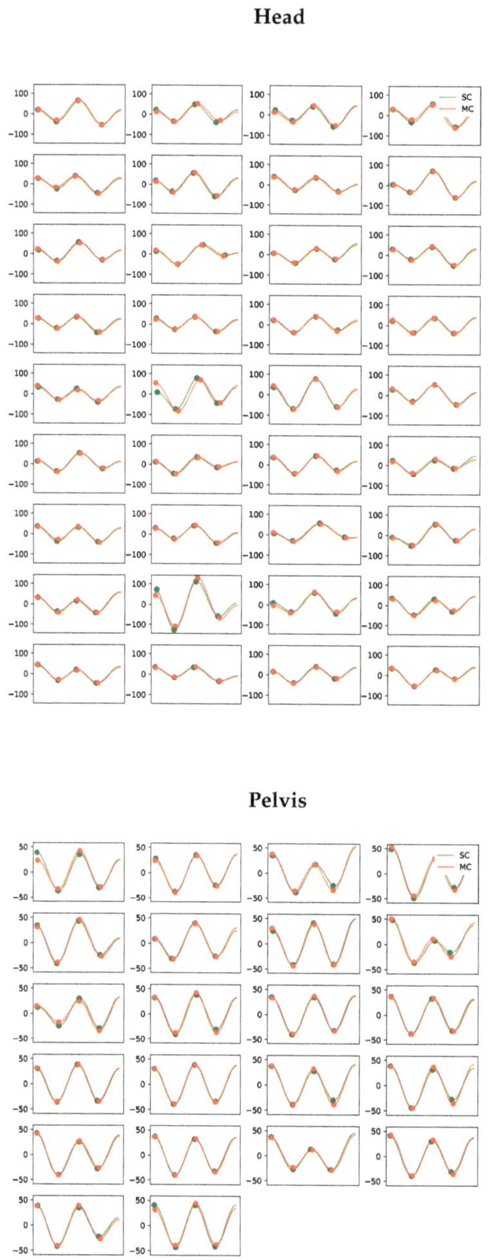

Figure A9. Vertical displacement signals per stride for the head and pelvis for horse 10. Each subplot contains the matched stride segments for the single-camera markerless system (SC) in green and the multi-camera marker-based system (MC) in red. The y-axis shows the vertical displacement in millimeters. The four dots on each curve indicate the positions of the two peaks and two valleys extracted using the approach in Section 2.6.2.

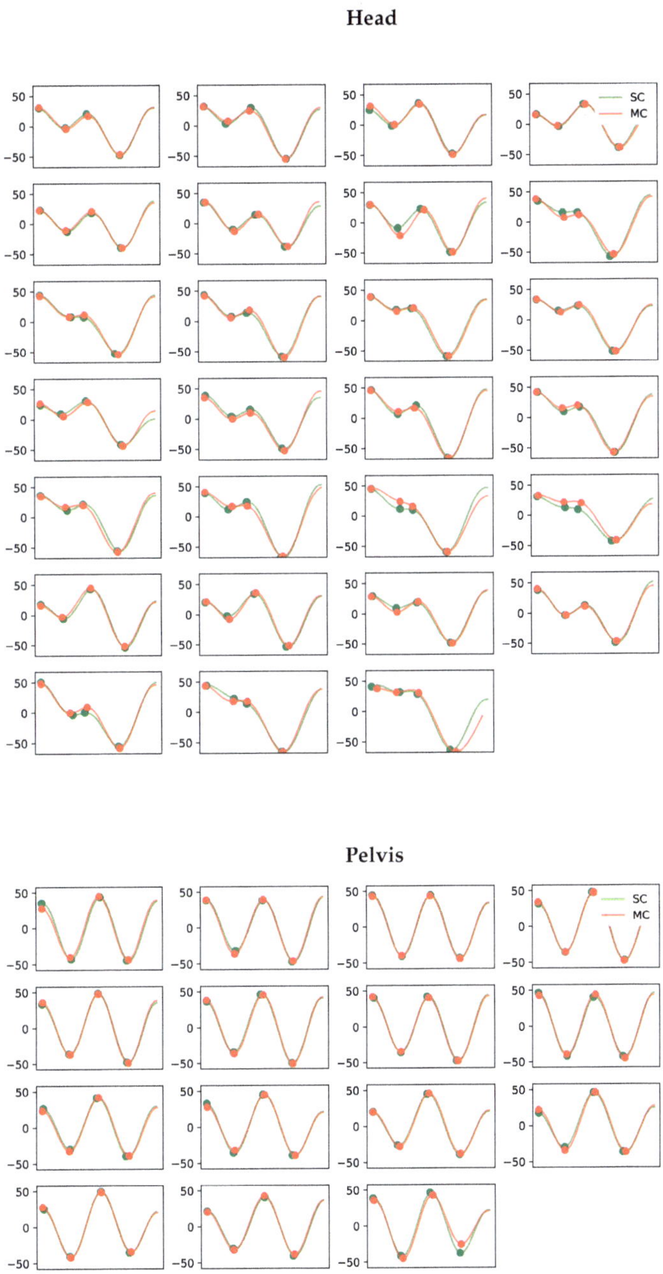

Figure A10. Vertical displacement signals per stride for the head and pelvis for horse 11. Each subplot contains the matched stride segments for the single-camera markerless system (SC) in green and the multi-camera marker-based system (MC) in red. The y-axis shows the vertical displacement in millimeters. The four dots on each curve indicate the positions of the two peaks and two valleys extracted using the approach in Section 2.6.2.

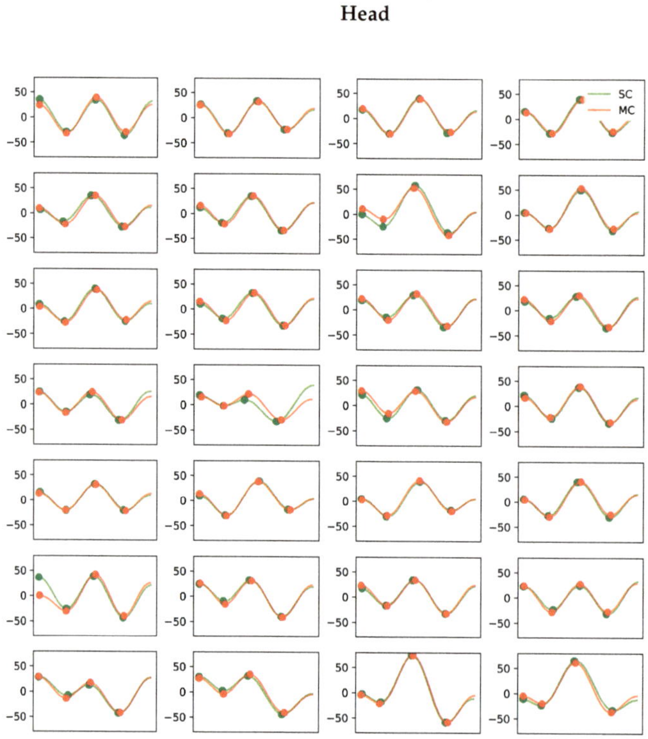

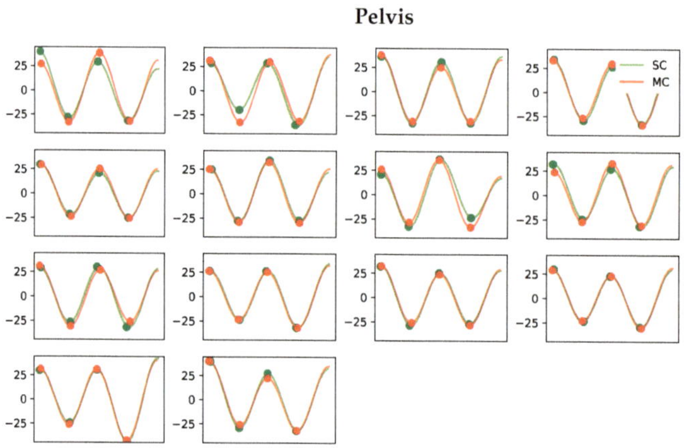

Figure A11. Vertical displacement signals per stride for the head and pelvis for horse 12. Each subplot contains the matched stride segments for the single-camera markerless system (SC) in green and the multi-camera marker-based system (MC) in red. The y-axis shows the vertical displacement in millimeters. The four dots on each curve indicate the positions of the two peaks and two valleys extracted using the approach in Section 2.6.2.

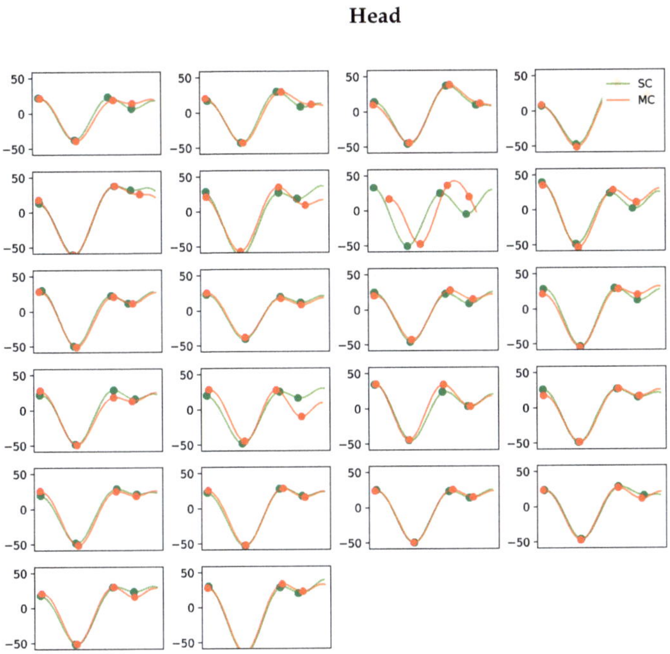

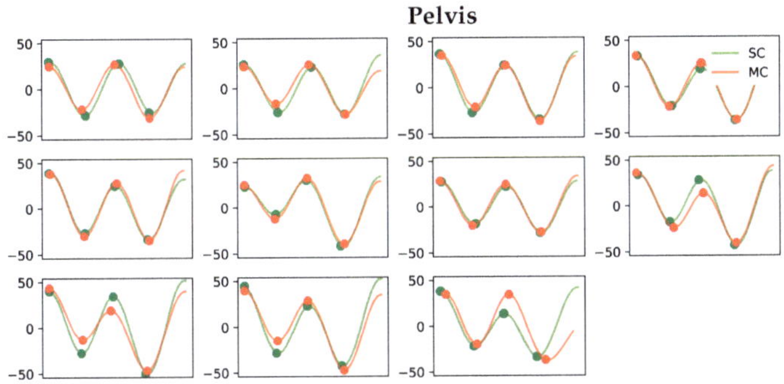

Figure A12. Vertical displacement signals per stride for the head and pelvis for horse 13. Each subplot contains the matched stride segments for the single-camera markerless system (SC) in green and the multi-camera marker-based system (MC) in red. The y-axis shows the vertical displacement in millimeters. The four dots on each curve indicate the positions of the two peaks and two valleys extracted using the approach in Section 2.6.2.

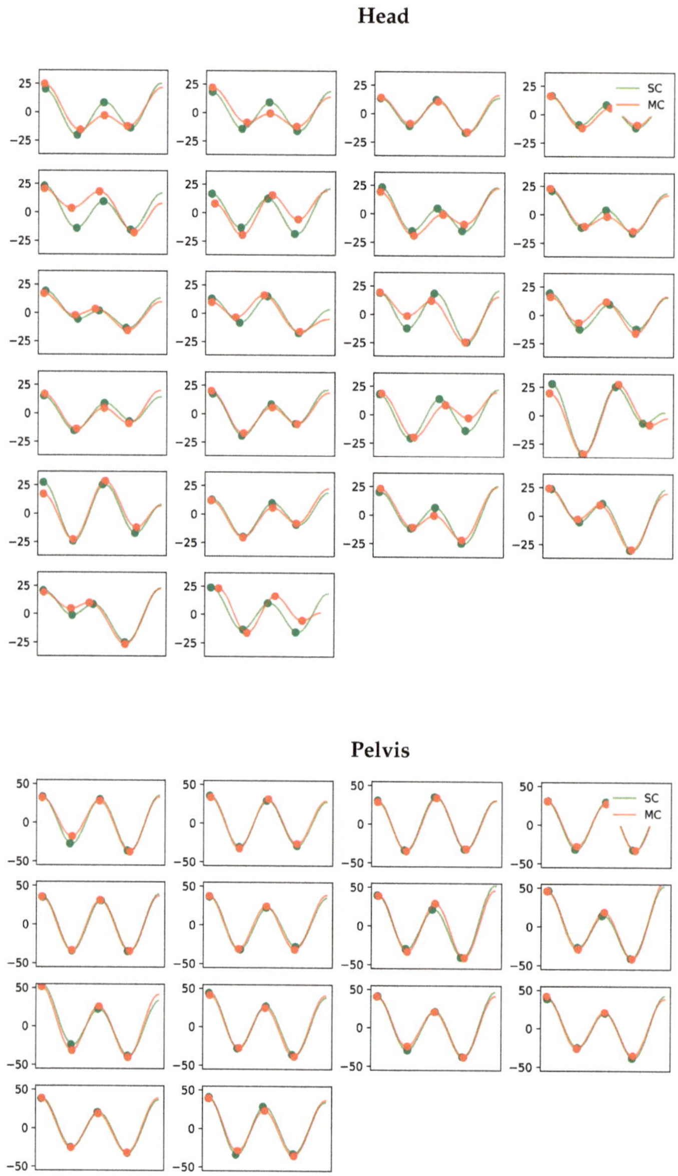

Figure A13. Vertical displacement signals per stride for the head and pelvis for horse 14. Each subplot contains the matched stride segments for the single-camera markerless system (SC) in green and the multi-camera marker-based system (MC) in red. The y-axis shows the vertical displacement in millimeters. The four dots on each curve indicate the positions of the two peaks and two valleys extracted using the approach in Section 2.6.2.

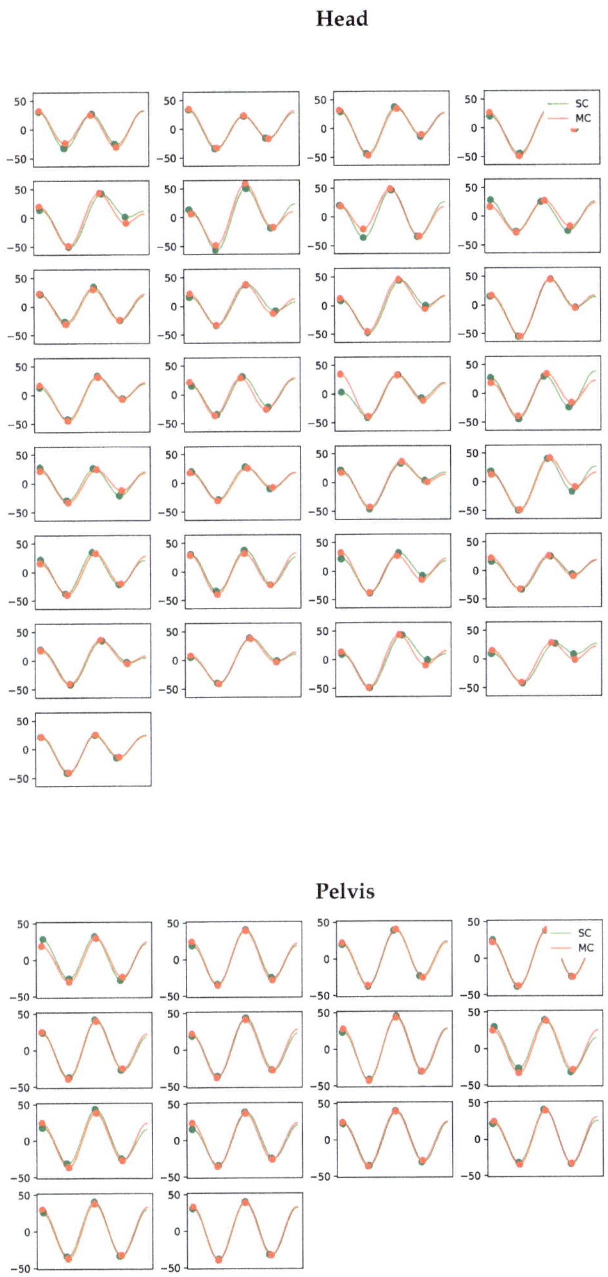

Figure A14. Vertical displacement signals per stride for the head and pelvis for horse 15. Each subplot contains the matched stride segments for the single-camera markerless system (SC) in green and the multi-camera marker-based system (MC) in red. The y-axis shows the vertical displacement in millimeters. The four dots on each curve indicate the positions of the two peaks and two valleys extracted using the approach in Section 2.6.2.

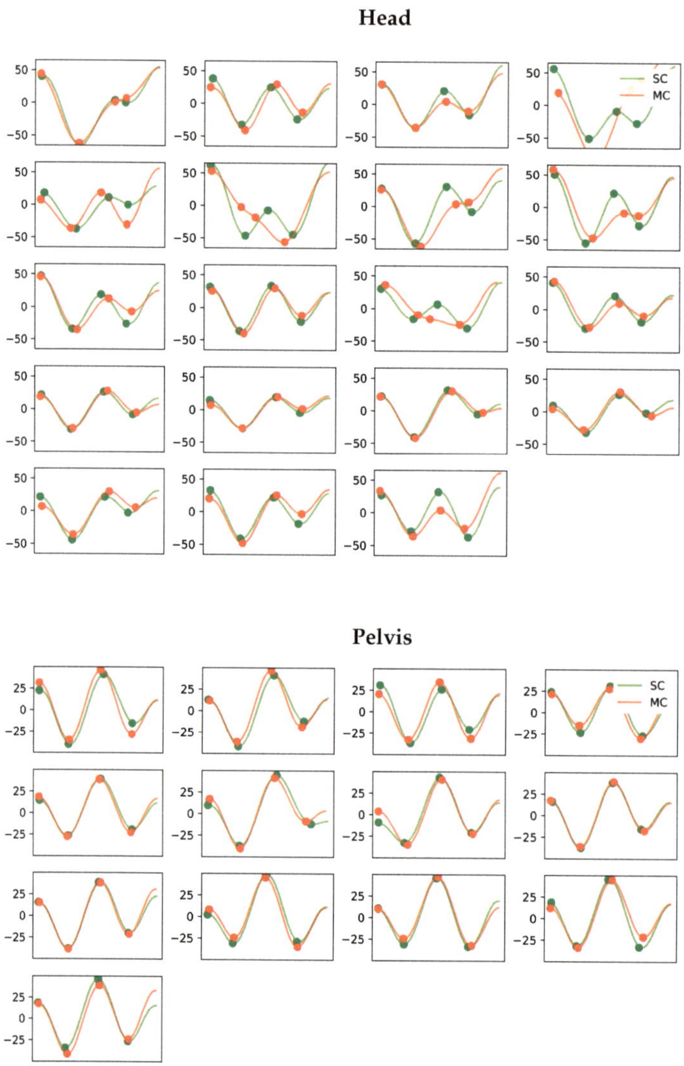

Figure A15. Vertical displacement signals per stride for the head and pelvis for horse 16. Each subplot contains the matched stride segments for the single-camera markerless system (SC) in green and the multi-camera marker-based system (MC) in red. The y-axis shows the vertical displacement in millimeters. The four dots on each curve indicate the positions of the two peaks and two valleys extracted using the approach in Section 2.6.2.

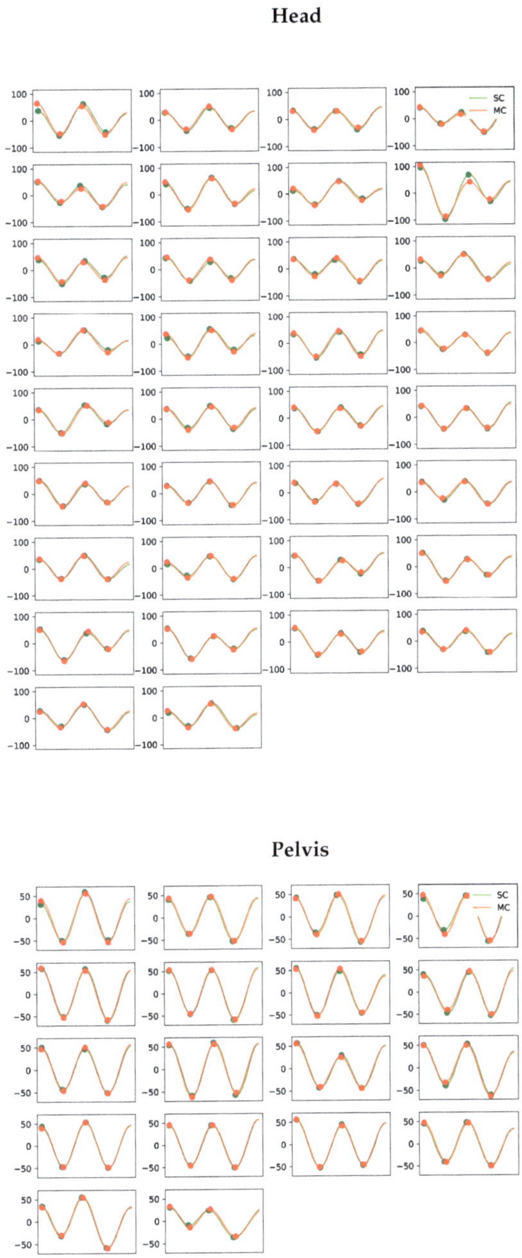

Figure A16. Vertical displacement signals per stride for the head and pelvis for horse 17. Each subplot contains the matched stride segments for the single-camera markerless system (SC) in green and the multi-camera marker-based system (MC) in red. The y-axis shows the vertical displacement in millimeters. The four dots on each curve indicate the positions of the two peaks and two valleys extracted using the approach in Section 2.6.2.

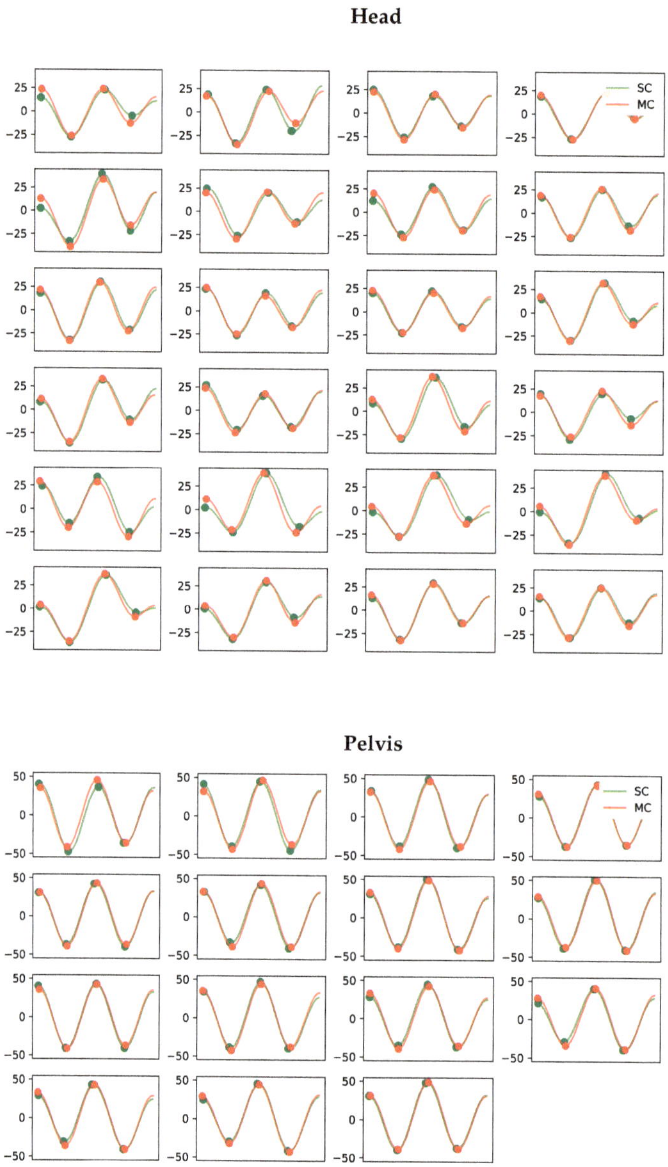

Figure A17. Vertical displacement signals per stride for the head and pelvis for horse 18. Each subplot contains the matched stride segments for the single-camera markerless system (SC) in green and the multi-camera marker-based system (MC) in red. The y-axis shows the vertical displacement in millimeters. The four dots on each curve indicate the positions of the two peaks and two valleys extracted using the approach in Section 2.6.2.

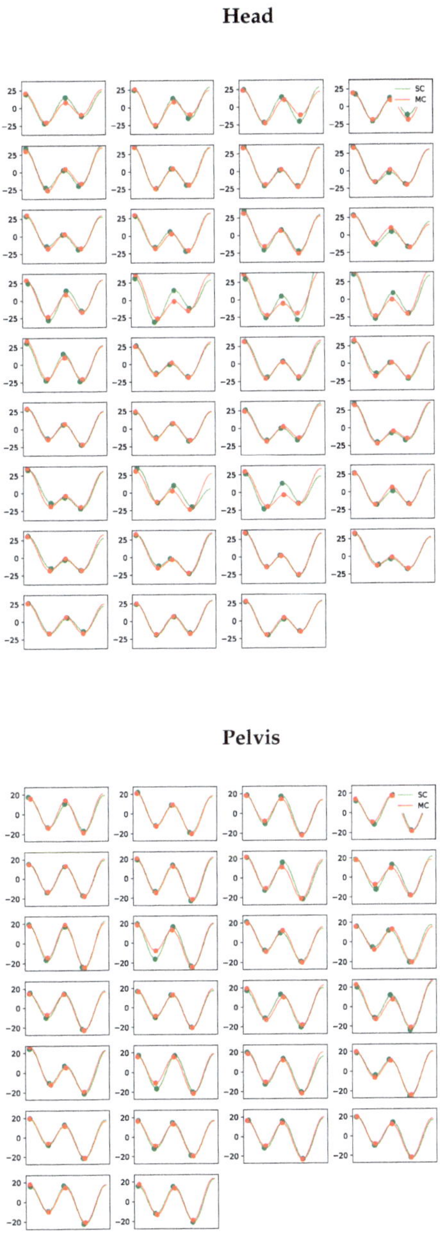

Figure A18. Vertical displacement signals per stride for the head and pelvis for horse 19. Each subplot contains the matched stride segments for the single-camera markerless system (SC) in green and the multi-camera marker-based system (MC) in red. The y-axis shows the vertical displacement in millimeters. The four dots on each curve indicate the positions of the two peaks and two valleys extracted using the approach in Section 2.6.2.

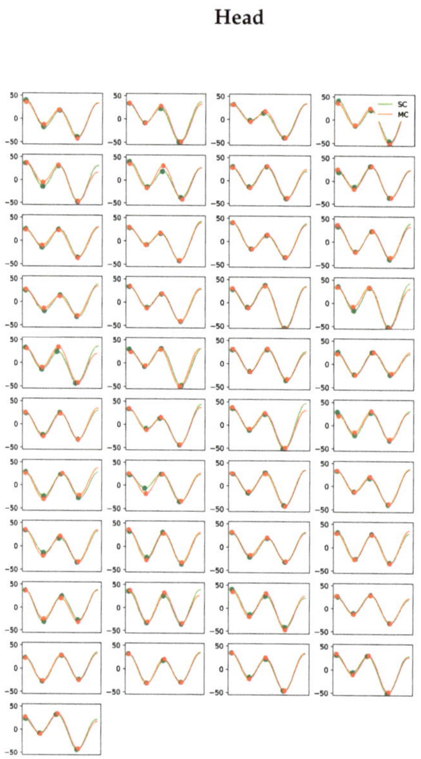

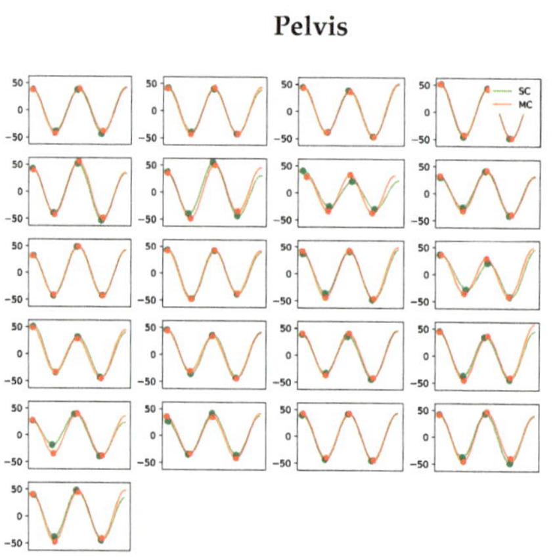

Figure A19. Vertical displacement signals per stride for the head and pelvis for horse 20. Each subplot contains the matched stride segments for the single-camera markerless system (SC) in green and the multi-camera marker-based system (MC) in red. The y-axis shows the vertical displacement in millimeters. The four dots on each curve indicate the positions of the two peaks and two valleys extracted using the approach in Section 2.6.2.

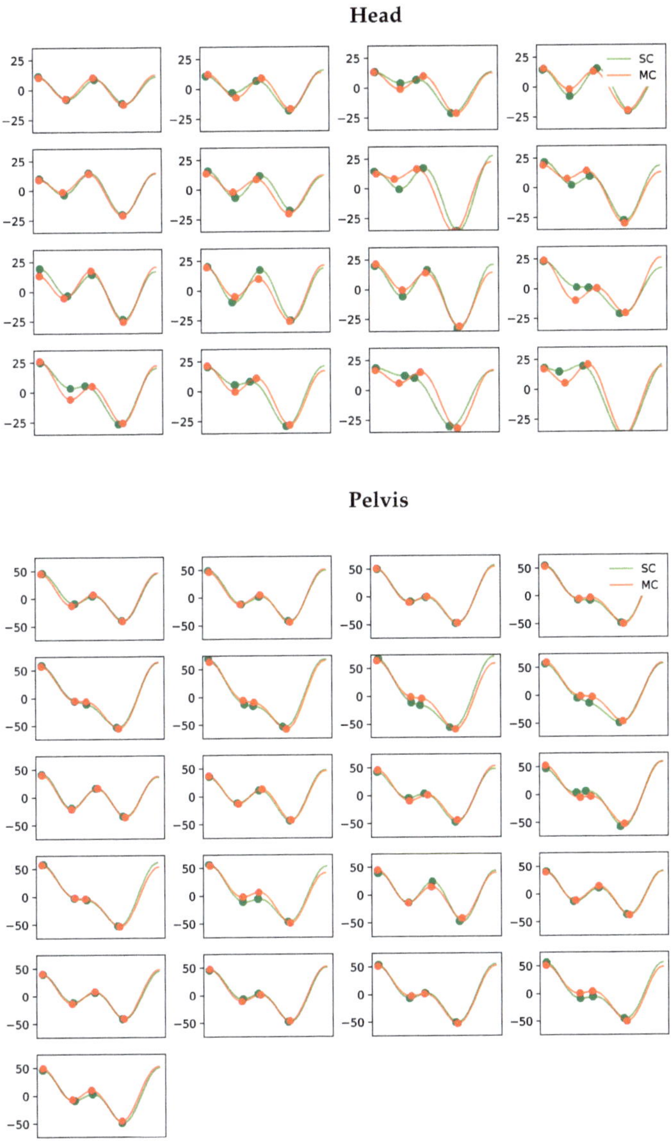

Figure A20. Vertical displacement signals per stride for the head and pelvis for horse 21. Each subplot contains the matched stride segments for the single-camera markerless system (SC) in green and the multi-camera marker-based system (MC) in red. The y-axis shows the vertical displacement in millimeters. The four dots on each curve indicate the positions of the two peaks and two valleys extracted using the approach in Section 2.6.2.

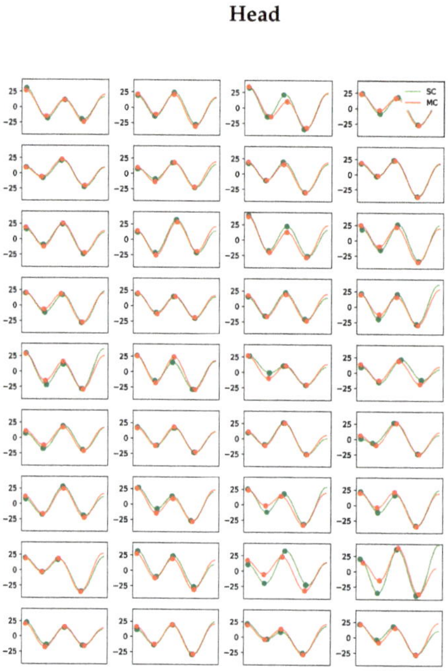

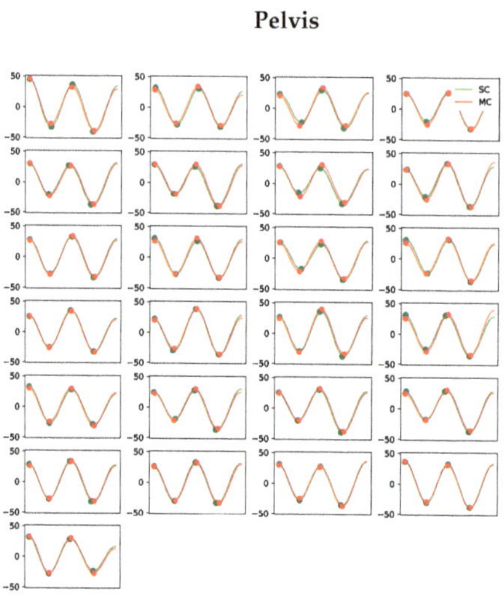

Figure A21. Vertical displacement signals per stride for the head and pelvis for horse 22. Each subplot contains the matched stride segments for the single-camera markerless system (SC) in green and the multi-camera marker-based system (MC) in red. The y-axis shows the vertical displacement in millimeters. The four dots on each curve indicate the positions of the two peaks and two valleys extracted using the approach in Section 2.6.2.

Head

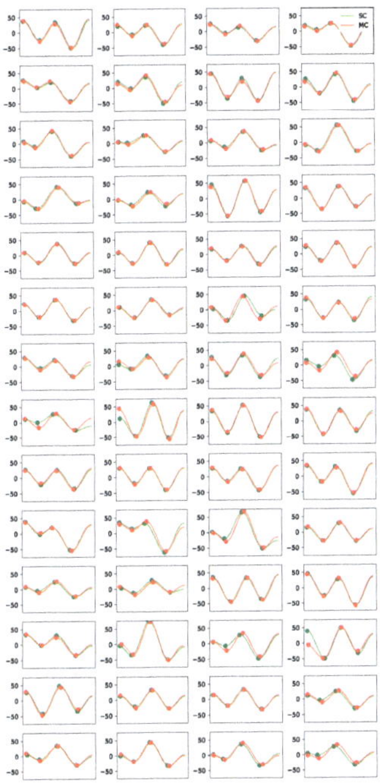

Pelvis

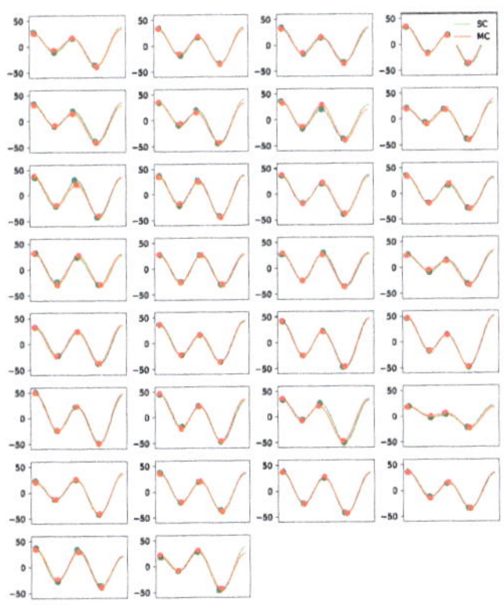

Figure A22. Vertical displacement signals per stride for the head and pelvis for horse 23. Each subplot contains the matched stride segments for the single-camera markerless system (SC) in green and the multi-camera marker-based system (MC) in red. The y-axis shows the vertical displacement in millimeters. The four dots on each curve indicate the positions of the two peaks and two valleys extracted using the approach in Section 2.6.2.

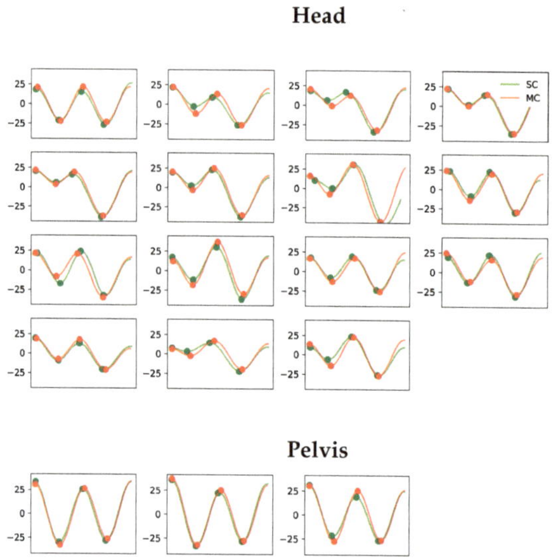

Figure A23. Vertical displacement signals per stride for the head and pelvis for horse 24. Each subplot contains the matched stride segments for the single-camera markerless system (SC) in green and the multi-camera marker-based system (MC) in red. The y-axis shows the vertical displacement in millimeters. The four dots on each curve indicate the positions of the two peaks and two valleys extracted using the approach in Section 2.6.2.

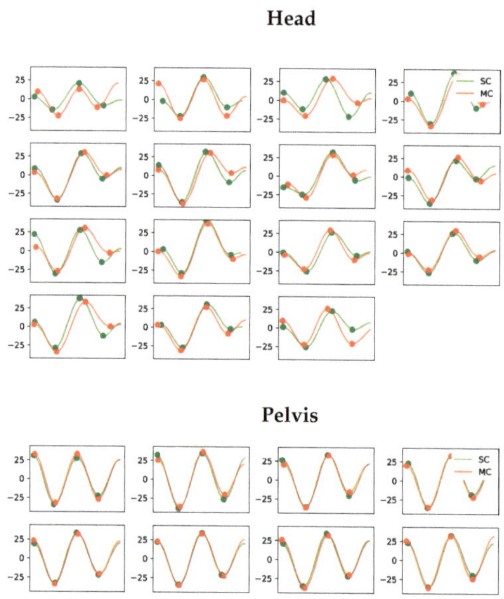

Figure A24. Vertical displacement signals per stride for the head and pelvis for horse 25. Each subplot contains the matched stride segments for the single-camera markerless system (SC) in green and the multi-camera marker-based system (MC) in red). The y-axis shows the vertical displacement in millimeters. The four dots on each curve indicate the positions of the two peaks and two valleys extracted using the approach in Section 2.6.2.

References

1. Roepstorff, C.; Gmel, A.I.; Arpagaus, S.; Bragança, F.M.S.; Hernlund, E.; Roepstorff, L.; Rhodin, M.; Weishaupt, M.A. Modelling fore- and hindlimb peak vertical force differences in trotting horses using upper body kinematic asymmetry variables. *J. Biomech.* **2022**, *137*, 111097. [CrossRef] [PubMed]
2. Bell, R.; Reed, S.K.; Schoonover, M.; Whitfield, C.; Yonezawa, Y.; Maki, H.; Pai, F.P.; Keegan, K.G. Associations of force plate and body-mounted inertial sensor measurements for identification of hind limb lameness in horses. *Am. J. Vet. Res.* **2016**, *77*, 337–345. [CrossRef] [PubMed]
3. Buchner, H.H.; Savelberg, H.H.; Schamhardt, H.C.; Barneveld, A. Head and trunk movement adaptations in horses with experimentally induced fore- or hindlimb lameness. *Equine Vet. J.* **1996**, *28*, 71–76. [CrossRef] [PubMed]
4. Parkes, R.S.; Weller, R.; Groth, A.M.; May, S.; Pfau, T. Evidence of the development of 'domain-restricted' expertise in the recognition of asymmetric motion characteristics of hindlimb lameness in the horse. *Equine Vet. J.* **2009**, *41*, 112–117. [CrossRef]
5. Holcombe, A.O. Seeing slow and seeing fast: Two limits on perception. *Trends Cogn. Sci.* **2009**, *13*, 216–221. [CrossRef]
6. Keegan, K.G.; Dent, E.V.; Wilson, D.A.; Janicek, J.; Kramer, J.; Lacarrubba, A.; Walsh, D.M.; Cassells, M.W.; Schiltz, P.; Frees, K.E.; et al. Repeatability of subjective evaluation of lameness in horses. *Equine Vet. J.* **2010**, *42*, 92–97. [CrossRef]
7. Hammarberg, M.; Egenvall, A.; Pfau, T.; Rhodin, M. Rater agreement of visual lameness assessment in horses during lungeing. *Equine Vet. J.* **2016**, *48*, 78–82. [CrossRef]
8. Arkell, M.; Archer, R.M.; Guitian, F.J.; May, S.A. Evidence of bias affecting the interpretation of the results of local anaesthetic nerve blocks when assessing lameness in horses. *Vet. Rec.* **2006**, *159*, 346–349. [CrossRef]
9. Mccracken, M.J.; Kramer, J.; Keegan, K.G.; Lopes, M.; Wilson, D.A.; Reed, S.K.; Lacarrubba, A.; Rasch, M. Comparison of an inertial sensor system of lameness quantification with subjective lameness evaluation. *Equine Vet. J.* **2012**, *44*, 652–656. [CrossRef]
10. Rhodin, M.; Egenvall, A.; Andersen, P.H.; Pfau, T. Head and pelvic movement asymmetries at trot in riding horses in training and perceived as free from lameness by the owner. *PLoS ONE* **2017**, *12*, 1–16. [CrossRef]
11. Müller-Quirin, J.; Dittmann, M.T.; Roepstorff, C.; Arpagaus, S.; Latif, S.N.; Weishaupt, M.A. Riding Soundness—Comparison of Subjective With Objective Lameness Assessments of Owner-Sound Horses at Trot on a Treadmill. *J. Equine Vet. Sci.* **2020**, *95*, 103314. [CrossRef]
12. Pfau, T.; Noordwijk, K.; Caviedes, M.F.S.; Persson-Sjodin, E.; Barstow, A.; Forbes, B.; Rhodin, M. Head, withers and pelvic movement asymmetry and their relative timing in trot in racing Thoroughbreds in training. *Equine Vet. J.* **2017**, *50*, 117–124. [CrossRef] [PubMed]
13. Pfau, T.; Parkes, R.S.; Burden, E.R.; Bell, N.; Fairhurst, H.; Witte, T.H. Movement asymmetry in working polo horses. *Equine Vet. J.* **2016**, *48*, 517–522. [CrossRef] [PubMed]
14. Scheidegger, M.D.; Gerber, V.; Dolf, G.; Burger, D.; Flammer, S.A.; Ramseyer, A. Quantitative Gait Analysis Before and After a Cross-country Test in a Population of Elite Eventing Horses. *J. Equine Vet. Sci.* **2022**, *117*. [CrossRef] [PubMed]
15. Lopes, M.A.; Eleuterio, A.; Mira, M.C. Objective Detection and Quantification of Irregular Gait With a Portable Inertial Sensor-Based System in Horses During an Endurance Race—A Preliminary Assessment. *J. Equine Vet. Sci.* **2018**, *70*, 123–129. [CrossRef]
16. Kallerud, A.S.; Fjordbakk, C.T.; Hendrickson, E.H.S.; Persson-Sjodin, E.; Hammarberg, M.; Rhodin, M.; Hernlund, E. Objectively measured movement asymmetry in yearling Standardbred trotters. *Equine Vet. J.* **2020**, *53*, 590–599. [CrossRef]
17. Maliye, S.; Voute, L.C.; Marshall, J.F. Naturally-occurring forelimb lameness in the horse results in significant compensatory load redistribution during trotting. *Vet. J.* **2015**, *204*, 208–213. [CrossRef]
18. Pfau, T.; Witte, T.H.; Wilson, A.M. A method for deriving displacement data during cyclical movement using an inertial sensor. *J. Exp. Biol.* **2005**, *208*, 2503–2514. [CrossRef] [PubMed]
19. Keegan, K.G.; Yonezawa, Y.; Pai, P.F.; Wilson, D.A. Accelerometer-based system for the detection of lameness in horses. *Biomed. Sci. Instrum.* **2002**, *38*, 107–112.
20. Bosch, S.; Bragança, F.M.S.; Marin-Perianu, M.; Marin-Perianu, R.; van der Zwaag, B.; Voskamp, J.; Back, W.; van Weeren, R.; Havinga, P. EquiMoves: A Wireless Networked Inertial Measurement System for Objective Examination of Horse Gait. *Sensors* **2018**, *18*, 850. [CrossRef] [PubMed]
21. Hardeman, A.M.; Bragança, F.M.S.; Swagemakers, J.H.; van Weeren, P.R.; Roepstorff, L. Variation in gait parameters used for objective lameness assessment in sound horses at the trot on the straight line and the lunge. *Equine Vet. J.* **2019**, *51*, 831–839. [CrossRef]
22. Serra Bragança, F.M.; Rhodin, M.; van Weeren, P.R. On the brink of daily clinical application of objective gait analysis: What evidence do we have so far from studies using an induced lameness model? *Vet. J.* **2018**, *234*, 11–23. [CrossRef] [PubMed]
23. Aurand, A.M.; Dufour, J.S.; Marras, W.S. Accuracy map of an optical motion capture system with 42 or 21 cameras in a large measurement volume. *J. Biomech.* **2017**, *58*, 237–240. [CrossRef] [PubMed]
24. LeCun, Y.; Bengio, Y. Convolutional networks for images, speech, and time series. *Handb. Brain Theory Neural Netw.* **1995**, *3361*, 1995.
25. Fukushima, K. Neocognitron: A hierarchical neural network capable of visual pattern recognition. *Neural Netw.* **1988**, *1*, 119–130. [CrossRef]
26. LeCun, Y.; Bengio, Y.; Hinton, G. Deep learning. *Nature* **2015**, *521*, 436–444. [CrossRef]

27. Azhand, A.; Rabe, S.; Müller, S.; Sattler, I.; Heimann-Steinert, A. Algorithm based on one monocular video delivers highly valid and reliable gait parameters. *Sci. Rep.* **2021**, *11*, 1–10. [CrossRef]
28. Wang, J.; Sun, K.; Cheng, T.; Jiang, B.; Deng, C.; Zhao, Y.; Liu, D.; Mu, Y.; Tan, M.; Wang, X.; et al. Deep high-resolution representation learning for visual recognition. *IEEE Trans. Pattern Anal. Mach. Intell.* **2020**, *43*, 3349–3364. [CrossRef] [PubMed]
29. Li, C.; Ghorbani, N.; Broomé, S.; Rashid, M.; Black, M.J.; Hernlund, E.; Kjellström, H.; Zuffi, S. hSMAL: Detailed Horse Shape and Pose Reconstruction for Motion Pattern Recognition. *arXiv* **2021**, arXiv:2106.10102.
30. Hatherley, J.J. Limits of trust in medical AI. *J. Med. Ethics* **2020**, *46*, 478–481. [CrossRef]
31. Girshick, R. Fast r-cnn. In Proceedings of the IEEE International Conference on Computer Vision, Santiago, Chile, 7–13 December 2015; pp. 1440–1448.
32. Long, J.; Shelhamer, E.; Darrell, T. Fully convolutional networks for semantic segmentation. In Proceedings of the IEEE Conference on Computer Vision and Pattern Recognition, Boston, MA, USA, 7–12 June 2015; pp. 3431–3440.
33. Bhat, G.; Lawin, F.J.; Danelljan, M.; Robinson, A.; Felsberg, M.; Gool, L.V.; Timofte, R. Learning what to learn for video object segmentation. In Proceedings of the European Conference on Computer Vision, Glasgow, UK, 23–28 August 2020; Springer: Berlin/Heidelberg, Germany, 2020; pp. 777–794.
34. Bragança, F.S.; Roepstorff, C.; Rhodin, M.; Pfau, T.; Van Weeren, P.; Roepstorff, L. Quantitative lameness assessment in the horse based on upper body movement symmetry: The effect of different filtering techniques on the quantification of motion symmetry. *Biomed. Signal Process. Control* **2020**, *57*, 101674. [CrossRef]
35. Keegan, K.G.; Yonezawa, Y.; Pai, F.; Wilson, D.A.; Kramer, J. Evaluation of a sensor-based system of motion analysis for detection and quantification of forelimb and hind limb lameness in horses. *Am. J. Vet. Res.* **2004**, *65*, 665–670. [CrossRef]
36. Pfau, T.; Boultbee, H.; Davis, H.; Walker, A.; Rhodin, M. Agreement between two inertial sensor gait analysis systems for lameness examinations in horses. *Equine Vet. Educ.* **2016**, *28*, 203–208. [CrossRef]
37. Bland, J.M.; Altman, D. Statistical methods for assessing agreement between two methods of clinical measurement. *Lancet* **1986**, *327*, 307–310. [CrossRef]
38. Keegan, K.G.; Kramer, J.; Yonezawa, Y.; Maki, H.; Pai, P.F.; Dent, E.V.; Kellerman, T.E.; Wilson, D.A.; Reed, S.K. Assessment of repeatability of a wireless, inertial sensor–based lameness evaluation system for horses. *Am. J. Vet. Res.* **2011**, *72*, 1156–1163. [CrossRef]
39. Wang, Y.; Li, J.; Zhang, Y.; Sinnott, R.O. Identifying lameness in horses through deep learning. In Proceedings of the ACM Symposium on Applied Computing, Virtual, 22–26 March 2021; pp. 976–985. [CrossRef]

animals MDPI

Article

Visually Assessing Equine Quality of Movement: A Survey to Identify Key Movements and Patient-Specific Measures

Annette G. Bowen [1,*], Gillian Tabor [2], Raphael Labens [1] and Hayley Randle [1]

[1] School of Agricultural, Environmental and Veterinary Sciences, Faculty of Science and Health, Charles Sturt University, Wagga Wagga, NSW 2678, Australia; rlabens@csu.edu.au (R.L.); hrandle@csu.edu.au (H.R.)
[2] Equestrian Performance Research Centre, Hartpury University, Gloucester GL19 3BE, Gloucestershire, UK; gillian.tabor@hartpury.ac.uk
* Correspondence: abowen@csu.edu.au

Simple Summary: Physiotherapy and rehabilitation is a burgeoning area of practice; to be evidence-based, it needs outcome measures designed for its focus on function. Based on frequency of use and rationale, this online survey aimed to identify a core group of in-hand assessments for equine movement. Additionally, the survey gathered information on how movement is currently monitored and opinions on the usefulness of modifying a patient-reported outcome measure for equine use. The survey attracted 81 participants and identified 24 key movements, including walk and trot on both firm and soft surfaces in a straight line and on a small circle, plus step back, hind leg cross-over, transitions and lunging at walk, trot and canter. Access to suitable surfaces and the training level of the horse and handler are the main barriers to using other movements. The majority (82%) of survey participants agreed or strongly agreed that a modified Patient-Specific Functional Scale would be useful for measuring complex movements. This knowledge of how equine clinicians are currently monitoring movement and using goal-setting will assist in designing a new outcome measure for quality of movement that includes both standardised and individualised measures.

Abstract: Outcome measures are essential for monitoring treatment efficacy. The lack of measures for quality of movement in equine physiotherapy and rehabilitation impairs evidence-based practice. To develop a new field-based outcome measure, it is necessary to determine movements most frequently observed during assessment of rehabilitation and performance management cases. An online survey of 81 equine sports medicine veterinarians and equine allied-health clinicians was conducted. The key movements identified included walk and trot on both firm and soft surfaces in a straight line and on a small circle, plus step back, hind leg cross-over, transitions and lunging at walk, trot and canter. The main barriers to observing some movements are access to suitable surfaces and the training level of the horse and handler. Subjective visual assessment of live or videoed horses was the most common method used to track progress of complex movements. The majority (82%) of survey participants agreed or strongly agreed that a modified Patient-Specific Functional Scale would be useful for measuring complex movements. Comments from all professions show a desire to have outcome measures relevant to their needs. This survey identified 24 in-hand movements, which can be used to form the foundation of a simple field-based outcome measure for quality of movement.

Keywords: equine physiotherapy; quality of movement; outcome measure; rehabilitation; goal setting

1. Introduction

Movement dysfunction causes horses significant suffering, therefore managing it efficiently is critically important. Because the body prioritises function over pain [1], addressing movement dysfunction is essential for positive animal welfare [2]. Movement dysfunction refers to poor quality of movement, and considers aspects such as whole body biomechanics, gait pattern, symmetry, motor-control, muscle activity and timing, willingness, and behaviours indicating discomfort [3,4]. Since physiotherapy is centred around improving function [5,6], physiotherapists are ideally placed to treat horses presenting with movement dysfunction.

Outcome measures that reflect client health status are essential for monitoring the safety and efficacy of treatment [7,8]. The absence of even a simple tool to quantify the functional change in response to treatment has allowed the use of non-evidence-based therapies to proliferate within the equine industry [9]. Ineffective treatments likely have negative welfare implications, wasting owners' time and money, while prolonging equine pain and dysfunction. Valid, reliable and relevant outcome measures that can be used in the field to assess quality of movement in horses and to monitor the success of equine physiotherapy and rehabilitation are needed [7,10].

Having been designed to grade lameness when walking and trotting in a straight line, existing lameness scales are too broad to adequately document subtle changes in quality of movement [3,11,12]. Given that these lameness scales are also subject to inconsistent applications by different practitioners [13–16], the lack of agreement between veterinary experts on the definition and measurement of lameness and asymmetry is not surprising [17]. Trot in a straight line, on its own, is insufficient to assess quality of movement due to the complexity and task-specific nature of movement [18]. Differences have been identified in hoof loading, spinal kinematics, body lean and asymmetry between different gaits, figures and surfaces [19–27]. Many movements tests are taught as an iterative assessment process [28]; however, it is currently unknown which ones are used most frequently in clinical practice, and if there is an established core group.

Instrumented gait analysis relying on inertia measurement units (IMUs) as used in the Equigait® (Cheshunt, UK) or Equinosis Q® (Columbia, IN, USA) system can objectively identify minute movement asymmetries. Despite acknowledging the value of IMUs, their data should be used as an aid to diagnosis [3,29], similar to medical imaging, and the clinical significance should be interpreted in conjunction with other assessments. While research using IMU's is rapidly advancing, in the authors' experience in the field, visual observation of movement still predominates, and this is routinely scored with subjective lameness grading scales.

While veterinarians need lameness scales to direct the clinical pathway for diagnosis, typically identifying a limb, severity and a pathoanatomical source [4,5], physiotherapists tend to use lameness scales as a triage tool. In addition to lameness scales there is also a place for a quality of movement outcome measure. Given that most horses are referred for physiotherapy with an established pathoanatomical diagnosis, the physiotherapists carry out a functional assessment to identify target tissues and directions for desensitising or strengthening (e.g., a cervical vertebral joint stiff into left lateral flexion, with hypertonicity of the right neck muscles and weak left neck muscles) [5].

Physiotherapists have a duty of care to ensure they provide quality practice; however, without outcome measures, decision-making is subject to bias and guesswork [30,31]. There is a strong desire from all stakeholders to have relevant outcome measures and research on the efficacy of equine physiotherapy [8,32,33]. However, current outcome measures designed for veterinarians that focus on lameness do not meet the needs of physiotherapists and equine clinicians working with rehabilitation and/or poor performance cases. Impairments are problems in body structure or function, while activity limitations refer to higher-level functions, such as complex whole-body movements [34]. Measures for both impairments and activity limitations are needed to accurately describe patient status [35]. While there are a variety of suitable equine impairment measures such as goniometry [36], palpation [37] and back profiles [38], there is currently a lack of outcome measures capable of monitoring activity limitations in horses. Without these, equine clinicians are left relying on subjective visual assessment and measures of impairment (e.g., passive range of movement), which should not be generalised to claim changes in whole-body movement.

For complex whole-body movements, goal setting is sometimes used in place of precise measures. In human physiotherapy, goal setting with the client is a vital part of client-centred care, and is used to monitor the long-term impact or value of care [39]. The Patient-Specific Functional Scale (PSFS) [40] (see Appendix A) is a patient-reported outcome measure used in human physiotherapy, which includes the client in scoring their ability to perform personally meaningful tasks. Part of the PSFS's popularity may be due to its adaptability for a large variety of movements or goals, compared to exhaustive list-style patient- or owner-reported outcome measures, which are often time-consuming and contain many irrelevant questions [41]. It should be possible to modify the PSFS for use by owners/riders and clinicians in equine physiotherapy and rehabilitation. Past publications shed little light on methods used in equine practice to measure complex movements; therefore, it is necessary to investigate how equine clinicians are currently using goals and monitoring complex movements.

To address these problems, we propose a new outcome measure be developed for equine quality of movement. The Equine Musculoskeletal Rehabilitation Outcome Score (TEMROS) identified domains for a composite rehabilitation outcome measure, noting outcome measures are lacking for the performance/functional capacity domain and suggesting developing a battery of movement tests [42]. The proposed outcome measure would be for use by equine clinicians working with horses undergoing rehabilitation or managing performance issues. Such horses may present with movement dysfunction, motion asymmetry, inconsistent, or subtle or mild lameness (e.g., AAEP < 2: Lameness that is difficult to observe at a walk or trot in a straight line but is present under certain circumstances [43]). It is currently unknown which movements clinicians believe to be most important or useful to include when assessing quality of movement in equine rehabilitation and performance. The proposed outcome measure would be a combination of a standardised battery of key movement tests (for simple routine movements) supplemented with a client-specific measure (for bespoke complex movements) that can be integrated into the assessment process.

This survey was an early investigative step in the development of a new field-based outcome measure. The primary aim of the survey was to identify which in-hand movements equine clinicians observe most frequently, and if there is a key group that could be taken forward to develop a new quality of movement outcome measure for use in equine physiotherapy and rehabilitation. Additionally, this study aimed to gather information on how complex movement is currently monitored and opinions on the usefulness of modifying the PSFS.

2. Materials and Methods

2.1. Subjects

For this study, equine clinicians were defined as equine sports medicine and rehabilitation veterinarians and qualified equine allied health professionals. Qualifications/syllabus of equine clinicians are heterogenous worldwide, and so it logically follows this would affect clinical practices. Therefore, it was decided to set tight inclusion criteria to try and achieve more homogeneity in qualification types and practice. The following inclusion criteria were applied: equine clinicians experienced in the areas of rehabilitation and performance, with at least an undergraduate degree in a relevant field (qualification names vary worldwide). Post-graduate training was desirable to try to achieve similarity in clinical reasoning and assessment processes due to comparable academic backgrounds.

There is an unknown number of equine clinicians with post-graduate qualifications worldwide. While it is challenging to ascertain the population, response rate and study power for web-based surveys, a detailed web-based investigation was conducted to attempt to estimate the sample frame; this suggested 21 professional associations could provide coverage of approximately 1000 equine clinicians. The *a priori* calculation of study power (95% CI, 5% error) yielded a requirement of 278 responses. However, based on the generally very low response to online surveys [44] and a previous online survey of a subgroup of this population gathering only 71 responses [32], a 90% CI and 10% margin of error were applied for this study, reducing the required minimum sample size to 64. It must be highlighted that this calculation is only an estimate—the results are largely descriptive and should be interpreted in the context of the participants, and not generalized too broadly. Additionally, the authors adhered to the Checklist for Reporting Results of Internet E-Surveys (CHERRIES) where possible [44].

Participant recruitment was via equine clinicians' professional associations (n = 21) who distributed the survey link through their member networks, e.g., Equine Sports Medicine and Rehabilitation Diplomats, Animal/Veterinary/Equine Physiotherapists and Animal Biomechanical Professionals (Chiropractors, Osteopaths), and flyers were posted on the associations' public Facebook® groups. Demographic information was collected on participant country of practice, qualifications, years of experience, current case load, and use of instrumented gait analysis. These details were used to determine eligibility for participation and to analyse variability in the sample's responses based on participant's background.

2.2. Data Collection

The questionnaire was conducted online using the Survey Monkey ® platform. Questions were reviewed by Charles Sturt University's (CSU) Spatial Data Analysis Network (SPAN), before being pilot-tested for user-friendliness by a small convenience sample of invited participants (n = 10). Pilot data were not included in the study results. Further revisions were made and the survey received ethical approval from Charles Sturt University, Human Research Ethics Committee (Protocol #H22082).

The questionnaire comprised 21 questions (7 open text, 2 closed-binary, 7 closed-Likert scale and 5 semi-closed) in three sections: 1—demographic details, 2—the frequency of movements used, and 3—how functional movement is currently monitored, with questions about goal setting, owner reported measures and the patient-specific-functional-scale. For Section 2, a list of 38 movements used during clinical assessment was compiled from published literature by the primary researcher (AB). To indicate how frequently each movement was used, participants had four possible responses: "always", "often", "sometimes" or "never". The PSFS was included as a display item alongside the questions relating to it. Open text questions allowed participants to provide a rationale for their answers. The full questionnaire and answer options are available in the Supplementary Materials.

The survey was designed to be completed in 15 to 20 min and was open for 6 weeks from 23 May to 4 July 2022 inclusive. Reminders were emailed regularly to the associations and posted on their social media pages to encourage participation by their members.

The survey's online landing page provided participant information and collected informed consent. Participation in the survey was voluntary and no incentives were offered. Anonymized survey data were received by the primary researcher (AB) and those requesting a summary of results were asked to directly email AB. The survey data were stored in accordance with the approved Human Research Ethics Application data management plan.

2.3. Data Analysis

Unusual responses were investigated before being included or excluded from the data, and the screened data were then collated by question in Microsoft Excel prior to being subjected to descriptive analysis. Jeffrey's Amazing Statistics Program (JASP version 16) was used for inferential analysis.

For descriptive analysis, mean and standard deviation (SD) were calculated for years of practice. Percentages were calculated for undergraduate and post-graduate qualifications, country of practice, workload with humans, equines and canines/other species, frequency of seeing performance management and rehabilitation cases, frequency of using simple video, kinematics, IMU or other devices, movements used "always" or "often" combined, use of formal goal setting, use of owner-reported measures, familiarity with and use of the

PSFS, opinion on usefulness of a modified PSFS for use by clinicians, owners (ADLs) and owners (complex movements), and participants based on background training. Mode was determined for the ordinal data relating to frequency of use of each movement.

For inferential analysis, Chi-squared tests were used to test for relationships between clinician background and the following: frequency of seeing rehabilitation cases, frequency of seeing performance cases, frequency of using simple video/kinematics/IMU/other devices, frequency of use of movement tests (then post hoc z scores manually calculated), use and familiarity with PSFS and opinion on usefulness of modified PSFS. Due to concerns on the violation of the normality assumption condition, the non-parametric Kruskal–Wallis test was used to test for relationships between clinician background and years of experience and proportion of work with human/equine/canine, plus between years' experience and familiarity with PSFS. Statistical significance was determined by $p < 0.05$. NVIVO was used to assist the qualitative analysis of themes from the open-ended questions.

3. Results

3.1. Responses

The questionnaire attracted 90 respondents; however, 9 were excluded for not meeting the inclusion qualifications and/or incomplete responses (completion rate 94%). Responses from 81 participants were therefore included in the analysis, of which 73 completed all questions (completeness rate of 90%). Not all participants responded to every question; the following results are presented based on the number of responses for each question. While it is impossible to calculate response rate when distributing surveys online, of the 52 addresses emailed, 50 were received. Several associations replied that they were unable to distribute surveys to their members due to internal policies, or requested payment. In response to this, the sample frame was revised down to 700 equine clinicians, the resultant sample size (90% CI, 10% error) being 62 participants. Reminders were emailed to active email addresses representing 19 associations and regularly posted on association Facebook pages (n = 14). Based on the estimated sample frame the approximate response rate was 13%.

3.2. Subjects' Background

Participants reported undergraduate qualifications in human physiotherapy (59%, n = 48), veterinary medicine (27%, n = 22), veterinary physiotherapy (10%, n = 8), human chiropractic (5%, n = 4), human osteopathy (5%, n = 4), and other (7%, n = 6) (zoology, biology, equine science, physical education, agriculture and manual therapy). Post-graduate qualifications included masters in veterinary/animal/equine physiotherapy (27%, n = 22), post-graduate diploma in veterinary/animal/equine physiotherapy (22%, n = 18), certificate or diploma in equine physiotherapy or rehabilitation (19%, n = 15), masters or post-graduate diploma in veterinary/animal/equine chiropractic (12%, n = 10), veterinary sports medicine and rehabilitation diploma (11%, n = 9), post-graduate diploma in animal biomechanical area (10%, n = 8), certificate or diploma in veterinary/animal/equine osteopathy (6%, n = 5), and other (14%, n = 11) (PhD, equine orthopaedics, equine surgery, veterinary acupuncture, equine biomechanics and rehabilitation, equine craniosacral therapy, equine anatomy and physiology, doctor of veterinary medicine, equine science).

Participants commonly held multiple qualifications, with 12% (n = 10) indicating more than one undergraduate qualification and 20% (n = 16) reporting more than one post-graduate qualification. Only 2% (n = 2) reported no post-graduate qualification.

Participants practiced as equine clinicians for a mean of 13.9 years (SD = 9.3). The majority of participants practiced in Australia (35%, n = 28), with 16% (n = 13) from the United Kingdom, 14% (n = 11) from the United States of America, 10% (n = 8) from New Zealand, 11% (n = 9) from mainland western European countries (Finland, Belgium, France, Germany, Italy, Netherlands and Sweden) and 13% (n = 10) from other countries (Ireland, Canada and South Africa).

All participants reported working with horses, with almost one-third, 29% (n = 17), focusing solely on horses, 57% (n = 46) also working with dogs or other species, and 64% (n = 52) having performed some work with human clients. As a proportion of their workload, horses ranged from 1 to 100%, humans from 0 to 99% and dogs or other species from 0 to 70%. For all participants, the mean proportion of work with equids was 58%, with humans 29% and with canids or other species 20%. The majority of participants, 80% (n = 65), saw horses for performance management either daily or weekly, while 77% (n = 62) saw horses for rehabilitation either daily or weekly (see Figure 1).

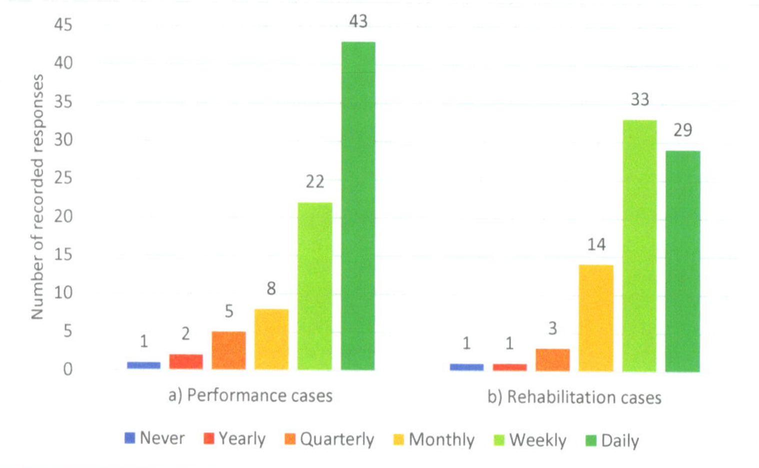

Figure 1. Frequency of participating equine clinicians seeing horses for (**a**) performance management and (**b**) rehabilitation (n = 81).

Simple video recordings were "always" or "often" used by 49% (n = 39) of participants while assessing quality of movement. Use of other technology was less frequent, with more than half "never" using kinematics, IMU's or other unnamed devices (see Figure 2).

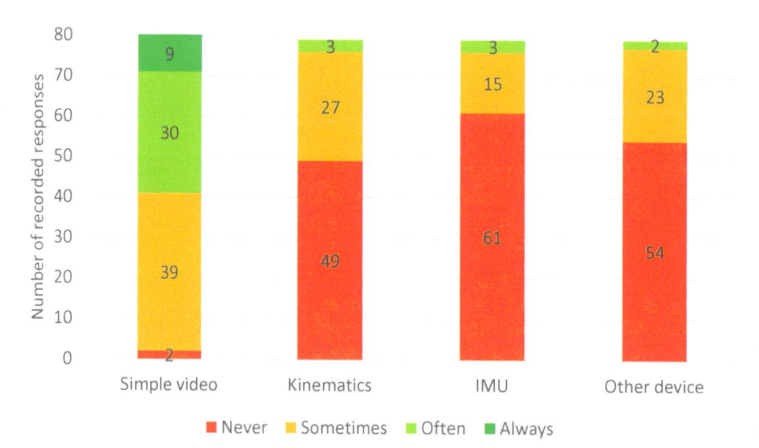

Figure 2. Frequency of participating equine clinicians using simple video (n = 80), kinematics (n = 79), Inertia Measurement Units (IMU) (n = 79) and other devices attached to the horse (n = 79) during assessment of quality of movement.

3.3. Essential Movement Tests

Movements on a firm surface were the most frequently used in-hand movement tests, with the use of inclines the least frequent. Movements are grouped by surface type (firm, soft or other) and displayed in the order used in the questionnaire; the cell containing the mode is highlighted/marked up (see Table 1).

Table 1. Frequency of use of in-hand movement tests when assessing equine quality of movement. Mode indicated with * and shaded (green for a mode of always, yellow for a mode of often, orange for a mode of sometimes and red for a mode of never), percentages < 50% shaded grey (n = 73).

Movement Test	Frequency of Use				Percentages of Often and Always Combined (%)
	Never	Sometimes	Often	Always	
Firm Surface					
Walk in a straight line—viewed from behind		4	8	61 *	95
Walk in a straight line—viewed from in front	1	6	7	59 *	90
Walk in a straight line—viewed side-on		9	15	49 *	88
Trot in a straight line—viewed from behind		8	17	48 *	89
Trot in a straight line—viewed from in front		10	17	46 *	86
Trot in a straight line—viewed side-on		14	27	32 *	80
Small circle (5–10 m) at the walk left and right rein	3	18	22	30 *	71
Small circle (5–10 m) at the trot left and right rein	4	23 *	23 *	23 *	63
Rein back/step back		20	14	39 *	73
Pivot/turn on the forehand left and right (aka hind leg cross-over, yielding the hind quarters)	5	21	15	32 *	64
Front leg cross-over/yielding the shoulders	11	28 *	15	19	47
Figure of 8/change of bend using tight turns (<5 m) in walk	17	31 *	19	6	34
Soft Surface					
Walk in a straight line—viewed from behind	4	15	38 *	16	74
Walk in a straight line—viewed from in front	4	16	38 *	15	73
Walk in a straight line—viewed side-on	5	18	37 *	13	68
Trot in a straight line—viewed from behind	3	16	41 *	13	74
Trot in a straight line—viewed from in front	3	20	38 *	12	68
Trot in a straight line—viewed side-on	3	22	39 *	9	66
Small circle (5–10 m) at the walk left and right rein	5	26	33 *	9	58
Small circle (5–10 m) at the trot left and right rein	7	23	35 *	8	59
Rein back/step back	8	26 *	26 *	13	53
Lunged on a circle (~15–20 m) at walk left and right rein	6	23	26 *	18	60
Lunged on a circle (~15–20 m) at trot left and right rein	7	21	26 *	19	62
Lunged on a circle (~15–20 m) at canter left and right rein	7	23	26 *	17	59
Other					
Walk up and down an incline	5	52 *	14	2	22
Lunge on an incline	36 *	33	3	1	5
Walk over pole/s	13	46 *	13	1	19
Trot over pole/s	16	47 *	9	1	14
Transition from halt to walk	7	21	23 *	22	62
Transition from walk to trot	4	24 *	24 *	21	62
Transition from trot to canter left/right lead on the lunge	4	30 *	26	13	53
Transition from canter to trot	3	32 *	26	12	52
Transition from trot to walk	3	25 *	22	23	62
Transition from walk to halt	6	24 *	21	22	59
Transition walk to halt on a diagonal line down incline	51 *	19	2	1	4
Transition halt to walk on a diagonal line up an incline	51 *	18	2	2	5
Dynamic mobilisations/baited stretches flexion/extension plane	2	14	31 *	26	78
Dynamic mobilisations/baited stretches lateral flexion and rotation left and right	1	15	30 *	27	78

Other movements suggested by participants fell into broad categories with some overlap: manual tests (n = 16 comments), particularly flexion tests (n = 4) and stimulating reflex movements (n = 5); balance (n = 13); neurological assessments (n = 12); lateral work (n = 5); under saddle (n = 2) and other (n = 10).

Rationales provided for the frequency of use of particular movements could be divided into factors related to the clinician (n = 16), the facilities (n = 13) or the horse (n = 12). Clinician factors describe un/familiarity with and preference for particular movements, as well as time limitations. Barriers to using movement tests included the facilities available, such as access to a level soft surface, inclines and poles, and horse factors such as the training level of the horse, age and discipline. Horse factors also covered the capability of the handler (n = 4) and that the clinicians' choice of movements to observe is needs-based (n = 10). For example, the differences between a young racehorse on a yard with only access to straight concrete and an older jumping horse at an equestrian centre.

3.4. Patient-Specific Measures

When asked if they use formal goal setting with clients, 64% (n = 47) of participants replied in the affirmative, and 36% (n = 26) replied no. In the open-ended question, the themes raised related to the type of goal (n = 21) (being clinical/problem list, task, short/long term, performance/competition), who was involved (n = 24) (client/owner/rider, trainer/coach and veterinarian), the method—SMART (n = 8), and use of realist timeframes or feasibility of the plan (n = 17). Five participants mentioned objective measurements (time, scoring tasks, IMU data, imaging), three raised the lack of objective measures and seven described informal subjective measurement of goals.

Owner-reported measures were indicated to be used by 74% (n = 54) of participants. When asked to specify, 7 participants provided outcome measures (three- or four-point grading systems), 18 reported quantitative measures (time/sets and repetitions, heart rate, flexi-curve, competition results) and the majority (n = 44) mentioned qualitative descriptions. Themes within the qualitative descriptions included subjective descriptions of movement quality (n = 29), observation of behaviour change (n = 18), lameness (n = 4) and third-party feedback (instructor, jockey/trainer/driver, dressage score or competition results).

The monitoring of complex functional movements was reported to be via clinician visual assessment (n = 27) including repeat video assessment (n = 23) and slow-motion video (n = 4), or owner subjective report (n = 19), with a small number mentioning measurements (n = 10) such as range of motion or workload and five reporting instrumented assessment techniques (IMU, Pain trace, FES).

In spite of 62% (n = 45) of participants reporting familiarity with the PSFS, only 21% (n = 15) confirmed using it. A further 36% (n = 26) of the participants were unfamiliar with the PSFS. Most of the participants, 82% (n = 58), agreed, of which 20% (n = 14) strongly agreed, that a modified equine version of the PSFS for use by clinicians to observe complex equestrian tasks would be useful. A similar trend was seen for usefulness of a modified equine version of the PSFS by owners/riders to observe both complex equestrian tasks and activities of daily living (ADLs) (see Figure 3).

Comments were mostly positive, with some neutral, while some raised limitations of using owners. Positive comments focused on how the PSFS can be individualised (n = 6). Key concerns around owners using the PSFS were the difficulty of grading movement (n = 10), owners being biased (n = 4) and the lack of compliance (n = 8).

General comments in the final open-ended question were overall positive, describing the study as useful work and expressing a desire for clinically relevant outcome measures. Concerns were raised about the scope of the challenge due to the sheer volume of variables that influence movement, and suggestions were made that the focus should be on developing outcome measures for clinicians rather than owners.

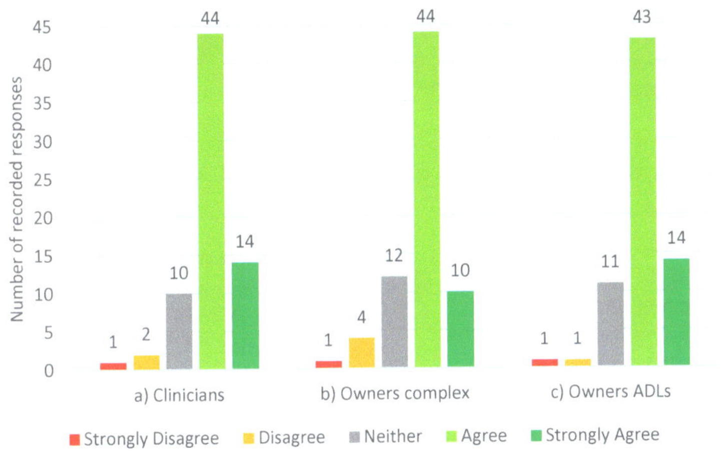

Figure 3. Participating equine clinicians' opinion on the statements; "a modified equine version of the Patient-Specific Functional Scale would be useful for: (**a**) clinicians to observe complex equestrian tasks (n = 71), (**b**) owners to report complex equestrian tasks (n = 71) and (**c**) owners to report activities of daily living (ADLs)" (n = 70).

3.5. Relationships between Variables Based on Background

Dividing participants based on undergraduate background resulted in 58% (n = 47) having a human physiotherapy background, 28% (n = 23) having a veterinary background and 15% (n = 11) having a mixed or other background.

There was a significant difference in years of experience between those with a veterinary background (19.21 years, SD = 9.7) and those with a human physiotherapy background (11.57 years, SD = 8.5)—$p = 0.003$.

The proportion of work with humans differed. Naturally, participants with a human physiotherapy background reported a larger percentage of work with humans (38%; SD = 31.82) than those from a mixed background (35%; SD = 36.83) or veterinary background (<1%; SD = 0.65) ($p < 0.001$). Those with a veterinary background attributed more of their workload to equines (88%; SD = 23.88), which significantly differed ($p < 0.001$) from the equine workload of those with a human physiotherapy background (45%; SD = 29.99) and those with a mixed background (55%; SD = 37.78).

Most participants saw rehabilitation and performance management cases regularly regardless of background discipline, be it rehabilitation ($\chi^2(10, N = 81) = 8.28, p = 0.602$) or performance management ($\chi^2(10, N = 81) = 4.122, p = 0.942$). There was no significant relationship between background and frequency of using simple video, kinematics or other devices; however, there was a statistically significant relationship ($p = 0.009$) between groups in relation to use of IMU sensors. Those with a veterinary background reported using IMU sensors "sometimes", which was more frequently than expected, as 11/22 (50%) of the veterinary background group "sometimes" or "often" used IMUs, while only 5/46 (11%) of the human physiotherapy background group "sometimes" or "often" used IMUs. In total, 2/11 (18%) of the mixed group "sometimes" or "often" used IMUs ($\chi^2(4, n = 79) = 13.485, p = 0.009$).

In relation to the frequency of use of different movements by background profession, there were several associations between variables; however, post hoc pair-wise comparisons revealed no pattern across "always" to "never" categories.

Veterinarians were more likely to be unfamiliar with the PSFS than allied health professionals, with a significant difference between groups ($p \leq 0.001$). Those with a physiotherapy background are both more likely to use the PSFS (14/39; $z = -2.72, p \leq 0.001$) and less likely to be unfamiliar with the PSFS (4/39; $z = 2.607, p \leq 0.001$). Those with a veterinary background are both more likely to be unfamiliar with the PSFS (18/22; z = 3.503, $p \leq 0.001$) and less likely to be familiar with but not use the PSFS than statistically expected (3/22; z = −2.065, $p \leq 0.001$).

There was no significant relationship between background and opinion on the usefulness of the PSFS by clinicians or owners. Those with fewer years of experience were more likely to be familiar with or use the PSFS (p = 0.043). All others relationships tested for, including for themes in the open-ended responses, found no significant difference.

4. Discussion

This survey is the first time equine clinicians have been asked about assessing quality of movement and, in contrast to existing lameness studies, this survey was multidisciplinary, consulting veterinarians and allied health professionals. In human medicine, siloed healthcare is being discouraged [39], and multidisciplinary practice is the future. Grading lameness is different to additionally assessing quality of movement; therefore, this list of key movements is a springboard to developing a unique outcome measure. There is little published research regarding quality of movement, including more complex movement, although Hobbs's scoping study [45] discusses it in relation to performance. Despite the professions having differing aims, these results demonstrate similarities between veterinarians and physiotherapists in the frequency of use of movements, which raises hopes regarding greater teamwork and complementary practice.

When the literature revealed no standardized set of movement tests for evaluating lameness or quality of movement, consulting a focus group of experts was considered, but it was decided a survey would canvas a larger audience and likely be more representative of field-based practice.

4.1. Participant Characteristics

The majority of participants saw equine performance management and rehabilitation cases either daily or weekly, thus regularly engaging with the type of horses this new outcome measure is intended for. In this sample, there was no difference between veterinarians and allied health professionals in seeing rehabilitation cases; however, that may be attributed to this survey targeting equine sports medicine and rehabilitation diplomats, not general veterinarians.

Simple video recordings are easily accessible via smart phones, compared to more expensive IMU systems, some of which are only available to veterinarians. It appears that many clinicians do not have access to instrumented gait analysis despite new systems becoming more readily available [46]. While the use of additional apps or software, e.g., to measure angles in videos, was not ascertained, the widespread use of video is a positive sign. Devices were reported to be used "sometimes" or "often", implying that they are not advantageous for assessing quality of movement with all equine clients. There was no significant relationship between those using devices and responses to other questions, such as preference for modifying the PSFS, suggesting access to technology did not bias participants.

4.2. Movement Test Preference

A list of the key movements most commonly used when assessing quality of movement has been collated from practicing equine clinicians. While previous studies had stated trot in a straight line was insufficient [23,47], a broader range of movements had not been defined. The movements listed are conducted in-hand, which helps bridge the gap between passive movements, or manually applied pressures, and a ridden assessment. These results support lists of common movements used for grading lameness [28], but refines those lists into movements used "always" or "often" to assess quality of movement.

Information on how complex movement is currently measured has been gathered, and although there were few objective outcome measures used for assessing complex movement, clinicians are keen for these to be developed further. Equine clinicians reported wanting to be more objective, and acknowledged the subjectivity and limitations of current assessment practices. This sentiment is in line with responses from veterinary physiotherapists in the United Kingdom [32], which highlighted the lack of objective measures, the level of understanding of the differences between subjective and objective measures, and the desire for more outcome measures to be designed for clinical practice, not just research.

The most commonly used movements and the barriers to assessment, while predictable, are now formally supported by survey evidence upgrading previously anecdotal assertions. A repeated theme in the comments was that assessment is an iterative process, with movements being chosen on a case-by-case basis. Despite this, within the frequently observed movements there appears to be a key group routinely used by equine clinicians. Several movements on a firm surface scored a mode of "always"; these are walk and trot in a straight line and on a small circle, step back and hind leg cross-over. In the context of fully assessing quality of movement and designing a suitable outcome measure, this seems a limited set of movements. In addition to the above "always"-observed movements, the larger subgroup that received a classification of "often" branches out to include different surfaces and gaits.

Movements scoring a mode of "never" or "sometimes" fit with the barriers mentioned previously, as these movement tasks require equipment (e.g., poles) or facilities (e.g., inclines) and a greater skill level from the horse and handler (e.g., front leg cross-over). Some clinicians described their assessment as restricted by industry expectations; for example, limited time per horse in racing stables, with the expectation to abbreviate assessment to palpation of the horse in the stable and not observing functional movements, in comparison to thoroughly assessing a dressage/sports horse all the way through being tacked up and ridden through specific movements reported by the rider as suboptimal.

Confining a new outcome measure to active in-hand movement tests avoids additional tack and rider related factors, or tests involving manual pressure (such as provoking balance reactions or stimulating muscular reflexes), which are difficult to standardise. Active in-hand movements are directed or guided by a cue, not by manual pressure. In addition, tools such as range of motion goniometers and palpation scales [37] already exist for hands-on assessment, along with the Ridden Horse Pain Ethogram [48], for assessing ridden behaviours. While acknowledging that pain, asymmetry, lameness, behaviour, and performance are inter-related constructs, this new outcome measure will focus on quality of movement or movement dysfunction. Dynamic mobilisation exercises were included in the survey and had a mode of "often"; however, while they are active in-hand movements, they differ from the other movement tests, as they are non-ambulatory and therefore should be excluded from further development within a new quality of movement outcome measure.

When asked to suggest other movement tests (or to identify any missing), participants' responses fell into categories of neurological tests (head high walking, tail pull), manual tests (weight shifting, resistance to displacement, hop test), reflexes (myotactic rounding response), manipulative assessments (flexion tests), three-leg balance, lateral work in-hand (which requires more advanced training in horse and handler to provide accurate pressure and release cues), under saddle active movements, and passive movements such as limb range of movement and back wiggle using the tail head. Participants also suggested observing movements the horse owner reported they are having issues with, such as tacking up, which are more behavioural assessments rather than quality of movement-related, but they are certainly a part of the observation phase of assessment and have been investigated by others, e.g., [49]. Many of the stimulated responses, passive, assisted or facilitated movements suggested can be influenced by the horse's motivation level and the applied external pressure, and are therefore difficult to standardise. Flexion tests have known issues with standardisation of force, time and individual horse response [50–53]; although they are not an accurate diagnostic tool [54], they are nonetheless still used to indicate areas of interest. However, it should be noted that the new outcome measure being designed is not intended for diagnosis, and flexion tests will not be included in it. Observing specific owner-reported movements comes under the remit of a modified PSFS, while balance and neurological tests are suitable for future research to create an equine neurological battery, similar to the canine FINFUN [55]. Reliable methods of monitoring canine functional movement are more advanced, with several condition specific outcome measures already in use e.g., neurological, arthritis, stifle and chronic pain [56].

Participants did not mention lunging (15–20 m circles) or cantering on the firm surface, only reporting small circles (5–10 m) at walk and trot. Due to its speed and biomechanics, canter places higher forces through the limbs, and cantering on a firm surface may pose an increased risk of exacerbating an issue and risk of slipping due to decreased traction on a smooth surface. Observing canter is useful, particularly for back pain and hindlimb lameness [57], but safety must always be considered first.

4.3. Patient-Specific Measure Preferences

The majority of therapists stated that they use formal goal-setting, sometimes with separate goals for owners and the clinician. However, without measurement, they are not outcome measures and lack the strong reliability, validity and sensitivity of systems such as goal attainment scaling (GAS) [58]. GAS helps with setting realistic goals [59]; being realistic was repeatedly mentioned in the survey responses. While SMART goals are supposed to be measurable, the achievement of many goals is often all or nothing [58]. No participants mentioned the use of GAS, nor any way of applying a weighting to reflect the importance or difficulty of the goal. However, GAS is time-consuming [60], which is one of the main reasons equine physiotherapists mention for not using objective measures [32].

The PSFS is a streamlined version of monitoring goals, with the 0–10 scoring being simpler for clients, but still incorporating discussion of what is realistic, and by setting what a 10/10 performance would look like, the individual's current ability and the steps necessary to bridge the gap are made clear. The PSFS is used in human physiotherapy, so it is unsurprising that fewer veterinarians had heard of the PSFS, and if a clinician is unfamiliar with an outcome measure, they are less likely to use it [61]. If all those involved in equine care embrace the new outcome measure, their ability to communicate with each other will be enhanced.

Equine clinicians are predominately using subjective methods to monitor complex movements, such as observation (live or video) and reported competition performance. Several participants stated they used objective measurements where possible, but admitted they were currently lacking. Many acknowledged that their approach taken to goal-setting and monitoring complex movements was informal, heavily reliant on subjective reports from the owner or the clinician's opinion, and not objectively measured or scored. When dealing with owners, a couple of participants mentioned using variations of a Likert grading scale (same/better/worse/different). Generally, these are simple to use as they indicate direction but not magnitude. The majority of participants supported the idea of modifying the PSFS for use with horses. Comments revealed that owners are not trusted to assess movement quality, yet for client-centred care, more education and involvement of owners is desirable [39].

4.4. Limitations and Further Research

The number of participants exceeded the a priori calculation of what was required to give the study acceptable power; nevertheless, sample size and self-selection bias must be acknowledged as potential limitations regarding the generalisability of the research findings reported in this study. The number of valid responses, from participants with comparable qualifications and experience in rehabilitation and performance management, would suggest that outcomes are associated with external validity. The number of participants attracted was similar to that in Tabor and Williams' [32] survey of veterinary physiotherapists in the United Kingdom, which used snowball sampling. Interest in the topic and survey fatigue likely contribute to the small participant numbers. Overall, the reach of the survey was limited by relying on third parties (professional associations) to distribute the link, and those parties not being personally invested or benefitting from ensuring distribution to all their members. Furthermore, some countries do not appear to have national associations, some members email address maybe incorrect, and some associations' rules around frequency of contacting members may mean potential participants only saw the link once, perhaps within a scheduled monthly e-newsletter. The high completion and completeness rates (94% and 90%) indicate strong engagement from those who chose to participate. The high average years of practice (13.9 years) and multiple qualifications support the participants having valuable clinical experience and knowledge that will inform their responses. Predictably, many of the participants also worked with humans, as in some countries this is a requirement to maintain their human physiotherapy registration. Even with restricting the inclusion criteria, there were over 30 different qualifications reported within this sample, with participants coming form 14 different countries. While the results of this study should be viewed through a descriptive lens, the coherence of the responses suggests similar assessment practices and challenges across the globe. Further research could look to replicate the findings with a broader population of equine physiotherapists and equine veterinarians.

This summary of the opinions of 81 equine clinicians advances previous knowledge by identifying a group of key movements to observe that can be taken forward as the foundation for a new quality of movement outcome measure. Despite the small number of objective measures in use, there is a strong desire for more robust outcome measures that can be integrated into practice. Future research efforts should focus on adapting the PSFS, currently in use in human medicine [62], for use with horses. Although research published on lameness has progressed substantially with instrumented techniques, there is still much that can be done to improve field-based visual observations of simple and complex movements.

5. Conclusions

An online survey of equine clinicians identified the most frequently observed in-hand movements, with a key group of 24 observed "always" or "often". The main limiting factors reported for assessments were the availability of different surfaces, and the horse and handler training level. Participants perceive benefits in modifying the Patient-Specific Functional Scale for monitoring complex movements. These movements will be taken forward for refinement as a battery of field-based quality of movement tests, accompanied by a modified PSFS for specific individual goals. Equine clinicians are keen for new outcome measures to be developed, but concerned that they need to be not only valid and reliable, but also user-friendly. Creating a new quality of movement outcome measure for horses undergoing performance management or rehabilitation will improve the ability to assess treatment efficacy, therefore enhancing evidence-based practice.

Supplementary Materials: The following supporting information can be downloaded at: https://www.mdpi.com/article/10.3390/ani13182822/s1, Questionnaire—Functional movement outcome measures in equine physiotherapy and rehabilitation.

Author Contributions: Conceptualisation, A.G.B., H.R., G.T. and R.L.; methodology, A.G.B., H.R., G.T. and R.L.; validation, A.G.B.; formal analysis, A.G.B.; investigation, A.G.B.; data curation, A.G.B.; writing—original draft preparation, A.G.B.; writing—review and editing, A.G.B., H.R., G.T. and R.L.; visualisation, A.G.B.; supervision, H.R., G.T. and R.L.; project administration, H.R. All authors have read and agreed to the published version of the manuscript.

Funding: This research was funded by an Australian Government Research and Training Program scholarship, which has no direct financial interest in the outcome of this investigation.

Institutional Review Board Statement: The study was conducted in accordance with the Declaration of Helsinki, and approved by the Human Research Ethics Committee of Charles Sturt University (protocol number: #H22082 date of approval: 22 May 2022).

Informed Consent Statement: Informed consent was obtained from all subjects involved in the study.

Data Availability Statement: Deidentified data are only available on request via Charles Sturt University, through Hayley Randle.

Acknowledgments: Gail Fuller; Survey Monkey® administrator for Charles Sturt University's (CSU) Spatial Data Analysis Network (SPAN). John Xie; reporting statistics advice, Quantitative Consulting Services, CSU.

Conflicts of Interest: The authors declare no conflict of interest. This study was conducted as part of AB's PhD program of research. The funders had no role in the design of the study; in the collection, analyses, or interpretation of data; in the writing of the manuscript; or in the decision to publish the results.

Appendix A

Name:__________________________ **Date:**____________________

Patient-Specific Functional Scale

This useful questionnaire can be used to help us tailor your care to your specific needs.

Please identify at least three important activities that you are unable to do OR are having difficulty with as a result of your problem. Write the activities you are unable to do OR are having difficulty with in the box below. Then use the scoring scale below to rate your ability to perform the activities you are having difficulty with.

Patient-Specific Activity Scoring Scale

(Unable to perform activity)	0	1	2	3	4	5	6	7	8	9	10	(Able to perform activity at the same level as before the injury/problem)

Activity	Initial Date 01/01/01	Date	Date	Date	Date
Ex. Getting into the car	7				
Ex. Trouble sleeping	9				
Ex. Bending, reaching	5				

EXAMPLE

For Patient Use:

Dates:								
Activity	Score		Score		Score		Score	
1.)								
2.)								
3.)								
4.)								
Total Scores:	Score	PT Initials	Score	PT Initials	Score	PT Initials	Score	PT Initials
	Eval		Progress Note		Progress Note		Discharge	

Physical Therapist Signature and Date:__________________________

For office use only:

Total score = sum of activity scores/number of activities
Minimum detectable change (90% CI) for average score = 2 points
Minimum detectable change (90% CI) for single activity score = 3 points
PSFS developed by: Stratford, P., Gill, C., Westaway, M., & Binkley, J. (1995). Assessing disability and change on individual patients: a report of a patient specific measure. Physiotherapy Canada, 47, 258-263. Reproduced with the permission of the authors.

RSV: 9/28/17

Figure A1. The Patient-Specific Functional Scale.

References

1. Hug, F.; Hodges, P.W.; Carroll, T.J.; De Martino, E.; Magnard, J.; Tucker, K. Motor adaptations to pain during a bilateral plantarflexion task: Does the cost of using the non-painful limb matter? *PLoS ONE* **2016**, *11*, e0154524. [CrossRef]
2. Mellor, D.J.; Beausoleil, N.J.; Littlewood, K.E.; McLean, A.N.; McGreevy, P.D.; Jones, B.; Wilkins, C. The 2020 five domains model: Including human-animal interactions in assessments of animal welfare. *Animals* **2020**, *10*, 1870. [CrossRef] [PubMed]
3. Dyson, S. Can lameness be graded reliably? *Equine Vet. J.* **2011**, *43*, 379–382. [CrossRef] [PubMed]
4. Goff, L. Physiotherapy assessment for the equine athlete. *Vet. Clin. N. Am. Equine Pract.* **2016**, *32*, 31–47. [CrossRef]
5. McGowan, C.M.; Cottriall, S. Introduction to equine physical therapy and rehabilitation. *Vet. Clin. N. Am. Equine Pract.* **2016**, *32*, 1–12. [CrossRef] [PubMed]
6. McGowan, C.M.; Goff, L. *Animal Physiotherapy: Assessment, Treatment and Rehabilitation of Animals*, 2nd ed.; John Wiley & Sons Incorporated: Chichester, UK, 2016.
7. Australian Physiotherapy Association. *Standards for Physiotherapy Practices*, 8th ed.; Australian Physiotherapy Association: Camberwell Victoria, Australia, 2011; p. 68.
8. Bergh, A. Outcome measures in animal physiotherapy. In *Animal Physiotherapy: Assessment, Treatment and Rehabilitation of Animals*, 2nd ed.; McGowan, C.M., Goff, L., Eds.; Wiley Blackwell: Chichester, UK, 2016; pp. 171–198.
9. Thirkell, J.; Hyland, R. A survey examining attitudes towards equine complementary therapies for the treatment of musculoskeletal injuries. *J. Equine Vet. Sci.* **2017**, *59*, 82–87. [CrossRef]
10. Duncan, E.A.S.; Murray, J. The barriers and facilitators to routine outcome measurement by allied health professionals in practice: A systematic review. *BMC Health Serv. Res.* **2012**, *12*, 96. [CrossRef]
11. Hardeman, A.; van Weeren, P.; Braganca, F.; Warmerdam, H.; Bok, H. A first exploration of perceived pros and cons of quantitative gait analysis in equine clinical practice. *Equine Vet. Educ.* **2021**, *34*, e438–e444. [CrossRef]
12. Gómez Álvarez, C.B.; Oosterlinck, M. The ongoing quest for a validated, universally accepted visual lameness grading scale. *Equine Vet. J.* **2022**, *55*, 5–8. [CrossRef]
13. Fuller, C.J.; Bladon, B.M.; Driver, A.J.; Barr, A.R.S. The intra- and inter-assessor reliability of measurement of functional outcome by lameness scoring in horses. *Vet. J.* **2006**, *171*, 281–286. [CrossRef]
14. Hewetson, M.; Christley, R.M.; Hunt, I.D.; Voute, L.C. Investigations of the reliability of observational gait analysis for the assessment of lameness in horses. *Vet. Rec.* **2006**, *158*, 852–858. [CrossRef] [PubMed]
15. Starke, S.D.; Oosterlinck, M. Reliability of equine visual lameness classification as a function of expertise, lameness severity and rater confidence. *Vet. Rec.* **2019**, *184*, 63. [CrossRef] [PubMed]
16. Clayton, H.M. *The Dynamic Horse; A Biomechanical Guide to Equine Movement and Performance*; Sport Horse Publications: Mason, MI, USA, 2004.
17. Van Weeren, P.R.; Pfau, T.; Rhodin, M.; Roepstorff, L.; Serra Bragança, F.; Weishaupt, M.A. What is lameness and what (or who) is the gold standard to detect it? *Equine Vet. J.* **2018**, *50*, 549–551. [CrossRef] [PubMed]
18. Dyson, S.; Greve, L. Subjective gait assessment of 57 sports horses in normal work: A comparison of the response to flexion tests, movement in hand, on the lunge, and ridden. *J. Equine Vet. Sci.* **2016**, *38*, 1–7. [CrossRef]
19. Rhodin, M.; Roepstorff, L.; French, A.; Keegan, K.G.; Pfau, T.; Egenvall, A. Head and pelvic movement asymmetry during lungeing in horses with symmetrical movement on the straight. *Equine Vet. J.* **2016**, *48*, 315–320. [CrossRef]
20. Logan, A.A.; Nielsen, B.D.; Robison, C.I.; Hallock, D.B.; Manfredi, J.M.; Hiney, K.M.; Buskirk, D.D.; Popovich, J.J.M. Impact of Gait and Diameter during Circular Exercise on Front Hoof Area, Vertical Force, and Pressure in Mature Horses. *Animals* **2021**, *11*, 3581. [CrossRef] [PubMed]
21. Byström, A.; Hardeman, A.; Braganca, F.; Roepstorff, L.; Swagemakers, J.-H.; van Weeren, P.; Egenvall, A. Differences in equine spinal kinematics between straight line and circle in trot. *Sci. Rep.* **2021**, *11*, 12832. [CrossRef]
22. Greve, L.; Dyson, S. What can we learn from visual and objective assessment of non-lame and lame horses in straight lines, on the lunge and ridden? *Equine Vet. Educ.* **2020**, *32*, 479–491. [CrossRef]
23. Greve, L.; Pfau, T.; Dyson, S.J. Thoracolumbar movement in sound horses trotting in straight lines in hand and on the lunge and the relationship with hind limb symmetry or asymmetry. *Vet. J.* **2017**, *220*, 95–104. [CrossRef]
24. Hardeman, A.; Serra Braganca, F.M.; Swagemakers, J.-H.; van Weeren, P.R.; Roepstorff, L. Variation in gait parameters used for objective lameness assessment in sound horses at the trot on the straight line and the lunge. *Equine Vet. J.* **2019**, *51*, 831–839. [CrossRef]
25. Marunova, E.; Hoenecke, K.; Fiske-Jackson, A.; Smith, R.K.W.; Bolt, D.M.; Perrier, M.; Gerdes, C.; Hernlund, E.; Rhodin, M.; Pfau, T. Changes in head, withers and pelvis movement asymmetry in lame horses as a function of diagnostic anaesthesia outcome, surface and direction. *J. Equine Vet. Sci.* **2022**, *118*, 104136. [CrossRef]
26. Pfau, T.; Stubbs, N.C.; Kaiser, L.J.; Brown, L.E.A.; Clayton, H.M. Effect of trotting speed and circle radius on movement symmetry in horses during lunging on a soft surface. *Am. J. Vet. Res.* **2012**, *73*, 10. [CrossRef] [PubMed]
27. Pfau, T.; Jennings, C.; Mitchell, H.; Olsen, E.; Walker, A.; Egenvall, A.; Tröster, S.; Weller, R.; Rhodin, M. Lungeing on hard and soft surfaces: Movement symmetry of trotting horses considered sound by their owners: Movement symmetry on hard and soft surfaces on the lunge. *Equine Vet. J.* **2016**, *48*, 83–89. [CrossRef] [PubMed]
28. Ross, M.W. Movement. In *Diagnosis and Management of Lameness in the Horse*, 2nd ed.; Ross, M.W., Dyson, S.J., Eds.; Elsevier: St Louis, MI, USA, 2011; pp. 64–80.

29. Pfau, T.; Roepstorff, L. To limp, or not to limp, is that the question? *Vet. J.* **2013**, *195*, 269–270. [CrossRef]
30. McGowan, C.M.; Stubbs, N.C.; Jull, G.A. Equine physiotherapy: A comparative view of the science underlying the profession. *Equine Vet. J.* **2007**, *39*, 90–94. [CrossRef] [PubMed]
31. Physiotherapy Board of Australia; Physiotherapy Board of New Zealand. *Physiotherapy Practice Thresholds in Australia and Aotearoa New Zealand*; Physiotherapy Board of Australia: Sydney, Australia, 2015; p. 37.
32. Tabor, G.; Williams, J. The use of outcome measures in equine rehabilitation. *Vet. Nurse* **2018**, *9*, 2–5. [CrossRef]
33. Doyle, A.; Horgan, N.F. Perceptions of animal physiotherapy amongst Irish veterinary surgeons. *Ir. Vet. J.* **2006**, *59*, 85–89. [CrossRef]
34. World Health Organisation. *Towards a Common Language for Functioning, Disability and Health: ICF the International Classification of Functioning, Disability and Health*; WHO: Geneva, Switzerland, 2002.
35. Abrams, D.; Davidson, M.; Harrick, J.; Harcourt, P.; Zylinski, M.; Clancy, J. Monitoring the change: Current trends in outcome measure usage in physiotherapy. *Man. Ther.* **2006**, *11*, 46–53. [CrossRef]
36. Adair, H.S.; Marcellin-Little, D.J.; Levine, D. Validity and repeatability of goniometry in normal horses. *Vet. Compend. Orthop.* **2016**, *29*, 314–319. [CrossRef]
37. Merrifield-Jones, M.; Tabor, G.; Williams, J. Inter- and intra-rater reliability of soft tissue palpation scoring in the equine thoracic epaxial region. *J. Equine Vet. Sci.* **2019**, *83*, 102812. [CrossRef]
38. MacKechnie-Guire, R.; MacKechnie-Guire, E.; Fairfax, V.; Fisher, D.; Fisher, M.; Pfau, T. The effect of tree width on thoracolumbar and limb kinematics, saddle pressure distribution, and thoracolumbar dimensions in sport horses in trot and canter. *Animals* **2019**, *9*, 842. [CrossRef]
39. Pantaleon, L. Why measuring outcomes is important in health care. *J. Vet. Intern. Med.* **2019**, *33*, 356–362. [CrossRef] [PubMed]
40. Stratford, P.; Gill, C.; Westaway, M.; Binkley, J. Assessing disability and change on individual patients: A report of a patient specific measure. *Physiother. Can.* **1995**, *47*, 258–263. [CrossRef]
41. Meakins, A. Outcome Measures Suck. Available online: https://www.thesports.physio/outcome-measures-suck/ (accessed on 20 May 2023).
42. Tabor, G.; Nankervis, K.; Fernandes, J.; Williams, J. Generation of domains for the equine musculoskeletal rehabilitation outcome score: Development by expert consensus. *Animals* **2020**, *10*, 203. [CrossRef]
43. AAEP Horse Show Committee. *Guide to Veterinary Services for Horse Shows*, 7th ed.; American Association of Equine Practitioners: Lexington, KY, USA, 1999.
44. Eysenbach, G. Improving the quality of Web surveys: The Checklist for Reporting Results of Internet E-Surveys (CHERRIES). *J. Med. Internet Res.* **2004**, *6*, e34. [CrossRef]
45. Hobbs, S.J.; St George, L.; Reed, J.; Stockley, R.; Thetford, C.; Sinclair, J.; Williams, J.; Nankervis, K.; Clayton, H.M. A scoping review of determinants of performance in dressage. *PeerJ* **2020**, *8*, e9022. [CrossRef]
46. Lawin, F.J.; Byström, A.; Roepstorff, C.; Rhodin, M.; Almlöf, M.; Silva, M.; Andersen, P.H.; Kjellström, H.; Hernlund, E. Is Markerless More or Less? Comparing a Smartphone Computer Vision Method for Equine Lameness Assessment to Multi-Camera Motion Capture. *Animals* **2023**, *13*, 390. [CrossRef] [PubMed]
47. Greve, L.; Pfau, T.; Dyson, S.J. Alterations in body lean angle in lame horses before and after diagnostic analgesia in straight lines in hand and on the lunge. *Vet. J.* **2018**, *239*, 1–6. [CrossRef]
48. Dyson, S.; Van Dijk, J. Application of a ridden horse ethogram to video recordings of 21 horses before and after diagnostic analgesia: Reduction in behaviour scores. *Equine Vet. Educ.* **2020**, *32*, 104–111. [CrossRef]
49. Dyson, S.; Bondi, A.; Routh, J.; Pollard, D.; Preston, T.; McConnell, C.; Kydd, J. Do owners recognise abnormal equine behaviour when tacking-up and mounting? A comparison between responses to a questionnaire and real-time observations. *Equine Vet. Educ.* **2021**, *34*, e375–e384. [CrossRef]
50. Nocera, I.; Sgorbini, M.; Gracia-Calvo, L.A.; Cacini, M.; Vitale, V.; Citi, S. A novel dynamometer for the standardisation of the force applied during distal forelimb flexion tests in horses. *Equine Vet. Educ.* **2021**, *33*, 484–488. [CrossRef]
51. Keg, P.R.; van Weeren, P.R.; Back, W.; Bameveld, A. Influence of the force applied and its period of application on the outcome of the flexion test of the distal forelimb of the horse. *Vet. Rec.* **1997**, *141*, 463–466. [CrossRef]
52. Armentrout, A.R.; Beard, W.L.; White, B.J.; Lillich, J.D. A comparative study of proximal hindlimb flexion in horses: 5 versus 60 seconds. *Equine Vet. J.* **2012**, *44*, 420–424. [CrossRef] [PubMed]
53. Starke, S.D.; Willems, E.; Head, M.; May, S.A.; Pfau, T. Proximal hindlimb flexion in the horse: Effect on movement symmetry and implications for defining soundness. *Equine Vet. J.* **2012**, *44*, 657–663. [CrossRef]
54. Ramey, D. Forelimb Flexion Tests. Musings by Dr Ramey. 2017. Available online: https://doctorramey.com (accessed on 30 August 2023).
55. Boström, A.F.; Hyytiäinen, H.K.; Koho, P.; Cizinauskas, S.; Hielm-Björkman, A.K. Development of the Finnish neurological function testing battery for dogs and its intra- and inter-rater reliability. *Acta Vet. Scand.* **2018**, *60*, 56. [CrossRef]
56. Wright, A.; Amodie, D.M.; Cernicchiaro, N.; Lascelles, B.D.X.; Pavlock, A.M.; Roberts, C.; Bartram, D.J. Identification of canine osteoarthritis using an owner-reported questionnaire and treatment monitoring using functional mobility tests. *J. Small Anim. Pract.* **2022**, *63*, 609–618. [CrossRef] [PubMed]
57. Barstow, A.; Dyson, S. Clinical features and diagnosis of sacroiliac joint region pain in 296 horses: 2004–2014. *Equine Vet. Educ.* **2015**, *27*, 637–647. [CrossRef]

58. Hurn, J.; Kneebone, I.; Cropley, M. Goal setting as an outcome measure: A systematic review. *Clin. Rehabil.* **2006**, *20*, 756–772. [CrossRef] [PubMed]
59. Turner-Stokes, L. Goal attainment scaling (GAS) in rehabilitation: A practical guide. *Clin. Rehabil.* **2009**, *23*, 362–370. [CrossRef]
60. Stevens, A.; Beurskens, A.; Koke, A.; Weijden, T.T.v.d. The use of patient-specific measurement instruments in the process of goal-setting: A systematic review of available instruments and their feasibility. *Clin. Rehabil.* **2013**, *27*, 1005–1019. [CrossRef]
61. Jette, D.U.; Halbert, J.; Iverson, C.; Miceli, E.; Shah, P. Use of standardized outcome measures in physical therapist practice: Perceptions and applications. *Phys. Ther.* **2009**, *89*, 125–135. [CrossRef] [PubMed]
62. Kyte, D.G.; Calvert, M.; van der Wees, P.J.; ten Hove, R.; Tolan, S.; Hill, J.C. An introduction to patient-reported outcome measures (PROMs) in physiotherapy. *Physiotherapy* **2015**, *101*, 119–125. [CrossRef] [PubMed]

animals

MDPI

Article

Locomotory Profiles in Thoroughbreds: Peak Stride Length and Frequency in Training and Association with Race Outcomes

Charlotte Schrurs [1,*], Sarah Blott [1], Guillaume Dubois [2], Emmanuelle Van Erck-Westergren [3] and David S. Gardner [1,*]

1 School of Veterinary Medicine & Science, University of Nottingham, Sutton Bonington, Loughborough LE12 5RD, UK
2 Arioneo Ltd., 94 Boulevard Auguste Blanqui, 75013 Paris, France
3 Equine Sports Medicine Practice, 83 Avenue Beau Séjour, 1410 Waterloo, Belgium
* Correspondence: charlotte.schrurs@nottingham.ac.uk (C.S.); david.gardner@nottingham.ac.uk (D.S.G.)

Simple Summary: Racehorses compete in short ('sprinters'); medium ('milers') or long distance ('stayers') races. Sprinters are thought to naturally have a shorter stride than stayers; but no study has objectively tested this theory. Here, using known race distance to categorize racehorses into one of the three aforementioned categories together with a stride tracking device that objectively measures locomotion; this study demonstrates that peak stride length in racehorses is a heritable trait that is different in sprinters versus stayers prior to them even racing at that distance. In training, sprinters took shorter strides of higher frequency and were faster to cover furlongs in race-speed training sessions from a standing start than stayers. These stride data were recorded during training sessions before the horses raced and thus categorised as 'sprinters' or 'stayers'. Stride length during training did not predict later racing success. This study provides the first objective insight into locomotory differences between sprinters and stayers. Such information when coupled with the trainer's experience/eye could help them choose the most suitable race for each individual horse; to benefit both its health and safety on the track.

Abstract: Racehorses competing in short (i.e., 'sprinters'), middle- or longer-distance (i.e., 'stayers') flat races are assumed to have natural variation in locomotion; sprinters having an innately shorter stride than stayers. No study has objectively tested this theory. Here, racehorses (n = 421) were categorised as sprinters, milers or stayers based on known race distance (n = 3269 races). Stride parameters (peak length and frequency) of those racehorses were collected from prior race-pace training sessions on turf (n = 2689; 'jumpout', n = 1013), using a locomotion monitoring device. Pedigree information for all 421 racehorses was extracted to three-generations. In training, sprinters had a shorter stride of higher frequency and covered consecutive furlongs faster than stayers ($p < 0.001$). Relatively short or longer stride did not predict race success, but stayers had greater race success than sprinters ($p < 0.001$). Peak stride length and frequency were moderately heritable (h^2 = 0.15 and 0.20, respectively). In conclusion, differences in stride were apparent between sprinters and stayers (e.g., shorter stride in sprinters) during routine training, even after accounting for their pedigree. Objective data on stride characteristics could supplement other less objectively obtained parameters to benefit trainers in the appropriate selection of races for each individual racehorse.

Keywords: horse; exercise; stride; performance; heritability

1. Introduction

In flat racing, Thoroughbreds compete in various types of races usually categorised as short (<1500 m), middle (1600–2500 m) or long (>2500 m) distance. Racehorses are usually considered to be naturally predisposed to one type of race distance, due to various physiological and morphological characteristics such as size, musculature [1], and stride [2,3]. Genetics is also important [4], although the precise contribution of genetics versus environmental variables which classify successful sprinters or stayers are relatively undefined. Nevertheless, subjective information is often used by many buyers and trainers of racehorses to assign them to become predominantly short or longer-distance performers. Even so, many racehorses initially race at shorter-distance, but subsequently perform better at longer-distances (i.e., 'sprinter-miler' or miler-stayer'). It is a common assumption and practice that racehorses are trained similarly, regardless of their labelling as a 'sprinter' or 'stayer'. In human sport, the training regimes of 100 m sprinters will contrast markedly to marathoners; short anaerobic bursts of speed requiring high muscular energy versus high aerobic capacity, efficient fuel utilization and fatigue resistance [5,6]. If trainers could complement their own assessment of a racehorses' best distance (i.e., subjective experience or their 'eye') with objectively obtained training data that classified the racehorses on locomotory characteristics that distinguished a sprinter from a stayer, then more specific training sessions could be implemented to increase the chances of better performance earlier in the racehorses' careers: horses would race at their appropriate distances and wastage could be reduced. Monitoring speed and stride length over time allows trainers to identify or anticipate musculoskeletal injuries early on during racehorse training [7].

Early determination of any type of racehorse involves complex decisions and multiple parameters. For example, shorter distance races (i.e., those at a distance of <7 furlongs or ~1400 m) require explosive speed and rapid, short strides to quickly reach maximum speed. Such a racehorse is often of shorter stature and greater muscularity, much like human sprinters. In contrast, racehorses that excel over longer-distance (>12 furlongs or ~2500 m) require stamina, often associated with leanness and longer, strides. Because such disparity in phenotype can underpin sports performance, genetic testing has grown in popularity across the racing industry [1,4]. Variation in single-nucleotide polymorphisms of the myostatin gene (MSTN), which controls muscle development, has shown that nearly all sprinters are homozygous ('C/C') at the MSTN locus, while heterozygous ('C/T') horses tend to favour middle-distance races (7–12 furlongs; 1400 m–2400 m). Racehorses homozygous ('T/T') appear better suited to longer distance races (>10 furlongs, 2000 m), according to previously obtained race performance [4,8,9].

It is axiomatic that in order to win any competition based on speed, the fastest individual will get to the finish line first. Racehorses increase speed firstly by increasing stride frequency (SF) up to a pace consistent with gallop (45+ kph) and then by increasing stride length (SL; 45–65+ kph) [3,10]. Therefore, in sprint races of shorter distance, the racehorse that is able to rapidly increase, or maintain a higher stride frequency, is more likely to achieve a higher speed and good performance. Over longer distances, longer stride becomes more important, alongside endurance capacity [11]. For decades, breeders and trainers have attempted to relate the physiological characteristics of racehorses during their training to their race-day performance [12]. Objective measurements of locomotory parameters have only recently become available for racehorse trainers, allowing them to potentially ascertain whether a young racehorse has a greater aptitude for sprinting or longer-distance races [3,13]. However, to date, no study has related race performance over multiple seasons with information on locomotory profile in training–do racehorses that have only raced in sprint races demonstrate an innately shorter stride early on in training? With the advent of smart devices that record multiple parameters in the equine athlete, the possibility for such an early insight into locomotory differences between sprinters, milers or stayers is now possible. A better understanding of individual horse stride characteristics could help racehorse professionals select suitable race distances, while also taking into account their own experience at placing racehorses in suitable meetings alongside other historical aspects of how racehorse conformation and pedigree information can influence such decisions. No study has specifically evaluated stride patterns in different types of racehorses (stratified by performance in short, middle or longer distance races) and retrospectively assessed locomotory profile in training in the same racehorses, considering their pedigree information, to account for the influence of genetics on racing outcomes.

Hence, in the present study, an observational study was conducted, using a fitness tracking device to study peak stride (length and frequency) in racing Thoroughbreds categorised according to the type of turf race they have participated in (sprint, mile or staying' race; based on distance) and their subsequent racing result (win/podium/top5). Using this classification of racehorses according to their race distance, we have retrospectively classified the training data of the same horses galloping at race-speed on turf to observe whether any differences in locomotory parameters were apparent in training sessions prior to and during subsequent races. We were further able to determine whether any training parameters within each category of racehorse could predict race performance. The primary hypothesis of the study is that racehorses categorised according to race distance (sprinter/miler/stayers) may be distinguished in training by having relatively short, medium or long stride, respectively when analysed at race speed (soft-medium-hard gallop session or 'jumpout'). Secondary hypotheses are: (1) sprinters-milers-stayers with relatively short or long stride within each category are more successful in their respective races, and (2) that locomotory parameters have moderate-to-high heritability. Finally, since many racehorses compete in different types of races (e.g., sprint, mile and/or staying race) we analysed the extent to which locomotory profiles (e.g., peak stride frequency, length) in training evolved over time within individual horses throughout the race season.

2. Materials and Methods

2.1. Databases

This retrospective, observational study used three large datasets, all including the same cohort of racehorses:

(1) racehorse training sessions: collected by means of a fitness tracker (the 'Equimetre'™) from a single racing yard (Ciaron Maher Racing) in Victoria, Australia
(2) racehorse pedigree information: publicly available and downloaded from https://www.pedigreequery.com (accessed 4 August 2022)
(3) race results: available upon subscription in Australia, with race data recorded and downloaded from http://www.racing.com (accessed 7 July 2022)

2.2. Designation of Racehorses according to Race Distance

A total of n = 421 racehorses participating in a total of n = 3269 races were included in this study. Races were categorised according to class of race. In Australia, Group and Listed races are those established by the Australian Racing Board to reflect the highest standard of racing for races run in Australia. Group 1 are the highest-class races, followed by Group 2, Group 3 and Listed races. In this study, the highest-class races (n = 347, 10.6% of total) comprised; Group 1 (n = 65 of 3269 races; 1.9 %), Group 2 (n = 55 races, 1.6%), Group 3 (n = 97 races, 2.9%) and Listed (n = 130 races, 3.9%), whereas all other races were classed as Uncategorised (n = 2922 races; 89.7%). Race distance was known from http://www.racing.com (accessed on 28 October 2022) and was classified for this particular study as a 'sprint' race <1600 m, 'mile race' 1601–2500 m or 'staying race' >2501 m. All races were conducted on turf between 20 March 2020 to 13 May 2022. Five types of racehorse were created: (1) pure sprinter–exclusively racing over sprint distance only (n = 265 horses, 1563 races); (2) sprinter-miler, competing predominantly in sprint but also some mile races (n = 81 horses, 775 races); (3) miler, pure mile races only (n = 22 horses, 167 races); (4) sprinter-miler-stayer, competing in all types of race (n = 37 horses, 327 races) and (5) stayer-miler, purely or predominantly racing at stayer distance with some mile races (n = 16 horses, 131 races). Racehorses were aged between 2–10 years of age at the time of racing and included males (colts/stallions; n= 33 average age, 2.93 ± 0.42 years), females (fillies/mares; n= 197, 3.88 ± 0.90 years), geldings (n = 174, 4.67 ± 1.42 years) or of unknown/unrecorded sex (n = 17, 3.76 ± 0.69 years). All race data were extracted online from http://www.racing.com, accessed on 28 October 2022. Other aspects of the dataset such as venue, track condition, carried weight, handicap, rating and prize money were recorded.

2.3. Training Data

Horses wore their regular tack and were exercised by a randomly allocated work rider, who varied according to individual training sessions. A tracking device ('Equimetre™', Arioneo, Ltd. Paris, France) was fitted to the girth prior to training by persons accustomed to using the device, as previously described [14]. The device recorded locomotory parameters (peak stride length and frequency) alongside speed (by GNSS) and cardiovascular parameters (peak HR), as previously described in detail [3]. The trainer determined the nature of each individual training session, directing the work-rider as appropriate. The Equimetre was not systematically placed on each horse for every individual training session, rather for specific sessions. From the GNSS (GPS + Glonass + Galileo) satellite data, speed (i.e., time taken to cover 200 m in seconds) recorded for each 200 m segment (at 200, 400, 600, 800, 1000, 1200 and 1400 m) was recorded. The fastest 200 m was then used to designate the session as soft, medium or hard gallop. All training sessions at gallop were conducted on turf. In addition, a separate dataset of 'jumpout' training sessions were available for analysis with similar logged data. These sessions aim to replicate race-day barrier trials and conditions. Horses of similar ability are grouped to 'race' simultaneously from starting gates for the duration of the training session. All jumpout sessions were also conducted on turf. All training data were collected between 7 April 2020 to 19 April 2022 and comprised a total of 2689 training sessions, with 12 (8–19) median (first-third interquartile range [IQR] per racehorse. From the exact date of training, together with the exact race date, the number of days prior to each race plus the interval in days between races could also be recorded for each horse. Final datasets were checked for artifacts and corrected accordingly in MS Excel. Environmental temperature and precipitation were recorded as potential covariates in any analyses. Using the hard outcome of race performance in races of known distance to classify five categories of racehorse from sprinter to stayer, then the same categorisation was applied retrospectively to all 421 racehorses during their gallop training sessions that occurred prior to, and during the two race seasons as recorded here (2020 to 2022).

2.4. Pedigree Data

For each individual racehorse, an online search was first conducted on the Thoroughbred Pedigree Database http://www.pedigreequery.com, accessed on 28 October 2022 to obtain a three generation pedigree for all 421 individual racehorses The resulting pedigree dataset consisted of n = 2690 horses from 629 sires (259 of which were founders), and 1628 dams (693 founders). Where racehorses were either not present or multiple racehorses with the same name existed, then data were cross-checked using a further database (Equineline.com). The data for each individual racehorse was then manually reverified on http://www.racing.com/horses/, accessed on 28 October 2022 for trainer, horse age, sex and racing profile. As a further check, using a random number generator in MS Excel (between 001–421), ten further racehorses were cross-checked for accuracy. The final three generation pedigree was used to estimate heritability.

2.5. Statistical Analysis

Any normally distributed descriptive data (e.g., peak stride length, stride frequency) are presented as mean (±1 standard deviation [SD]). Similar data that were not normally distributed or categorical are presented as median (1st–3rd interquartile range) or as percentage (of total number) for categorical variables. Data distribution was checked either by standard tests (e.g., Shapiro–Wilk test) or checking of residuals post analysis. If necessary, data was log-transformed ($\log_{10}$) to normalise the distribution of the data prior to analysis. For some analyses, where assumptions for analysis of variance (ANOVA) could not be met due to occasional missing data (e.g., artefacts removed or no data present), linear mixed models (restricted maximum likelihood; REML) were used with the main effect of interest fitted as a fixed effect and HorseID or racecourse fitted as random effects. This statistical model assumes that occasional missing data are distributed at random amongst fixed effects. Other potentially confounding factors that were not part of the design but may influence outcome, as assessed by univariate analysis ($p < 0.10$) were included as co-variates (e.g., interval between race days, temperature, precipitation). Estimates of heritability were generated using a sparse inverse relationship matrix ('ainv') generated for all 421 racehorses and their three-generation pedigree. Combining the pedigree file with phenotypic outcomes such as stride length in an animal model (i.e., using REML) allowed us to obtain variance parameters and narrow sense heritability estimates (additive genetic variance; Genstat v21, VSNi, Rothampsted, Harpenden, UK). Approximate standardised error (SE) for h^2 was obtained using the delta method, which uses a Taylor's expansion to get the variance of a function of a parameter ($Var(f(x)) = Var(x) \times (f'(x))^2$). Estimates were obtained after adjusting for age and including the type of racehorse (e.g., sprinter versus stayer) as fixed effects. Significant variation in the proportion of wins/placing according to the type of racehorse ('sprinter versus stayer') was analysed by logistic regression fitting win, top3 or top5 as individual binomial outcomes (yes/no) and type of horse as a fixed effect adjusted for any significant confounding variables (age of horse, track condition, race class). All data were analysed using Genstat v22 (VSNi Ltd., Rothampsted, Harpenden, UK). Statistical significance was accepted at $p < 0.05$.

3. Results

3.1. Racing Data and Performance

Within each category, racehorses participated in a similar number of races: (pure sprinter, 4 [1–8] races); sprinter-miler, 7 [1–14] races; miler, 6 [1–11] races; sprinter-miler-stayer, 8 [1–12] races; stayer, 7 [2–12] races, median [1st–3rd IQR]. Sprinters were significantly younger than milers, who were younger than stayers at the time of racing: (pure sprinter, 3.6 ± 0.9 years; sprinter-miler, 4.6 ± 1.2 years; miler, 4.8 ± 1.3 years; sprinter-miler-stayer, 4.9 ± 1.0 years; stayer, 6.6 ± 1.3 years mean ± 1 SD). Average prize money won according to the class of the race was significantly different between race classes, (Group 1, $93,898 ± 85,880; Group 2, $38,955 ± 42,618; Group 3, $28,573 ± 29,159; Listed, $27,012 ± 33,646; Uncategorised, $9847 ± 12,938). For $n = 35$ of 3268 races the final position was unknown. Overall, 508 races were won by 255 different racehorses, 331 different racehorses achieved a top three placing in a total of 2175 races and 375 of 421 racehorses were placed top five in a total of 1668 races. The remainder were unplaced. Racehorses therefore either won or were placed top three or top five in 15.5, 36.4 or 51.0% of races, which varied significantly according to the type of horse (Table 1). 'Stayers' were less common, competed in fewer races but were more successful than sprinters (Table 1). Race distance (meters) was not different ($p > 0.05$) between different class of race (Group 1, 1712 ± 664; Group 2, 1624 ± 427; Group 3, 1564 ± 501; Listed, 1762 ± 653; Uncategorised, 1566 ± 571 m).

Table 1. Race performance stratified by type of horse.

	All (n = 3269)	Sprinter (n = 1671)	Sprinter-Miler (n = 874)	Miler (n = 167)	Sprinter-Miler-Stayer (n = 408)	Stayer (n = 149)	* p-Value
Wins (%)	508 (15.5)	234 (14.0)	134 (15.3)	27 (16.2)	74 (18.1)	39 (26.2)	<0.001
Top3 (%)	1190 (36.4)	593 (35.5)	299 (34.2)	60 (35.9)	166 (40.7)	72 (48.3)	<0.001
Top5 (%)	1668 (51.0)	823 (49.3)	422 (48.3)	89 (53.3)	239 (58.6)	95 (63.8)	<0.001

Values are number meeting criteria for each row (proportion [%] of total races in each column). Data as per Racing.com racing records in Victoria, Australia (n = 421 different racehorses, n = 3269 different races). * analysed by logistic regression (see Section 2.5 in Methods).

3.2. Training Data and Locomotory Performance

All sessions were effectively 'race-pace', as illustrated in Table 2, with horses covering a furlong (200 m) in 10–12 s, achieving speeds of up to 67 kph, with peak stride frequencies and length increasing with speed and indicative of race-pace efforts, as previously described. However, when categorised according to the type of racehorse, then significant differences were apparent; sprinters *per se* had significantly shorter peak stride length and higher frequency than stayers, with a gradual change between intermediary categories (Table 3).

The expected increments in peak stride length and frequency with harder training sessions were observed across all categories of racehorse (Table 3).

Table 2. Descriptive characteristics of the training dataset.

	Soft Gallop (n = 635)	Medium Gallop (n = 579)	Hard Gallop (n = 585)	p-Value
Best 0–200 m (s)	11.6 ± 0.1	11.3 ± 0.1	10.8 ± 0.4	<0.001
Max speed (kph)	62.5 ± 0.9	64.2 ± 0.8	66.8 ± 1.4	<0.001
Peak stride frequency (stride/s)	2.37 ± 0.08	2.40 ± 0.00	2.45 ± 0.08	<0.001
Peak stride length (ms)	7.35 ± 0.24	7.48 ± 0.24	7.63 ± 0.27	<0.001

Values are Mean ± 1SD for continuous data recorded by 'Equimetre' in Australia (n = 421 different racehorses, n = 1799 different training sessions). Data were available throughout the year. Training intensity (soft/med/hard gallop) was calculated from the cohort based upon the fastest furlong (200 m interval) for each session and slower intensities (slow/med/hard canter) were excluded. Such data was restricted to training sessions conducted on turf track surfaces. Data were analysed by one-way ANOVA, blocking for the individual horse to account for multiple training sessions conducted by the same horse.

Table 3. Peak stride frequency and length in race-speed training efforts categorised by type of racehorse.

	Sprinter	Sprinter-Miler	Miler	Sprinter-Miler-Stayer	Stayer	* p-Value
Training distance (m)	4924 ± 1146 ^{a}	4987 ± 1232 ^{ab}	4993 ± 1192 ^{ab}	5167 ± 1240 ^{b}	5333 ± 1148 ^{ab}	0.018
'Work' distance (m)	1802 ± 380 ^{a}	1912 ± 479 ^{b}	1968 ± 479 ^{b}	2124 ± 565 ^{c}	2292 ± 650 ^{c}	<0.001
			Peak stride frequency (strides/sec)			
Soft Gallop	2.39 ± 0.07 ^{a}	2.36 ± 0.07 ^{b}	2.38 ± 0.08 ^{bc}	2.35 ± 0.08 ^{bc}	2.28 ± 0.06 ^{c}	Type horse, <0.001 Train intensity, <0.001 Interaction, 0.03
Medium Gallop	2.41 ± 0.07	2.39 ± 0.07	2.38 ± 0.08	2.37 ± 0.06	2.29 ± 0.08	
Hard Gallop	2.46 ± 0.08 *	2.43 ± 0.08 *	2.46 ± 0.05 *	2.41 ± 0.06 *	2.34 ± 0.05 *	
			Peak stride length (meters)			
Soft Gallop	7.31 ± 0.23 ^{a}	7.41 ± 0.23 ^{ab}	7.37 ± 0.21 ^{b}	7.41 ± 0.24 ^{bc}	7.60 ± 0.20 ^{c}	Type horse, <0.001 Train intensity, <0.001 Interaction, 0.07
Medium Gallop	7.44 ± 0.24	7.50 ± 0.22	7.52 ± 0.30	7.56 ± 0.22	7.77 ± 0.24	
Hard Gallop	7.61 ± 0.28 *	7.67 ± 0.27 *	7.54 ± 0.20 *	7.67 ± 0.24 *	7.88 ± 0.08 *	

Values are Mean ± 1SD for continuous data recorded by 'Equimetre' in Australia (n = 421 different racehorses, n = 1799 different training sessions). Horse profile (sprinter, miler, stayer) was determined based on race distance and subcategories (pure sprinter/miler, sprinter-miler, sprinter-miler-stayer) were formed according to the nature/proportion of the races for every individual horse (see Methods). Data were available throughout the period before (not more than three months) and during racing. Data were analysed by restricted maximal likelihood (REML) for the main effect of type of racehorse, with each individual racehorse included as a random effect, adjusting for significant covariates (age and weight of the horse). ^{a,b,c} Values within a row with differing superscripts are significantly different at $p < 0.05$, with Bonferroni correction for multiple testing. * Significant effect of training intensity (hard versus soft gallop).

In further data, for 378 of the 421 horses where speed and locomotory information were available for pre-race 'jumpout' training sessions (n = 1013); that is, starting from a standing start in stalls, then the best time to cover any 200 m (furlong) from the first to the fifth furlong at 1000 m, then speed gradually became slower for all categories of horse, as expected, but was always significantly faster for retrospectively designated sprinters versus stayers (Figure 1a). In addition, peak stride frequency was higher (Figure 1b), stride length was shorter (Figure 1c) and peak recorded speed was higher (Figure 1d) in sprinters versus stayers. During the course of two racing seasons, we described whether locomotory parameters changed within individual racehorses of each category (sprinters to stayers; Figure 2). Whilst significant variability with individual training session from the first to tenth (relatively few horses completed ≥10, data censured at n = 10 training sessions) existed for peak stride length (Figure 2a) and peak speed (a slight increment; Figure 2c), the effect sizes were relatively small and not consistent, suggesting little evolution of locomotory parameters (i.e., no effect for peak stride frequency, Figure 2b,d).

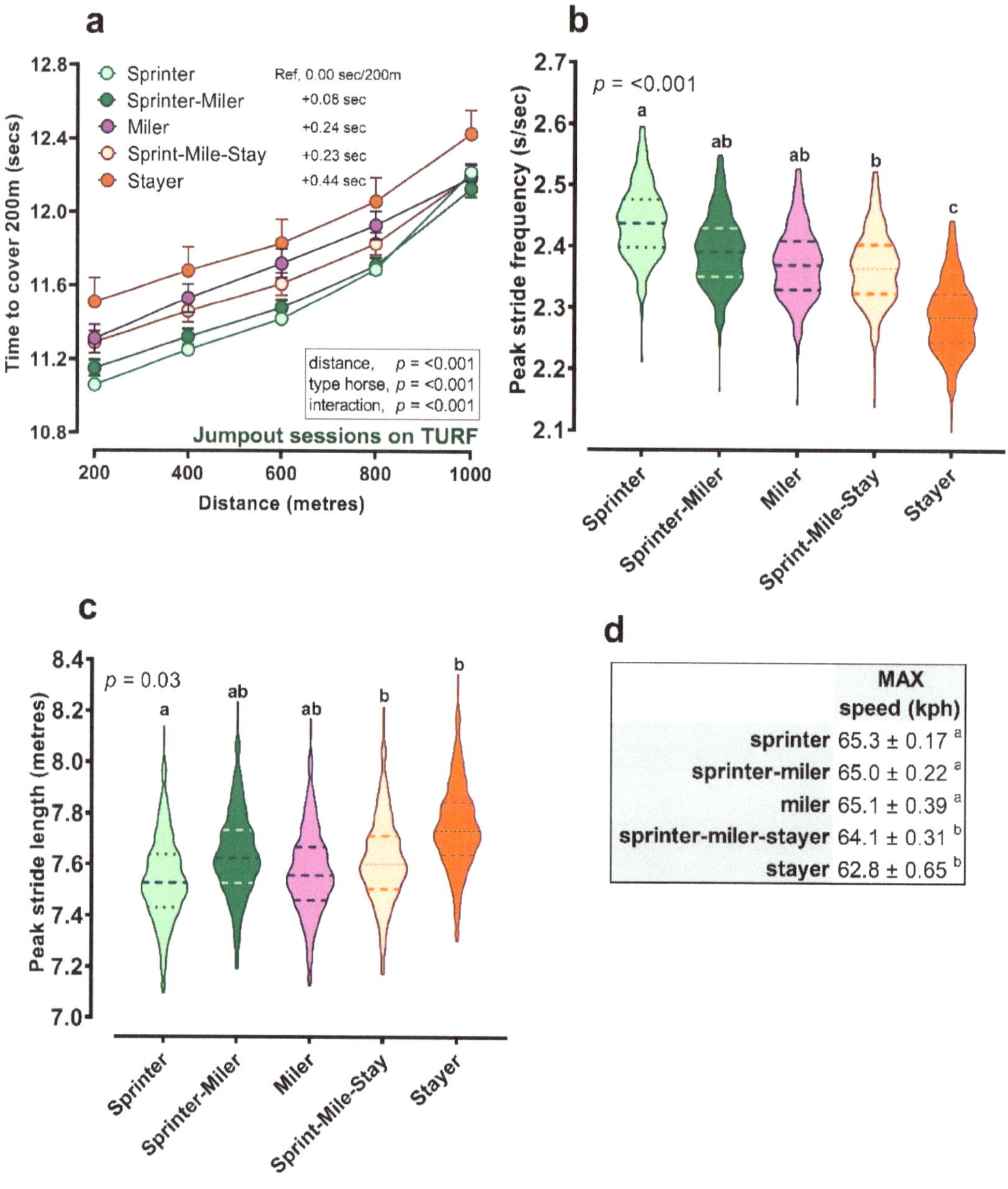

Figure 1. Training data during jumpout for different types of racehorse. (**a**) data are estimated marginal means ± SEM for consecutive 200 m segments (**b**) data are for all horses' peak stride frequency or (**c**) peak stride length during jumpout training sessions, (**d**) mean ± 1SD speed, according to category of racehorse. All data obtained from an 'Equimetre' used at a single racing yard in Victoria, Australia (n = 378 different racehorses, n = 1013 different 'jumpout' training sessions). Type of racehorse applied retrospectively to training data after competing in races of known distance. Data analysed by Restricted Maximal Likelihood (REML), as described previously (e.g., see Table 3). Differing superscripts are significantly different at $p < 0.05$.

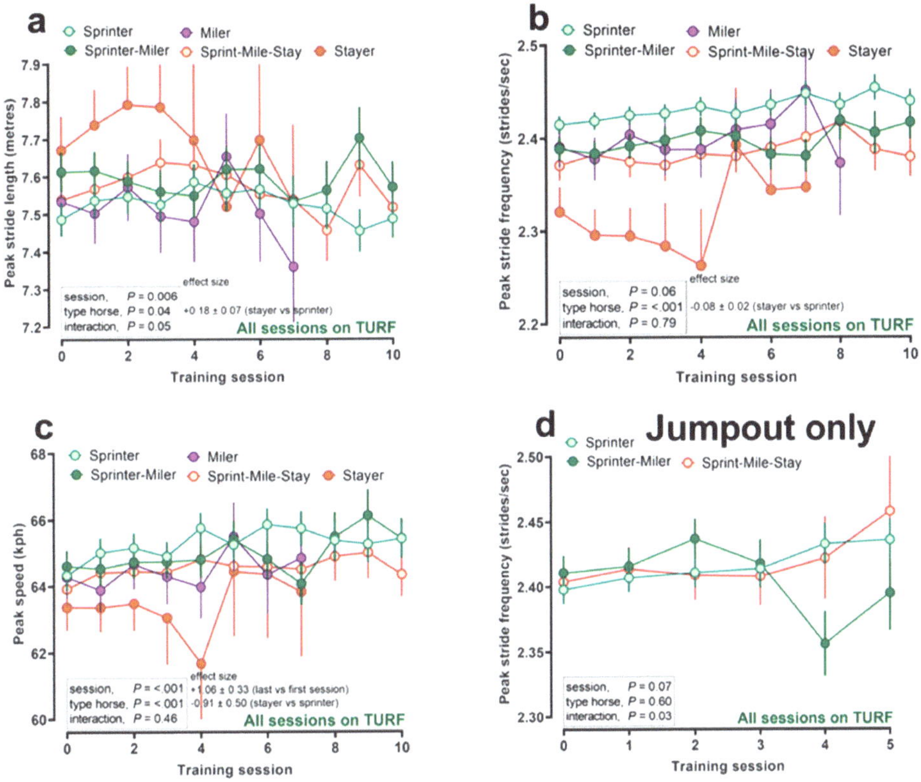

Figure 2. Evolution of locomotory parameters throughout the training season. Change in locomotory parameter with number of training sessions ('session') for each type of racehorse ('type horse'). Racehorses were categorised based on competing in races of known distance, as described in Methods. (**a**–**d**) data are estimated marginal means ± SEM for consecutive training sessions (x-axis) over the course of two racing seasons, adjusting for age of racehorse and interval between training sessions. Individual racehorse, year/training month were included as random effects. Data were obtained using an appropriately fitted 'Equimetre' device from a single racing yard in Victoria, Australia.

3.3. Training Data, Type of Racehorse and Predicting Race Outcome

Combining locomotory data during training for each individual racehorse with their race outcomes (win or top three 'podium') suggested that colts were more likely to win than geldings, with the chance of winning a group race declining as the class of race increased (Figure 3a). There was a trend for racehorses with longer peak stride length (i.e., stayers) to have an increased chance of winning and finishing in the top 3, regardless of race class and racehorse type (Figure 3b).

3.4. Heritability of Stride Parameters and Peak Heart Rate

After accounting for pedigree, which incorporates all traits with high genetic potential that were not recorded in our dataset (e.g., height, musculature etc . . .) then the difference in stride parameters recorded during training, according to the type of racehorse, was maintained (e.g., sprinters having shorter stride with higher frequency than stayers; Table 4).The estimates of narrow-sense heritability were significant (as determined by change in the log^2 deviance ratio when pedigree information was included or not) and the values of h^2 were low to moderate (Table 4). The heritability of peak heart rate was however not significantly different across racehorse categories (Table 4).

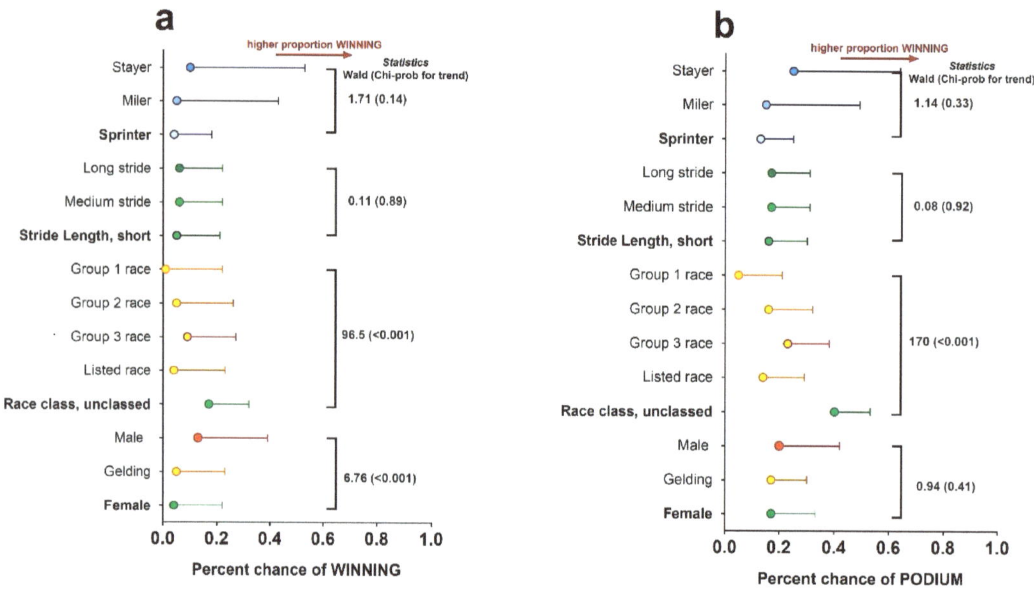

Figure 3. Predicting race wins or podium places on training data. Predicting race wins or podium places on training data. Data are predicted mean ± SEM for (**a**) winning a race (left graph) or (**b**) achieving a top three placing (right graph). Predicted means were obtained by integrating known race outcome data from Racing.com (Victoria, Australia; n = 421 different racehorses, n = 3269 different races) with training data (only gallop on turf) for the same horses before and during two race seasons (n = 1799 different training sessions). Data were analysed with race outcome (e.g., win or top three) as the variable of interest fitting sex of horse, race class, stride length and age as fixed effects in the model. Since the same horse completed multiple training sessions and multiple races then the individual horse was fitted as a random effect using Generalised Linear Mixed Models (GLMM). Statistics for main effects are indicated on the right on the graph with associated Wald statistic and χ^2 probability. Statistical significance was accepted at $p < 0.05$.

Table 4. Heritability (h^2) of locomotory and peak heart rate during race-speed training efforts categorised by type of racehorse.

	Sprinter	Sprinter-Miler	Miler	Sprinter-Miler-Stayer	Stayer	Heritability	* p-Value
Peak stride frequency (stride/s)	2.43 ± 0.01^{a}	2.39 ± 0.01^{b}	2.38 ± 0.01^{b}	2.37 ± 0.01^{b}	2.31 ± 0.02^{c}	0.20 ± 0.15	<0.001
Peak stride length (meters)	7.45 ± 0.02^{a}	7.54 ± 0.03^{ab}	7.49 ± 0.05^{ab}	7.53 ± 0.04^{b}	7.62 ± 0.06^{ab}	0.18 ± 0.14	0.003
Peak heart rate (beats/min)	217 ± 0.6^{a}	216 ± 0.8^{a}	214 ± 1.6^{a}	215 ± 1.2^{a}	215 ± 1.8^{a}	0.19 ± 0.15	0.08

Values are Mean ± 1SE for continuous data recorded by 'Equimetre' in Australia (n = 421 different racehorses with three-generation pedigree). Horse profile (sprinter, miler, stayer) was determined based on race distance and subcategories (pure sprinter/miler, sprinter-miler, sprinter-miler-stayer) were formed according to the nature/proportion of the races for every individual horse (see Methods). Data are averaged values for each horse from all available gallop sessions (n = 1699). Data were analysed and heritability estimated by REML analysis of an Animal Model. SE for Heritability (h^2) was calculated using the delta method. Values within a row with differing superscripts are significantly different at $p < 0.05$, with Bonferroni correction for multiple testing. * Overall p-value for comparison between groups of main effect.

4. Discussion

This study has directly, and objectively, outlined how differences in locomotory profile (short, medium or long peak stride length/frequency) are already apparent in sprinter versus stayer racehorses, during race-speed training sessions. Indeed, during mock-races from a standing start, i.e., 'jumpout' sessions, sprinters also achieved higher speeds than stayers. Nevertheless, racehorses with relatively short or long stride within sprint or stayer categories, respectively did not predict race performance (i.e., winning or podium position). However, we are able to report for the first time that locomotory parameters of racehorses have moderate heritability. Therefore, the study provides evidence to support our primary hypothesis, that racehorses can be distinguished in training by having relatively short, medium or long stride. Whilst locomotory parameters have moderate heritability, locomotory parameters in individual racehorses do not appear to alter considerably during the course of a race season. Hence, we suggest that differences in locomotory profiles are tangible for each type of racehorse (e.g. sprinter, miler, stayer), necessitating unique stride and speed aptitudes for the required distance. Race-day performance remains complex and may be influenced by a multitude of factors including sex of the horse, stride and to some extent pedigree as described in this study.

4.1. Racing Data and Performance

In Australia, horses race all year long with the season running from August to July, including a period of 'spell or detraining'. A spell or period of detraining refers to an extended period, usually 6 to 8 weeks, during which a racehorse is given a rest in the paddock. This break is dependent on the number of race starts completed during that year [15]. Thoroughbreds begin racing at the age of two and often progress from relatively shorter to longer distances (~above 1600 m) as their stamina and musculature develops, usually when they reach the age of three [16]. Previous research has shown that 2 year old racehorses are more suited to shorter races than any other age group [4,17,18]. Older racehorses, between 4 to 5 years of age, are therefore more likely to race over longer distances (i.e., 1600–3200 m) [19]. These trends were consistent with the ages observed across the three racehorse profiles (sprinter, miler or stayer) in this study; younger horses tend to be sprinters, whilst milers and stayers were significantly older.

Racehorses being trained in Australia are predominantly sprinters. 39% of Group races in Australia are run over less than 1400 m compared with 23% in both the UK and Ireland [20–22]. This may be partially explained by the fact that, in some racing nations, a premium is allocated to horses participating in shorter distance races, as the prizemoney/class of the races tends to be higher than other race distances. Sprinters largely characterised our dataset; we observed a much higher proportion of sprinters with both race and training data than stayers (according to a race distance classification established by [23]). This is not surprising considering the strong selection for early speed which characterizes the Australian racing industry. However, there has been a surge of global initiatives to boost and encourage the breeding of stayers to counteract this phenomenon [24]. Evoking greater prestige and higher prize money, some examples of long-standing stayers' race include The Epsom Derby (UK; 2420 m), Prix de L'Arc de Triomphe (France; 2400 m), Breeders' Cup Classic (USA; 2000 m) and the Melbourne Cup (Australia; 3200 m).

The limited number of pure stayers in our dataset nevertheless presented the highest proportion of race wins, compared to other categories of racehorse. Stayers were significantly older, were possibly more mature and of better 'quality' and thus retained to race or were better placed in suitable races given greater knowledge about their optimal characteristics. Younger, less talented and successful horses may also have dropped out of the yard and thus dataset. To an extent, therefore, perhaps such longer distance races are comprised of more appropriately placed and better racehorses. Additionally, in longer distance races, there is more opportunity for jockeys or trainers to utilize racing tactics [25].

Interestingly, a racehorse's peak racing age was previously suggested to be 4.45 years [26], a two-year difference with the stayers in this study.

4.2. Training Data and Locomotory Performance

Racehorse athletic careers generally only span a few years, during which racing opportunities can be limited [15]. Opting for a race distance that matches the individual horse's characteristics and racing ability could markedly contribute to increasing its chance of winning. Therefore, trainers subjectively determine individual racehorse locomotory profile (sprinter, miler or stayer) early on in their training in order to ideally target the most appropriate exercise program and maximize their racing performance. Yet, a racehorse's ability to gallop over five furlongs for a sprint race, as opposed to twenty for a stayer's race, will differ significantly in terms of locomotion strategy. As they approach peak speeds, individual horses will either naturally increase their peak stride length or frequency. Over shorter distances, the requirements for acceleration and speed are pivotal, but as the distance increases, then efficiency of stride and stamina become more important. Stride length, rather than frequency is the main determining parameter to achieve higher maximal speeds [3]. During standard gallop training sessions, our results revealed clear locomotory differences: sprinters had shorter stride length of a higher frequency than stayers. It is conceivable that the effect of warm up, if different between sprinters and stayers (not to our knowledge) may have exerted some effect on these stride characteristics, as previously evidenced in showjumpers [27]. Fatigue can also cause racehorses to lose a stable stride frequency [28], triggering a decrease in stride length [29]. We were unable to account for such aspects in our study, but in-field biomarking of fatigue through spot-sampling of blood could reveal important differences that could be trained in.

In preparation for racing, racehorses are often exposed to 'jump-out' training sessions, which consist of grouping horses of similar age/level, to start from barrier stalls and to race against each other under timed conditions. This race-day simulation exercise is different to official race-day barrier trials [30], but, from the horses' perspective, is akin to a race. Unsurprisingly, speeds recorded during such sessions were among the highest recorded in our dataset yet were still significantly higher for sprinters compared to milers/stayers. Thus, in both regular training sessions and race-speed simulation sessions, sprinters and stayers could be clearly differentiated on stride characteristics. Nevertheless, we did not note any significant evolution of stride characteristics through incremental training sessions over the course of two race seasons (~10 training sessions per horse). Such differences are likely small for any individual horse and it is likely that a very large dataset would be required to observe significant differences to validate the evolution of stride over a racehorse's career. Previous research has suggested that a typical racehorse improves its race time by approximately 10 (horse) lengths in sprints of <1 mile and up to 15 lengths for middle-longer distance races (≥1 mile) from the age of 2 to 4.5 years [26]. Hypothetically speaking, a proportion of this improvement could be attributed to alterations in the speed or efficiency of locomotion, although this was not measured in that study.

4.3. Training Data, Type of Racehorse and Predicting Race Outcome

Racehorse success on the track results from a complex combination of genetics [31], nutrition [32] and training [33]. Such factors determine the expression of physical traits specific to the athletic demands of the sport. In Thoroughbreds, muscle strength, speed and endurance have been identified as traits that favour superior performance at various race distances [34]. In this study, colts (i.e., younger male horses not gelded) had higher odds of winning than geldings. This aligns with previous research which identified some of the non-genetic factors that affect racehorse performance: sex, age, class of race, track condition, handicap weight and distance [35], and suggests that younger 'entire' male horses have the greatest chance of winning a race. Such an observation is also at odds with the fact that, in our dataset, the few stayers, who were older, had more race success. Perhaps the greater competition between horses in sprint races, the predominant race category in our dataset, is primarily won by colts as opposed to geldings. In stayer races, primarily competed in by older mares and geldings, and for obvious reasons very few entire males, then such differences are not apparent.

Thoroughbreds present unique musculoskeletal characteristics compared to other breeds. Notably, they have a large mass of skeletal muscle, low body-fat proportion and a greater percentage of fast twitch muscle fibres [36]. The composition of muscle fibre type, namely in the propulsive gluteal muscles, evolves with age and training, progressively improving stamina [37]. Previous work on racehorse wither height, has also revealed interesting insights. In mature horses, wither height was positively correlated with racing performance [38] and stride length [39]. The relationship between conformation and stride variables in foals aged 6–8 months has also been studied: increased speed was attained by longer stride length in heavier foals and higher stride frequency in taller foals [40]. The effect of training on performance has also been examined. [37] outlined that training strategies targeting both strength and endurance concurrently impinge on performance when compared to training programmes aimed at optimizing either one or the other [37]. This is explained by the fact that strength for acceleration is required for a sprint race. Strength is associated with an increased muscle mass, a shift from slow twitch to fast twitch muscle fibres and an increase in ATP utilisation. As a result, adaptations for sprinters would be disadvantageous for stayers as they rely on slow twitch muscle fibres and aerobic metabolism.

In Standardbreds and Thoroughbreds, after three years of training, changes in the trotting strides were observed: stride length, stride duration and swing phase increased [41]. Training plays an important role in the development of the above parameters [42]. Our findings highlighted a tendency of increased odds of winning and/or finishing in the top 3 in horses displaying a longer stride length. Similarly, in harness trotters, a test performed on the track showed that performing horses presented the highest maximal stride frequency and a long stride length [43].

4.4. Heritability of Stride Parameters and Peak Heart Rate

For the last three centuries, Thoroughbreds have been intensely bred for their elite athleticism, stamina and aptitude for speed. Racehorse pedigree information is registered in The General Studbook, 1791 [44] and can be traced back to their original ancestry. The Thoroughbred genetic pool is narrow and emerges from three foundation stallions (Arab, Barb and Turk) and approximately 30 foundation mares (UK) [45–47]. Since then, the continuity of the breed has become ever more controlled and refined. For example, English and Irish breeding industries focused on producing distinctive types of horses from precocious, fast, 2-year-old sprinters, 'classic' middle-distance runners or horses with enhanced stamina suitable for less popular 'classics' races such as the St Leger (United Kingdom; 2900 meters). Heritability of any given trait refers to the percentage of the parental trait that could effectively be transmitted to its offspring. Calculations on narrow-sense heritability estimates (h^2) for specific traits such as stride length aim to estimate the strength of genetic determinants for the particular characteristic (human height being highly heritable at 0.85), with the remainder being non-genetic, additive, environmental effects such as trainer, rider, track, etc. In flat racing, heritability of performance has been estimated as relatively low with wide confidence intervals, e.g., h^2 between 0.15 to 0.55 [35,48]. The heritability of locomotory characteristics (speed, stride length and frequency) has been estimated previously in French saddle horses and was considered to increase with pace (e.g., from walk [$h^2 = 0.23$], trot, canter through to gallop [$h^2 = 0.52$]) [49]. In this study of racing thoroughbreds, heritability of peak stride length and frequency was moderate ($h^2 = 0.15$–0.20), suggesting that 15–20% of the variation in locomotion in Thoroughbreds is due to the particular genes each racehorse inherited, with the remaining 80–85% of the variation due to environmental (non-genetic) factors. Since peak heart rate was consistently measured in our training data, we thought it interesting to also assess its heritability, despite previous papers indicating that between-individual variability is likely high [3,50,51]. Nevertheless, similar to locomotory characteristics heritability of peak HR was moderate (h^2 = 0.19).

Finally, it should be recognized that the study is a convenience sample of racehorses having used an 'Equimetre' intermittently, but in a repeatable fashion in training. The study is retrospective and observational. One test of our data would be to prospectively assign racehorses based on stride characteristics in training to being a sprinter or stayer and observe whether greater success in that category was achieved. Other factors that could influence stride but were not recorded consistently such as different warm-up protocols or accumulated fatigue were not taken into account. Since many racehorses compete in different types of race (e.g., sprinter or mile, mile or staying race) it would be interesting to analyse the extent to which locomotion (e.g., peak stride frequency, length) evolves over the course of a racehorse's career for different profiles (sprinter, miler, stayer).

5. Conclusions

In conclusion, this study demonstrates that locomotory differences exist (peak stride length, frequency) between various types of racehorse (sprinters, milers and stayers). Stride characteristics measured at the onset of training can predict aptitude to racing in a given category, regardless of the potential progress obtained with training. Peak stride length is a moderately heritable trait that can be bred for. Considering heritability of stride along with objective locomotory data and other aspects (i.e., preferred ground, going), may also help trainers choose early on what type of training (short, middle- or long-distance work outs) or which race to enter (distance, profile, going etc ...). Such a hybrid approach using data alongside experience may contribute to improved welfare on the track and prolong racing careers.

Author Contributions: Conceptualization, D.S.G.; methodology, D.S.G.; software, C.S., D.S.G. and S.B.; validation, G.D.; formal analysis C.S., D.S.G. and S.B.; investigation, C.S. and D.S.G.; resources, G.D.; data curation, G.D.; writing—original draft preparation, C.S. and D.S.G.; writing—review and editing, C.S., D.S.G., E.V.E.-W., G.D. and S.B.; visualization, D.S.G.; supervision, D.S.G.; project administration, D.S.G.; funding acquisition, C.S. All authors have read and agreed to the published version of the manuscript.

Funding: This research received no external funding.

Institutional Review Board Statement: The animal study protocol was approved by the Institutional Review Board (or Ethics Committee) of the University of Nottingham (protocol code 3270 201029). Ethical review and approval were waived for this study. As the study is retrospective and observational no experimental protocols were conducted that required ethical oversight.

Informed Consent Statement: Arioneo works with racehorse trainers who collect data from individual horses (anonymized for analysis) that are owned by private individuals. No personal information was collected for any individual.

Data Availability Statement: All data were collected by Arioneo Ltd. The race results and pedigree information are publicly available at http://www.racing.com, accessed on 28 October 2022 and http://www.pedigreeenquiry.com, accessed on 28 October 2022, whilst the training data were previously collected as part of routine recording by the racing yard, who shared the data with the external company (Arioneo Ltd.) that manufactures the data logging device (the 'Equimetre'). Anonymised training data available at http://www.arioneo.com, accessed on 28 October 2022.

Acknowledgments: No direct funding was granted for this study, but Charlotte Schrurs received part-funding towards her fees from the University of Nottingham, Arioneo Ltd. and the Royal Belgian Benevolent Society. The authors acknowledge the help of Roger Payne and David Baird (VSNi, Ltd.) and the Genstat user community (genstat@jiscmail.ac.uk) for invaluable help establishing, coding and running the Animal Model. The authors would also like to thank the trainers and sports performance analysts at Ciaron Maher Racing for sharing their data, insights and knowledge on the training of their racehorses. This study would not have been possible without their participation. All authors would particularly like to express their appreciation to Joshua Kadlec-Cavanagh.

Conflicts of Interest: Charlotte Schrurs is self-funding her Ph.D. David S. Gardner and Sarah Blott are funded by The School of Veterinary Medicine and Science, University of Nottingham. Guillaume Dubois is an employee of Arioneo Ltd. and had no influence on the reporting of results as presented. Emmanuelle Van Erck-Westergren is an Equine Sports Medicine specialist and consultant for Arioneo Ltd.

References

1. Tozaki, T.; Sato, F.; Hill, E.W.; Miyake, T.; Endo, Y.; Kakoi, H.; Gawahara, H.; Hirota, K.-I.; Nakano, Y.; Nambo, Y. Sequence variants at the myostatin gene locus influence the body composition of Thoroughbred horses. *J. Vet. Med. Sci.* **2011**, *73*, 1108030597. [CrossRef] [PubMed]
2. Hellander, J.; Fredricson, I.; Hertén, G.; Drevemo, S.; Dalin, G. Galloppaktion I—Basala gangartsvariabler i relation till hästens hastighet. *Sven. Vet.* **1983**, *35*, 75–82.
3. Schrurs, C.; Dubois, G.; Patarin, F.; Cobb, M.; Gardner, D.S.; Van Erck-Westergren, E. Cardiovascular and locomotory parameters during training in Thoroughbred racehorses: A multi-national study. *Comp. Exerc. Physiol.* **2022**, *18*, 185–199. [CrossRef]
4. Hill, E.W.; Gu, J.; Eivers, S.S.; Fonseca, R.G.; McGivney, B.A.; Govindarajan, P.; Orr, N.; Katz, L.M.; MacHugh, D. A sequence polymorphism in MSTN predicts sprinting ability and racing stamina in thoroughbred horses. *PLoS ONE* **2010**, *5*, e8645. [CrossRef]
5. Kusy, K.; Zielinski, J. Sprinters versus long-distance runners: How to grow old healthy. *Exerc. Sport Sci. Rev.* **2015**, *43*, 57–64. [CrossRef] [PubMed]
6. Thompson, M. Physiological and biomechanical mechanisms of distance specific human running performance. *Integr. Comp. Biol.* **2017**, *57*, 293–300. [CrossRef] [PubMed]
7. Wong, A.S.; Morrice-West, A.V.; Whitton, R.C.; Hitchens, P.L. Changes in Thoroughbred speed and stride characteristics over successive race starts and their association with musculoskeletal injury. *Equine Vet. J.* 2022, *in press*. [CrossRef]
8. Binns, M.; Boehler, D.; Lambert, D. Identification of the myostatin locus (MSTN) as having a major effect on optimum racing distance in the Thoroughbred horse in the USA. *Anim. Genet.* **2010**, *41*, 154–158. [CrossRef]
9. Tozaki, T.; Miyake, T.; Kakoi, H.; Gawahara, H.; Sugita, S.; Hasegawa, T.; Ishida, N.; Hirota, K.; Nakano, Y. A genome-wide association study for racing performances in Thoroughbreds clarifies a candidate region near the MSTN gene. *Anim. Genet.* **2010**, *41*, 28–35. [CrossRef]
10. Clayton, H.M. Horse species symposium: Biomechanics of the exercising horse. *J. Anim. Sci.* **2016**, *94*, 4076–4086. [CrossRef]
11. Deuel, N.R.; Park, J.-J. The gait patterns of Olympic dressage horses. *J. Appl. Biomech.* **1990**, *6*, 198–226. [CrossRef]
12. Saastamoinen, M.T.; Barrey, E. Physiological Traits. In *The Genetics of the Horse*; CAB International: Cambridge, MA, USA, 2000; p. 439.
13. Schrurs, C.; Dubois, G.; Van Erck-Westergren, E.; Gardner, D.S. Does sex of the jockey influence racehorse physiology and performance. *PLoS ONE* **2022**, *17*, e0273310. [CrossRef] [PubMed]
14. Ter Woort, F.; Dubois, G.; Didier, M.; Van Erck-Westergren, E. Validation of an equine fitness tracker: Heart rate and heart rate variability. *Comp. Exerc. Physiol.* **2021**, *17*, 189–198. [CrossRef]
15. Velie, B.; Wade, C.; Hamilton, N. Profiling the careers of Thoroughbred horses racing in Australia between 2000 and 2010. *Equine Vet. J.* **2013**, *45*, 182–186. [CrossRef]
16. Huggins, M. *Flat Racing and British Society 1790–1914: A Social and Economic History*; Routledge: London, UK, 2014.
17. Farries, G.; McGettigan, P.; Gough, K.; McGivney, B.; MacHugh, D.; Katz, L.; Hill, E. Genetic contributions to precocity traits in racing Thoroughbreds. *Anim. Genet.* **2018**, *49*, 193–204. [CrossRef]
18. Hill, E.W.; Ryan, D.P.; MacHugh, D.E. Horses for courses: A DNA-based test for race distance aptitude in thoroughbred racehorses. *Recent Pat. DNA Gene Seq. Discontin.* **2012**, *6*, 203–208. [CrossRef]
19. Butler, J.A.; Colles, C.M.; Dyson, S.J.; Kold, S.E.; Poulos, P.W. *Clinical Radiology of the Horse*; John Wiley & Sons: Hoboken, NJ, USA, 2017.
20. Racing Australia. Australian Group Races. Available online: http://www.racingaustralia.com.au (accessed on 1 August 2022).
21. Horse Racing Ireland. Irish Pattern Races, Listed Races and Premier Handicaps. 2017. Available online: https://www.goracing.ie/ (accessed on 3 August 2022).
22. British Horseracing Authority. UK Flat Pattern. 2017. Available online: https://www.britishhorseracing.com (accessed on 1 September 2022).
23. Rooney, M.F.; Hill, E.W.; Kelly, V.P.; Porter, R.K. The "speed gene" effect of myostatin arises in Thoroughbred horses due to a promoter proximal SINE insertion. *PLoS ONE* **2018**, *13*, e0205664. [CrossRef]
24. Webb-Carter, C. *A Study into British Stayers and Staying Races*; The Thoroughbred Breeders' Association: Newmarket, UK, 2015.
25. Sobczynska, M. Genetic correlations between racing performance at different racing distances in Thoroughbreds and Arab horses. *Czech J. Anim. Sci.* **2006**, *51*, 523. [CrossRef]
26. Gramm, M.; Marksteiner, R. The effect of age on thoroughbred racing performance. *J. Equine Sci.* **2010**, *21*, 73–78. [CrossRef]
27. Tranquille, C.; Walker, V.; Hodgins, D.; McEwen, J.; Roberts, C.; Harris, P.; Cnockaert, R.; Guire, R.; Murray, R. Quantification of warm-up patterns in elite showjumping horses over three consecutive days: A descriptive study. *Comp. Exerc. Physiol.* **2017**, *13*, 53–61. [CrossRef]

28. Johnston, C.; Gottlieb-Vedi, M.; Drevemo, S.; Roepstorff, L. The kinematics of loading and fatigue in the Standardbred trotter. *Equine Vet. J.* **1999**, *31*, 249–253. [CrossRef] [PubMed]
29. Wickler, S.; Greene, H.; Egan, K.; Astudillo, A.; Dutto, D.; Hoyt, D. Stride parameters and hindlimb length in horses fatigued on a treadmill and at an endurance ride. *Equine Vet. J.* **2006**, *38*, 60–64. [CrossRef] [PubMed]
30. The Rules of Racing of Racing Victoria. Available online: https://www.racingvictoria.com.au/the-sport/racing/~{}/media/1c929fd13ebf4ea998c579b5333fd438.ashx (accessed on 1 August 2022).
31. Gaffney, B.; Cunningham, E. Estimation of genetic trend in racing performance of thoroughbred horses. *Nature* **1988**, *332*, 722–724. [CrossRef]
32. Hintz, H.F. Nutrition and equine performance. *J. Nutr.* **1994**, *124*, 2723S–2729S. [PubMed]
33. Morrice-West, A.V.; Hitchens, P.L.; Walmsley, E.A.; Wong, A.S.; Whitton, R.C. Association of Thoroughbred Racehorse Workloads and Rest Practices with Trainer Success. *Animals* **2021**, *11*, 3130. [CrossRef] [PubMed]
34. Kay, J.; Vamplew, W. *Encyclopedia of British Horse Racing*; Routledge: London, UK, 2012.
35. Hintz, R.L. Genetics of performance in the horse. *J. Anim. Sci.* **1980**, *51*, 582–594. [CrossRef] [PubMed]
36. Kearns, C.; McKeever, K.H.; Abe, T. Overview of horse body composition and muscle architecture: Implications for performance. *Vet. J.* **2002**, *164*, 224–234. [CrossRef]
37. Rivero, J.L. A scientific background for skeletal muscle conditioning in equine practice. *J. Vet. Med. Ser. A* **2007**, *54*, 321–332. [CrossRef]
38. Dolvik, N.; Klemetsdal, G. Conformational traits of Norwegian cold-blooded trotters: Heritability and the relationship with performance. *Acta Agric. Scand. Sect. A-Anim. Sci.* **1999**, *49*, 156–162. [CrossRef]
39. Galisteo, A.; Cano, M.; Morales, J.; Vivo, J.; Miró, F. The influence of speed and height at the withers on the kinematics of sound horses at the hand-led trot. *Vet. Res. Commun.* **1998**, *22*, 415–424. [CrossRef]
40. Leach, D.; Cymbaluk, N.F. Relationships between stride length, stride frequency, velocity, and morphometrics of foals. *Am. J. Vet. Res.* **1986**, *47*, 2090–2097. [PubMed]
41. Drevemo, S.; Dalin, G.; Fredricson, I.; Björne, K. Equine locomotion: 3. The reproducibility of gait in Standardbred trotters. *Equine Vet. J.* **1980**, *12*, 71–73. [CrossRef] [PubMed]
42. Miró, F.; Santos, R.; Garrido-Castro, J.; Galisteo, A.; Medina-Carnicer, R. 2D versus 3D in the kinematic analysis of the horse at the trot. *Vet. Res. Commun.* **2009**, *33*, 507–513. [CrossRef] [PubMed]
43. Barrey, E.; Auvinet, B.; Couroucé, A. Gait evaluation of race trotters using an accelerometric device. *Equine Vet. J.* **1995**, *27*, 156–160. [CrossRef]
44. Weatherby, S. *An Introduction to a General Stud Book*; Weatherby and Sons: London, UK, 1791.
45. Cunningham, E.; Dooley, J.; Splan, R.; Bradley, D. Microsatellite diversity, pedigree relatedness and the contributions of founder lineages to thoroughbred horses. *Anim. Genet.* **2001**, *32*, 360–364. [CrossRef] [PubMed]
46. Bower, M.A.; Campana, M.; Whitten, M.; Edwards, C.J.; Jones, H.; Barrett, E.; Cassidy, R.; Nisbet, R.; Hill, E.; Howe, C. The cosmopolitan maternal heritage of the Thoroughbred racehorse breed shows a significant contribution from British and Irish native mares. *Biol. Lett.* **2011**, *7*, 316–320. [CrossRef]
47. Wallner, B.; Palmieri, N.; Vogl, C.; Rigler, D.; Bozlak, E.; Druml, T.; Jagannathan, V.; Leeb, T.; Fries, R.; Tetens, J. Y chromosome uncovers the recent oriental origin of modern stallions. *Curr. Biol.* **2017**, *27*, 2029–2035.e25. [CrossRef]
48. Langlois, B. Heritability of racing ability in Thoroughbreds—A review. *Livest. Prod. Sci.* **1980**, *7*, 591–605. [CrossRef]
49. Barrey, E.; Desliens, F.; Blouin, C.; Langlois, B. Heritabilities of gait characteristics: Application for breeding in dressage. In Proceedings of the Conference on Equine Sports Medicine and Science 2002, the Elite Dressage and Three-Day-Event Horse, Saumur, France, 19–21 October 2002.
50. Couroucé, A.; Chrétien, M.; Valette, J. Physiological variables measured under field conditions according to age and state of training in French Trotters. *Equine Vet. J.* **2002**, *34*, 91–97. [CrossRef]
51. Betros, C.; McKeever, K.; Kearns, C.; Malinowski, K. Effects of ageing and training on maximal heart rate and VO_2max. *Equine Vet. J.* **2002**, *34*, 100–105. [CrossRef]

animals

MDPI

Article

Electromyographic and Kinematic Comparison of the Leading and Trailing Fore- and Hindlimbs of Horses during Canter

Lindsay B. St. George [1,*], Hilary M. Clayton [2], Jonathan K. Sinclair [1], Jim Richards [3], Serge H. Roy [4] and Sarah Jane Hobbs [1]

1 Research Centre for Applied Sport, Physical Activity and Performance, University of Central Lancashire, Preston PR1 2HE, UK; sjhobbs1@uclan.ac.uk (S.J.H.)
2 Department of Large Animal Clinical Sciences, Michigan State University, East Lansing, MI 48824, USA
3 Allied Health Research Unit, University of Central Lancashire, Preston PR1 2HE, UK
4 Delsys/Altec Inc., Natick, MA 01760, USA; sroy@delsys.com
* Correspondence: lbstgeorge@uclan.ac.uk

Simple Summary: The muscular adaptations that facilitate the differing biomechanical functions of the leading (Ld) and trailing (Tr) limbs during canter in horses remains largely unknown. We conducted the first comparative study of muscle activation and movement within the leading and trailing fore- (F) and hindlimbs (H) during overground canter. Surface electromyography and three-dimensional motion capture data were collected from the right fore- and hindlimbs, as well as the splenius muscle, of ten horses ridden in left- and right-lead canter, when the limbs functioned as TrF/TrH and LdF/LdH, respectively. The TrH is first to make ground contact and exhibited significantly greater gluteal activation than LdH to stabilize the more extended hip joint and to generate greater limb retraction and a strong forward push-off during stance. Then, during TrF and LdH diagonal support, bilateral splenius activation occurred, possibly to counteract downward head and neck movement. The LdF was the last to make contact and was more protracted than the TrF through greater elbow flexion during swing, but triceps activity did not significantly differ between forelimbs. Inter-limb differences in movement and muscle activity provide an objective justification for working the horse equally on both canter leads to promote balanced muscular development.

Abstract: This study compared muscle activity and movement between the leading (Ld) and trailing (Tr) fore- (F) and hindlimbs (H) of horses cantering overground. Three-dimensional kinematic and surface electromyography (sEMG) data were collected from right triceps brachii, biceps femoris, middle gluteal, and splenius from 10 ridden horses during straight left- and right-lead canter. Statistical parametric mapping evaluated between-limb (LdF vs. TrF, LdH vs. TrH) differences in time- and amplitude-normalized sEMG and joint angle–time waveforms over the stride. Linear mixed models evaluated between-limb differences in discrete sEMG activation timings, average rectified values (ARV), and spatio-temporal kinematics. Significantly greater gluteal ARV and activity duration facilitated greater limb retraction, hip extension, and stifle flexion ($p < 0.05$) in the TrH during stance. Earlier splenius activation during the LdF movement cycle ($p < 0.05$), reflected bilateral activation during TrF/LdH diagonal stance, contributing to body pitching mechanisms in canter. Limb muscles were generally quiescent during swing, where significantly greater LdF/H protraction was observed through greater elbow and hip flexion ($p < 0.05$), respectively. Alterations in muscle activation facilitate different timing and movement cycles of the leading and trailing limbs, which justifies equal training on both canter leads to develop symmetry in muscular strength, enhance athletic performance, and mitigate overuse injury risks.

Keywords: equine; surface electromyography; sEMG; biomechanics; optical motion capture; gait analysis; forelimb; intralimb coordination; lead

1. Introduction

In quadrupeds, an asymmetrical gait is one in which the footfalls of one or both contralateral limb pairs occur as couplets, which implies an unequal time interval between left and right footfalls [1]. The limbs contacting the ground before and after the shorter time interval are called the trailing (Tr) and leading (Ld) limbs, respectively [1–3]. Canter and gallop are common asymmetrical gaits in horses. When the leading limbs are on the same side of the body in the fore- and hindlimb pairs, the gait is said to have a transverse sequence, whereas a rotary canter/gallop has the leading limbs on opposite side for the two limb girdles [1]. In cantering horses, both the fore (F) and hind (H) limb footfalls occur as couplets, and the order of limb contacts typically follows a transverse sequence [1]. Additionally, movements of the LdH and TrF are synchronized [1,4–9]. The footfall pattern is: TrH, LdH-TrF, then LdF [4–9]. Based on the leading forelimb, the horse is said to be cantering on the left lead or the right lead [4,5,7,8].

The canter represents an important gait due to its frequent and essential use in equestrian competition and training [4,10]. It is the gait employed during show jumping competition [11], and the development of a quality canter has been described as one of the most important aspects of jump training programmes [12]. Dressage horses perform four variations of the canter (collected, working, medium, extended) as well as the execution of half pass, canter pirouettes, and flying lead changes [8,9]. Furthermore, research has determined that canter is the only trait evaluated during performance testing that is highly correlated with future performance in both dressage and show jumping [13,14]. Despite the importance of this gait for sport horse training and competition, relatively few studies have focussed on canter within the equine biomechanics literature [10]. Of these studies, the differing functional demands of the leading and trailing fore- and hindlimbs during canter have been quantified [4,5,15,16], but the underlying differences in muscle function that facilitate these differences remain largely unknown.

During canter, the leading limb is often referred to as the "swinging" limb and is brought more forward during swing phase, while the trailing limb is generally referred to as the "supporting" or "propelling" limb [4,15]. These definitions have been supported by kinetic [5,15,17] and kinematic [4,16] studies. The "supporting" trailing limbs exhibit the greatest propulsive forces [5,15], with the TrF also experiencing the greatest vertical impulse and vertical loading of approximately 1.5 times the horse's body weight [5]. The trailing limbs have been reported to show significantly more retraction [4,16], which Back et al. [4] link to their closer orientation to the centre of mass (COM). The trailing limbs also show greater metacarpophalangeal (MCPJ) [4,16] and metatarsophalangeal joint (MTPJ) extension during stance [4] that is associated with greater vertical limb loading [18]. In contrast, the "swinging" LdF and LdH exhibit the greatest braking forces combined with minimal propulsive forces, which is related to their functions of controlling the lowering of the COM during the stance phase and subsequently raising of the COM prior to the suspension phase [5,15]. Significantly greater protraction has been observed in the leading limbs [4,16], which is driven by significantly greater hip and elbow flexion throughout the stride cycle [4,16]. The differences in movement, intralimb timing and coordination, and loading between leading and trailing limbs during canter [4,5,16] indicate that horses should be worked regularly on the left and right canter leads to strengthen the muscles symmetrically and thus reduce the risk of fatigue and injury. However, further research is required to quantify the actions of muscles that facilitate these kinetic and kinematic differences between leading and trailing limbs during canter.

Surface electromyography (sEMG) has been used in several studies to quantify muscle function during walk and trot [19–25]. However, relatively few studies have used sEMG to study muscle function during treadmill [19,26] or overground [27,28] canter. One study used sEMG to study between-limb differences in muscular function during canter [28]. In this study St. George et al. [28] provided a proof of principle for appropriate sEMG signal processing, developed using the known differences between LdH and TrH loading and movement during canter [4,5,15,16]. Biceps femoris muscle activity, measured using average rectified values (ARV) and integrated EMG (iEMG), was significantly greater in the LdH than TrH. This finding led the authors to suggest that biceps femoris must work eccentrically with greater force to stabilise the hip and stifle joints of the LdH [28], which experience greater limb loading [5]. This study provided preliminary insight into differences in muscle function related to biomechanical changes during canter. However, to our knowledge, no studies have compared both the movement and underlying muscle activation of leading and trailing fore- and hindlimbs within the same horse during overground canter. This information would have real-world applications for equestrians, as understanding the differing neuromuscular demands between leading and trailing limbs during canter could aid in the identification of muscular imbalances and the design of training programs to improve muscular symmetry and athletic performance.

Thus, the aim of this study was to measure and compare muscle function and movement between the leading and trailing fore- and hindlimbs during overground canter using sEMG and three-dimensional (3D) motion capture. In addition, head and neck movement represents an active element of the fundamental gait mechanism during canter [29,30], so we evaluated splenius activation in the context of LdF and TrF movement cycles. Within the forelimbs, it was hypothesized that the TrF, which experiences the greatest vertical limb loading across all limbs [5], would exhibit greater joint flexion/extension during stance and greater muscular activity across the stride cycle than the LdF. Within the hindlimbs, it was hypothesized that greater protraction [4] and vertical limb loading [5], experienced by the LdH, would be associated with greater joint flexion/extension and greater muscular activity across the stride when compared to the TrH.

2. Materials and Methods

Ethical approval for this study was obtained from the University of Central Lancashire's Animal Projects Committee (RE/13/04/SH). Written informed consent was obtained from all horse owners and riders prior to data collection.

2.1. Horses and Horse Preparation

Data were collected from 10 riding horses (mean $\pm$ SD age: 10.6 $\pm$ 2.4 years, height: 160.9 $\pm$ 8.0 cm, sex: 5 mares, 5 geldings, breed: 7 Warmblood, 1 Thoroughbred, 1 Irish Sports Horse, 1 Arabian $\times$ Welsh Cob). All horses were in work/training at the time of the study and were physically fit. Six (n = 6) horses had competed at a minimum level of British Showjumping Foxhunter up to 1.60 m international show jumping classes. Four (n = 4) horses had lower-level eventing and show jumping competition experience at jump heights ranging from 0.8 to 1.0 m. Our study focusses on movement and muscle activity within the general riding horse population, so lameness evaluations were not conducted by a veterinarian, and all horses were believed to be sound by their owner/rider. Horses were ridden by their normal rider, each with 14–20 years riding experience and having competed at a minimum level of 1.0 m unaffiliated show jumping. Prior to data collection, horses completed a short warm up of approximately 15 min in walk, trot, and canter at the rider's discretion. Following warm up, kinematic markers and sEMG sensors were attached over pre-determined anatomical locations and to pre-prepared skin over superficial muscles, respectively. Spherical retro-reflective markers (25 mm diameter) were attached over anatomical landmarks on each horse's right fore- and hindlimb, as described by St. George et al. [31].

Surface EMG sensors (Trigno, Delsys Inc. Natick, MA, USA) were unilaterally positioned over prepared skin on the right side of each horse to record from the long head of triceps brachii (triceps), middle gluteal (gluteal), vertebral head of biceps femoris (biceps), and splenius muscles. The reader is referred to St. George et al. [31] for detailed descriptions of sensor site locations for each muscle. Prior to data collection, hair was removed from sensor sites and thoroughly cleaned with isopropyl alcohol. A small amount of saline solution was applied to the electrode bars to act as an electrolytic solution before sensors were adhered to prepared skin using a combination of Delsys Adhesive Surface

Interface Strips (Delsys Inc., Natick, MA, USA) and strips of double-sided tape [31]. Sensors were positioned on the muscle belly, with the electrodes oriented perpendicular to the underlying muscle fibre direction [32,33].

2.2. Equipment Set Up

Eight infrared Qualisys Oqus cameras (Qualisys AB, Goteborg, Sweden) were positioned side-by-side in a linear configuration and an extended calibration was conducted to enable the collection of data from multiple strides. The calibration volume was approximately 8 m in length, and ground poles were placed parallel to and approximately 4.5 m from the cameras to define the optimal capture volume for horse/rider combinations.

2.3. Data Collection Protocol

The sEMG and 3D kinematic data were collected from the right side of the horse at 2088 Hz and 232 Hz, respectively, during ridden canter trials. Unilateral sEMG and kinematic data were collected during right- and left-lead canter in a random order. The right forelimb and hindlimb functioned as LdF and LdH during right lead canter and as TrF and TrH during left lead canter. Kinematic and sEMG data were collected synchronously using an external trigger system (Delsys Trigger Module, Delsys Inc. Natick, MA, USA) and Qualisys Track Manager software (version 2018.1, Qualisys AB, Goteborg, Sweden).

A ridden static trial was initially recorded with each horse standing in the centre of the optimal capture volume. Canter trials were then collected, with each horse being ridden through the optimal capture volume (adjacent to the placing poles) at their preferred canter velocity. A minimum of six canter trials were collected for each horse, with three trials collected from randomised left- and right-lead canter. A trial was deemed successful when the horse maintained the canter and correct canter lead and remained within the optimal capture volume.

2.4. Data Processing and Analysis

2.4.1. Kinematic Data Processing and Analysis

Kinematic data were tracked in Qualisys Track Manager (version 2018.1, Qualisys AB, Goteborg, Sweden), and then, both sEMG and kinematic data were imported into Visual3D (version 2020.07.4, C-Motion Inc., Germantown, MD, USA) for further signal processing and data analysis. Kinematic data were interpolated (maximum gap: 10 frames) and low-pass filtered (Butterworth 4th order) with a cut-off frequency of 12 Hz, as determined using residual analysis. For each horse, a rigid-body segment model of the right fore- and hindlimb was created—in accordance with the method described by Hobbs et al. [34]—and applied to all dynamic trials from the corresponding horse. Sagittal plane joint angles were calculated based on the static trial using the cardan sequence x, y, z. Flexion/extension was defined as rotation around the segment coordinate system x-axis, with the flexor side defined as caudal for shoulder, carpal, stifle, MTPJ, and MCPJ joints and as cranial for elbow, hip, and tarsal joints. Joint angular velocity was calculated as the first derivative of joint angular displacement. To calculate pro-retraction angles, fore- and hindlimb segments were defined using markers on the proximal end of the scapular spine and the tuber coxae as the respective proximal ends and the corresponding lateral hoof wall marker (approximately over the centre of rotation of the distal interphalangeal joint) as the distal end. Fore- and hindlimb pro-retraction angles were calculated in relation to a body reference segment, defined using a marker placed between the tubera sacrale and a virtual landmark, projected from the tubera sacrale marker to a point directly above the marker on the scapular spine.

Fore- and hindlimb hoof impact and lift-off events were calculated using the method described by Holt et al. [35] and were applied to kinematic and sEMG signals. Successive right hindlimb impact events were used to segment canter strides, irrespective of whether the hindlimb functioned as LdH or TrH. Discrete spatiotemporal variables were calculated for each canter stride, including fore- and hindlimb stance duration, stride duration, and stride velocity, which was calculated as the first derivative of the tubera sacrale marker coordinates within the laboratory coordinate system (y-axis) averaged over each canter stride. To correct for conformational differences between horses, joint angle data were normalised to the corresponding joint angles from each horse's static trial and are thus presented as angular changes from the standing position [36,37].

2.4.2. sEMG Data Processing and Analysis

Raw sEMG signals were differentially amplified by a factor of 909, a CMRR of >80 dB and internal Butterworth high-pass (20 ± 5 Hz cut-off, >40 dB/dec) and low-pass filters (450 ± 50 Hz, >80 dB/dec). During post-processing, signals were DC-offset removed, high-pass filtered using a Butterworth 4th order filter with a 40 Hz cut-off frequency [28,38], and full-wave rectified. The ARV was calculated from full-wave-rectified signals from each muscle, using stride duration as the time interval, and normalised relative to the maximum ARV value observed across all strides within each horse and muscle [28]. Prior to normalisation, outlier ARV data were detected and removed using the method described by St. George et al. [31]. Muscle activity onset and offset events were calculated using the double threshold method for equine sEMG signals [31]. The timing threshold was defined as 5% of the average stride duration across all horses, and the amplitude threshold was defined as 5% of the peak amplitude of each individual sEMG signal. Onset and offset events and the resultant activity duration for each muscle were normalised to the percentage of each respective canter stride duration. Timing of peak amplitude for each stride was detected from enveloped (10 Hz) signals and normalized to the percentage of each respective canter stride [31].

For the analysis of continuous sEMG data, full-wave-rectified signals were enveloped using a Butterworth low-pass filter (4th order, 25 Hz cut-off) and normalised to a reference voluntary contraction (RVC). The RVC was defined as the maximum sEMG amplitude value observed across all canter strides within each horse and muscle. Prior to normalisation, peak amplitude values from each canter stride were checked for outliers to ensure that sEMG signals were normalised to a value that accurately reflected the maximum activity observed during canter [31]. The normalisation techniques for ARV and continuous sEMG data permitted examination of the proportional difference between leading and trailing limb muscle function.

2.5. Statistical Analysis

Descriptive statistics (mean ± SD) were calculated for discrete kinematic and sEMG variables within each limb. sEMG data from the triceps and splenius were grouped according to the LdF and TrF movement cycles, with the biceps and gluteal grouped according to LdH and TrH movement cycles. Differences in discrete measurements between leading and trailing fore- and hindlimbs (LdH/LdF vs. TrH/TrF) were analysed using within-subjects linear mixed effects models, with limbs modelled as fixed factors and with random intercepts by participants included, whilst adopting the restricted maximum likelihood method. Linear mixed effects models were undertaken using SPSS software (version 28.0.1.1. (15), IBM Corp., Armonk, NY, USA). In addition, one-dimensional Statistical Parametric Mapping (SPM) was used to analyse differences between leading and trailing fore- and hindlimbs using continuous, time-series data from normalised sEMG, joint angle, and joint angular velocity data, which were time normalised to 101 data points per gait cycle. SPM was undertaken within MATLAB 2019b (MATLAB, MathWorks, Natick, USA), using source code available at http://www.spm1d.org/ (accessed on 16 April 2023).

3. Results

3.1. Kinematic Differences between Leading and Trailing Fore- and Hindlimbs

Kinematic and sEMG data from 67 left-lead and 64 right-lead canter strides were analysed and are presented here. Descriptive statistics for discrete kinematic data are presented as mean ± SD in Table 1. Forelimb stance duration was significantly longer for the TrF compared to the LdF ($p < 0.05$). Stride duration, stride velocity, and hindlimb stance duration did not significantly differ between canter leads and the measured leading and trailing limbs.

Table 1. Mean ± standard deviation for stride velocity (m/s) and measured temporal kinematic variables. Data are grouped according to left and right canter lead, where the measured limbs function as TrF/TrH and LdF/LdH, respectively. Differences between canter leads and the associated leading and trailing limbs are presented for each variable as p values.

Variable	Canter Lead/Limb		p Value
	Left Lead TrH or TrF	Right Lead LdH or LdF	
Stride velocity (m/s)	4.41 ± 0.42	4.42 ± 0.40	0.729
Stride duration (s)	0.59 ± 0.02	0.59 ± 0.02	0.641
Forelimb stance duration (s)	0.29 ± 0.02	0.27 ± 0.02	0.018 *
Hindlimb stance duration (s)	0.32 ± 0.03	0.32 ± 0.04	0.786

* Between-limb differences are significant at the 0.05 level. Abbreviations: leading forelimb (LdF), leading hindlimb (LdH), trailing forelimb (TrF), trailing hindlimb (TrH).

Group-averaged joint angle–time curves and SPM results for joint angle and joint angular velocity data from the fore- and hindlimbs are presented in Figures 1 and 2, respectively. In the forelimbs, the LdF was more protracted and less retracted than the TrF ($p < 0.001$), and the TrF elbow joint was more extended in late stance ($p < 0.001$). The MCPJ was less flexed during mid-swing ($p = 0.02$) and the elbow was more extended during late swing ($p < 0.001$) in the TrF compared to the LdF. The shoulder angle was more flexed in the TrF than the LdF during the late swing phase ($p = 0.016$) and during the majority of stance ($p < 0.001$). SPM results for forelimb joint angular velocity data (Figure 2) showed no significant differences between the LdF and TrF ($p > 0.05$) except for peak protraction velocity, which was faster in the TrF than the LdF ($p < 0.001$).

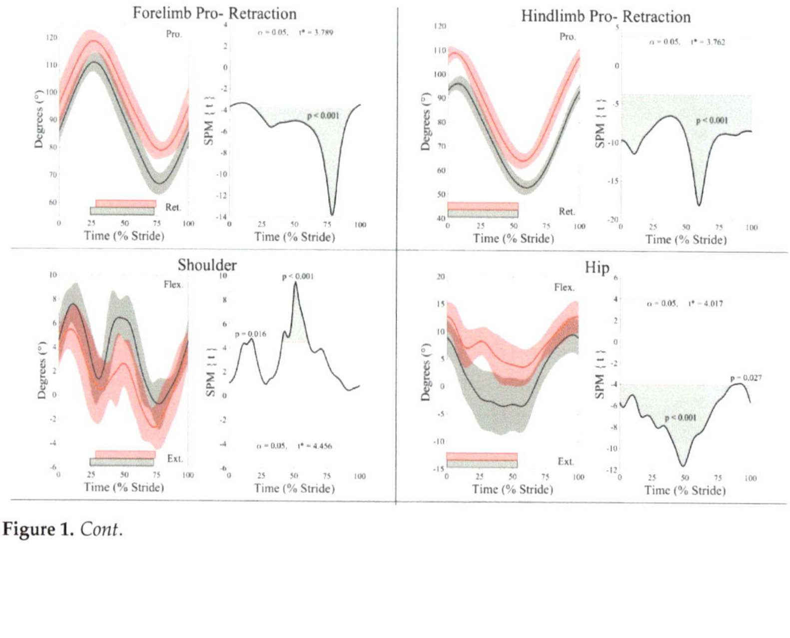

Figure 1. *Cont.*

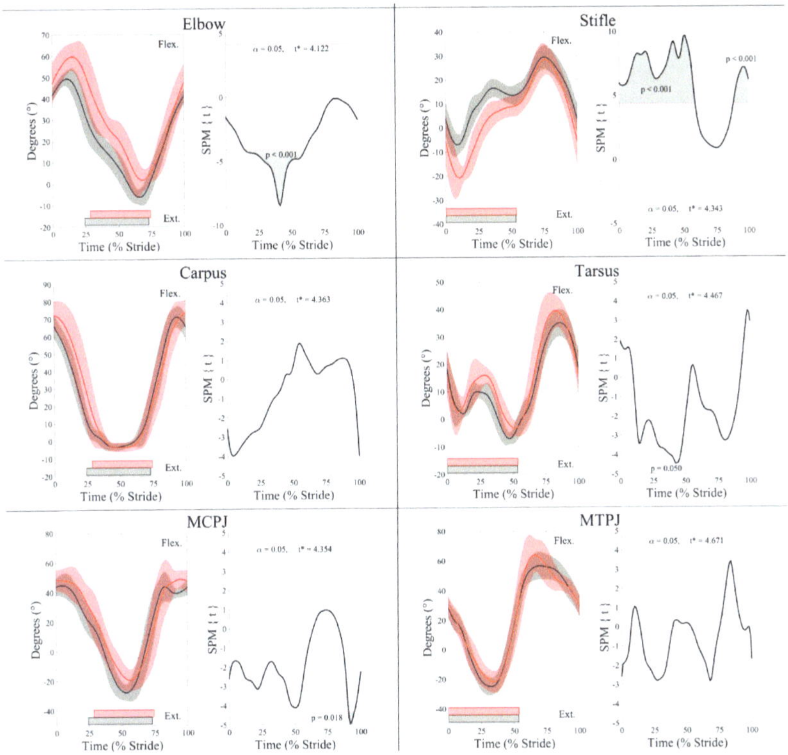

Figure 1. SPM results for normalized sagittal plane joint angles (°) from the leading (red) and trailing (black) fore- and hindlimbs across the group of horses (n = 10). For each kinematic variable, left-side graphs illustrate mean (solid line) and standard deviation (shaded area) data, and right-side graphs illustrate the paired samples t-test SPM results (black solid line) and the critical thresholds (α, t*) for significance (red dashed line), with grey shaded areas indicating regions/data clusters with statistically significant differences between limbs. p values for each data cluster are presented. The joint angle graphs include horizontal bars that represent stance phase duration from their respective leading (red bars) and trailing (black bars) limbs. Data are time-normalized to stride duration, calculated using corresponding impacts of the leading or trailing hind limb.

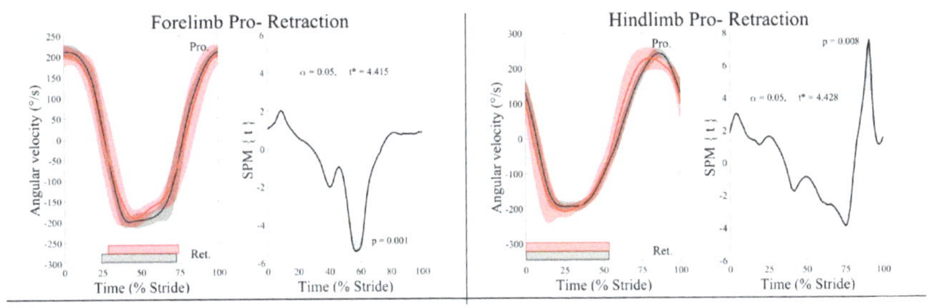

Figure 2. *Cont.*

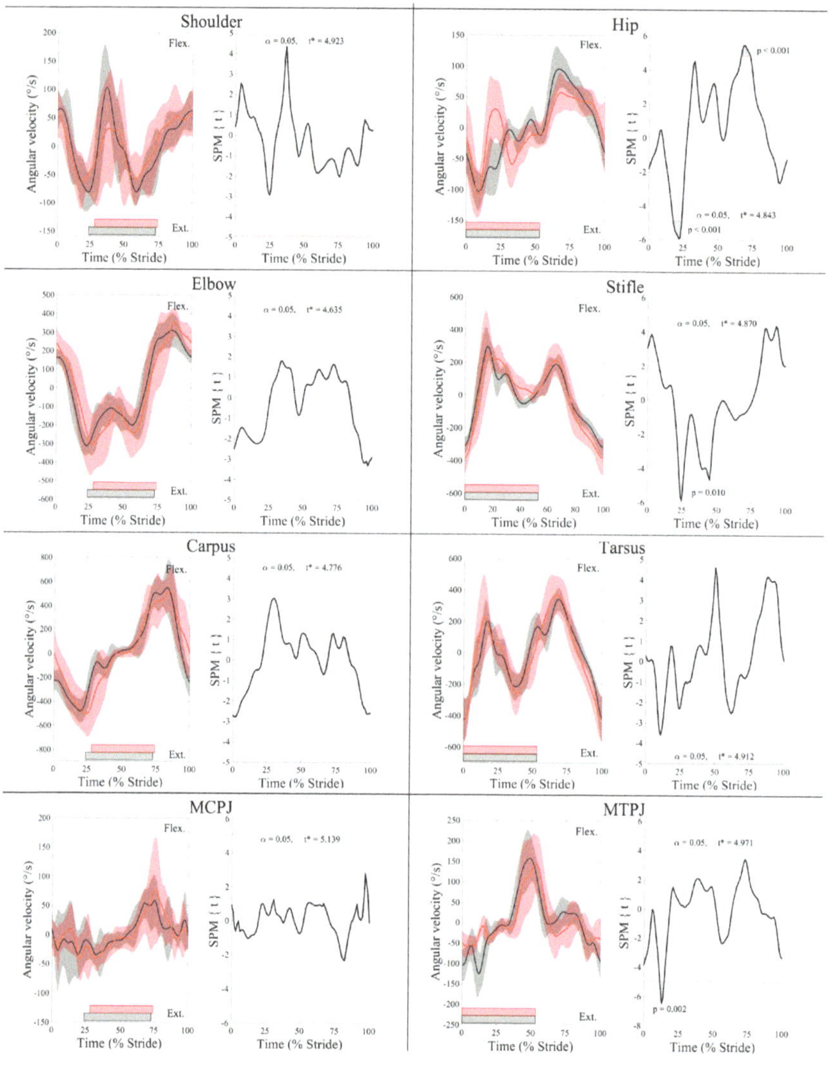

Figure 2. SPM results for normalized sagittal plane joint angular velocity (°/s) from the leading (red) and trailing (black) fore- and hindlimbs across the group of horses (n = 10). For each kinematic variable, left-side graphs illustrate mean (solid line) and standard deviation (shaded area) data and right-side graphs illustrate the paired samples t-test SPM result (black solid line) and the critical thresholds (α, t*) for significance (red dashed line), with grey-shaded areas indicating regions/data clusters with statistically significant differences between limbs. p values for each data cluster are presented. The joint angular velocity graphs include horizontal bars that represent stance phase duration from their respective leading (red bars) and trailing (black bars) limbs. Data are time-normalized to stride duration, calculated using corresponding impacts of the leading or trailing hindlimb.

As with the forelimbs, in the hind limbs, the LdH was more protracted and less retracted than the TrH ($p < 0.001$) (Figure 1). The TrH hip joint was more extended than the LdH throughout stance ($p < 0.001$) and less flexed throughout swing ($p < 0.05$). In contrast, the stifle joint was more flexed in the TrH than the LdH in late swing ($p < 0.001$) and during stance ($p < 0.001$). In late stance, peak tarsal extension was greater in the TrH than the

LdH ($p = 0.05$). Peak angular velocity of hind limb retraction and hip extension were faster for TrH than LdH in late swing ($p < 0.01$) (Figure 2). The TrH exhibited a short period of significantly faster angular velocity of hip, stifle, and MTPJ extension at approximately mid-stance ($p < 0.05$) (Figure 2).

3.2. Surface Electromyography Data

Descriptive statistics for discrete sEMG data are presented as mean ± SD in Table 2. In addition, the average phasic activation patterns of each muscle—derived from sEMG activity onset and offset events—together with the stance phases of the leading and trailing fore- and hindlimbs are illustrated in Figure 3. In the forelimbs, discrete (Table 2, Figure 3) and continuous sEMG data (Figure 4) from triceps did not significantly differ between the LdF and TrF ($p > 0.05$). There was a significant phasic shift in the splenius activation pattern, in which LdF activity onset, offset, and peak amplitude occurred earlier in the stride cycle than TrF ($p < 0.05$), with non-significant differences in ARV and activity duration observed between limbs ($p > 0.05$) (Table 2, Figure 3). This phasic shift in splenius activation was observed in continuous sEMG waveforms, where SPM results (Figure 4) showed significant differences in splenius activity during late-swing and late-stance phase of the forelimbs ($p < 0.05$). In the hindlimbs, ARV and activity duration of the TrH gluteal were greater ($p < 0.05$) than the LdH (Table 2, Figure 3). Activation offset of the LdH biceps occurred later in the stride cycle than the TrH ($p < 0.05$), but activity duration was not significantly affected by this ($p > 0.05$) (Table 2, Figure 3). SPM results for hindlimb muscles showed no significant differences between the LdH and TrH ($p > 0.05$) (Figure 4).

Table 2. Mean ± standard deviation for discrete sEMG variables from each superficial muscle of interest. Data are grouped according to leading (LdF/LdH) and trailing (TrF/TrH) fore- and hindlimbs. Differences between limbs are presented for each variable as *p* values.

Muscle	Variable	Limb		*p* Value
		TrH	LdH	
Biceps femoris	ARV (%)	62.7 ± 20.3	80.2 ± 14.9	0.179
	Activity duration (% stride)	46.9 ± 13.7	47.5 ± 14.9	0.822
	Peak amplitude (% stride)	16.5 ± 5.9	16.7 ± 7.2	0.541
	Activity offset (% stride)	31.9 ± 7.8	36.2 ± 6.5	0.018 *
	Activity onset (% stride)	93.5 ± 6.5	94.3 ± 5.7	0.287
Middle gluteal	ARV (%)	77.6 ± 14.1	66.3 ± 19.4	0.046 *
	Activity duration (% stride)	54.8 ± 13.8	48.6 ± 14.5	0.024 *
	Peak amplitude (% stride)	13.6 ± 5.2	16.7 ± 8.2	0.163
	Activity offset (% stride)	32.6 ± 7.5	33.5 ± 7.5	0.340
	Activity onset (% stride)	84.2 ± 7.3	88.2 ± 9.6	0.069
		TrF	LdF	
Triceps brachii	ARV (%)	72.5 ± 18.2	68.5 ± 19.7	0.179
	Activity duration (% stride)	66.4 ± 14.4	56.5 ± 18.0	0.234
	Peak amplitude (% stride)	40.4 ± 13.9	35.9 ± 13.7	0.531
	Activity onset (% stride)	101.8 ± 9.4 §	109.1 ± 9.7 §	0.061
	Activity offset (% stride)	56.6 ± 6.5	56.6 ± 9.9	0.368

Table 2. *Cont.*

		TrH	LdH	
Splenius	ARV (%)	75.8 ± 17.0	64.8 ± 17.7	0.322
	Activity duration (% stride)	51.1 ± 10.3	57.2 ± 12.5	0.192
	Peak amplitude (% stride)	59.0 ± 11.4	32.3 ± 15.2	0.000 *
	Activity onset (% stride)	42.7 ± 25.9	103.7 ± 14.0 §	0.002 *
	Activity offset (% stride)	81.2 ± 7.0	60.7 ± 10.0	0.029 *

* Between-limb differences are significant at the 0.05 level. Abbreviations: average rectified value (ARV), leading forelimb (LdF), leading hindlimb (LdH), trailing forelimb (TrF), trailing hindlimb (TrH). Note that only activity onset and offset events from the main activation burst (as presented in Figure 3) of each muscle are presented here. § Values > 100% reflect activity onsets that spanned the end to the beginning of the stride cycle and so activity onsets < 20% for these muscles were normalized to permit direct comparisons between horses, strides, and limbs.

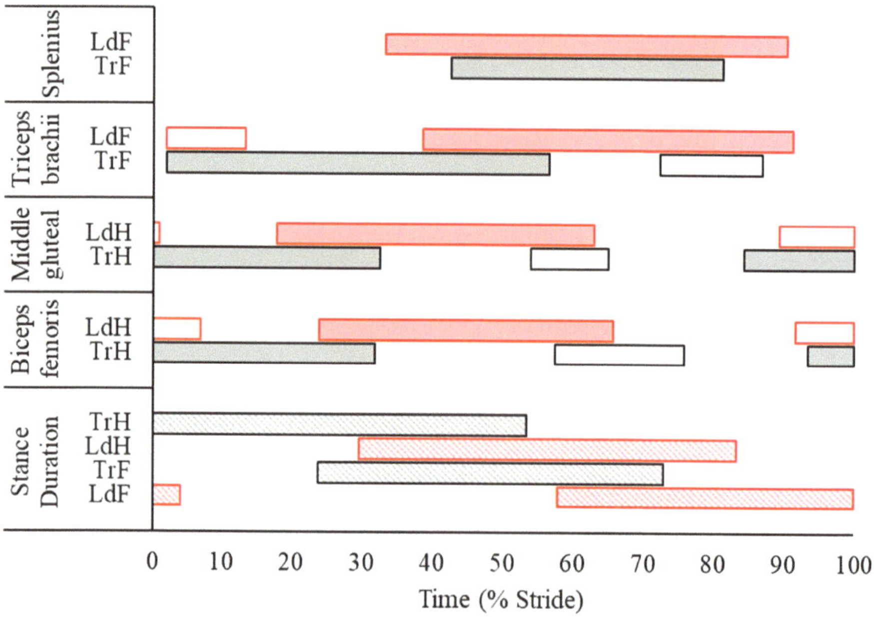

Figure 3. Average phasic muscular activation patterns of the studied muscles across $n = 10$ horses during the canter stride cycle, calculated using average sEMG activity onset and offset events from the leading (LdF) and trailing (TrF) forelimbs, and the leading (LdH) and trailing (TrH) hind limbs. Data are time-normalized to canter stride duration, calculated using impacts of the TrH. To present data from a complete stride cycle, a composite stride was constructed by time shifting the leading (LdF/LdH) limb data using the time ratio between TrH–LdH advanced placement and TrH stance duration (55.5%) presented by Clayton [9] for overground, medium canter. Red and black horizontal bars represent stance phase duration (diagonal stripe fill) and muscle activity duration from the leading (LdF, LdH) and trailing (TrF, TrH) fore- and hindlimbs, respectively. Solid horizontal bars represent the consistent, main burst of muscular activity, whereas unfilled horizontal bars represent intermittent muscular activity across measured strides.

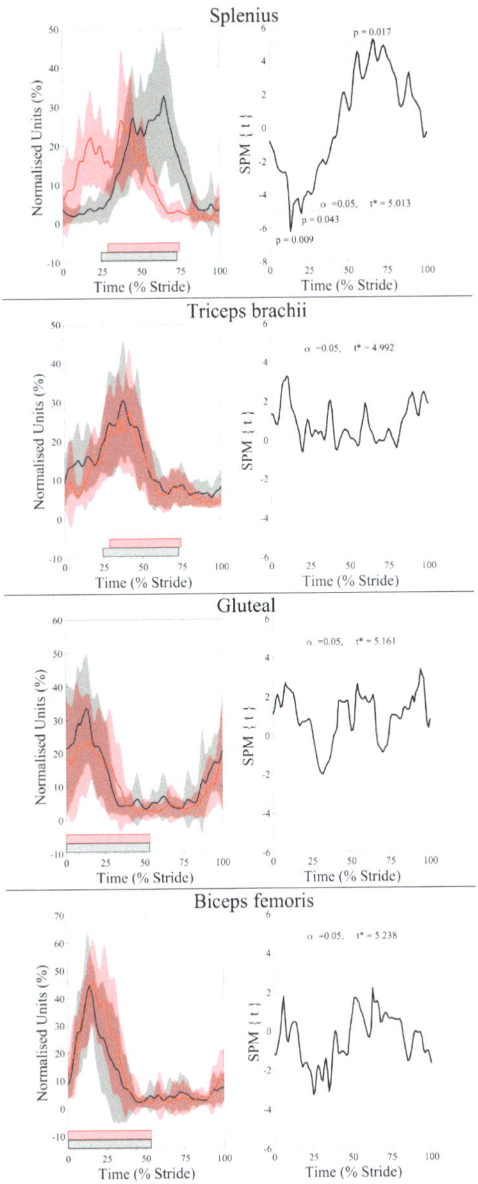

Figure 4. SPM results for time- and amplitude-normalized sEMG data across the group of horses (n = 10) for studied superficial muscles of the leading (red) and trailing (black) fore- and hindlimbs across the group of horses (n = 10). Left-side graphs illustrate mean (solid line) and standard deviation (shaded area) sEMG data, and right-side graphs illustrate the paired samples t-test SPM result (black solid line) and the critical thresholds (α, t*) for significance (red dashed line), with grey shaded areas indicating regions/data clusters with statistically significant differences between conditions. p values for each data cluster are presented. Horizontal bars represent stance phase duration from the respective leading (red bars) and trailing (black bars) limbs. Data are time-normalized to stride duration, calculated using corresponding impacts of the leading or trailing hindlimb.

4. Discussion

In this study, we combined sEMG and motion capture to conduct the first comparative study of muscle activation and movement within the leading and trailing fore- and hindlimbs during ridden, overground canter. In the forelimbs, the TrF showed greater shoulder flexion and greater elbow extension in midstance, but the triceps muscle, which acts across both joints, showed a non-significant trend for greater ARV and activity duration within this limb. Thus, our hypothesis that the TrF would exhibit greater joint flexion/extension during stance phase and greater muscular activity across the stride cycle than the LdF can be partially accepted. We also investigated splenius activation in the context of LdF and TrF movement cycles and found a significant phasic shift for earlier activation within the LdF stride cycle, with non-significant differences in ARV and activity duration observed between limbs. In the hindlimbs, we observed significantly greater LdH protraction and hip flexion during swing and significantly greater stifle extension during stance but with significantly less gluteal activity across the stride cycle compared to the TrH. Thus, our hypothesis that the LdH would exhibit greater joint flexion/extension and muscular activity across the stride than TrH was also partially accepted.

4.1. Electromyographic and Kinematic Differences between Leading and Trailing Forelimbs

In comparison to the LdF, the more vertically loaded TrF [5,17] exhibited a significantly greater retraction angle, with greater shoulder flexion and elbow extension during stance. In contrast, the LdF had significantly greater protraction driven by significantly greater elbow flexion during swing. These kinematic findings agree with the between-limb differences reported in previous studies of horses cantering overground [16] and on a treadmill [4] at faster speeds than were studied here. Although we observed significantly greater MCPJ flexion in the LdF during swing, which agrees with these studies [4,16], they also reported significantly greater maximal MCPJ extension in the TrF during stance, which was observed in our data but did not reach statistical significance. Since TrF is the limb with the highest peak vertical force at canter [5,15,17], the significantly longer TrF stance duration that was observed here but not in a previous study [4] may be a strategy to provide the necessary impulse over a longer time with a lower peak load [17,39]. This may suggest that, at the speed studied here, differences in limb loading were modulated by significant alterations in stance duration and non-significant alterations in peak MCPJ extension, which exhibits a linear relationship with limb force [18]. However, further research using ground reaction force (GRF) data is required to confirm this. As such, methodological differences—in particular, differences in canter speed and the study of overground vs. treadmill locomotion—may explain discrepancies in temporal findings and MCPJ kinematics between studies.

Crevier-Denoix et al. [16] is the only known study to measure and compare joint angular velocity of the forelimbs during canter measured on turf and synthetic surfaces, but only reported data from the MCPJ and carpal joints. In accordance with this study, they found no significant differences in carpal joint angular velocity or peak MCPJ extension velocity during stance on either surface but reported significantly greater peak MCPJ flexion velocity of the LdF than the TrF during late stance, on the turf surface only [16]. In agreement with Crevier-Denoix et al. [16], we did not observe significant differences in MCPJ flexion velocity during canter on a synthetic surface. Thus, despite some discrepancies in temporal findings and MCPJ kinematics between studies, our overall findings agree with previous research comparing kinematics of the LdF and TrF during canter [4,16] and corroborate their functional roles as the "swinging" and "supporting" limbs, respectively [4].

Harrison et al. [19] noted that, during walk and trot, most FL muscles display peak EMG activity at the hoof impact event but noted two different peaks at mid-stance and in early swing during canter. This agrees with phasic activity patterns observed in this study for the triceps, in which a main burst of activity was consistently observed from late-swing to mid-late stance, with a second shorter and less frequently observed burst following FL lift-off (Figure 3). Thus, our findings support the suggestion by Harrison et al. [19] that this additional burst at the beginning of swing may reflect the need for active muscle contraction to aid passive forces, produced by the tendons and ligaments, in the generation of greater joint torques that are required to sustain a steady canter gait. Triceps activity did not differ significantly between LdF and TrF, but subtle differences in sEMG amplitude and phasic activation patterns appear to reflect the facilitation of significantly different movement cycles between forelimbs. Earlier, albeit non-significant, triceps activation within the TrF corresponded with significantly earlier and decreased peak limb protraction and elbow flexion and earlier hoof impact, and vice versa in the LdF. Non-significant differences in ARV may also reflect the differing functions of each limb during stance phase, where triceps activation is possibly more related to stabilization of the shoulder and elbow joints against the greater vertical forces experienced by the TrF and against the high braking forces experienced by the LdF [5,15]. We suggest that future studies examine co-contraction of the biceps brachii and triceps brachii, which has previously been described as important for joint stability, positional control of the limb, and mitigation of shear loading during stance phase at canter [19]. Therefore, studies examining the synergistic activity of biceps brachii and triceps brachii may provide further insight into the neuromuscular strategies of the LdF and TrF during canter.

We observed significantly different phasic activity patterns of the splenius between the LdF and TrF movement cycles, offering some insight into splenius activity in relation to ipsilateral forelimb movement during canter. Splenius activity onset occurred from mid-swing to mid-stance phase during the LdF movement cycle and from early-stance to early-swing phase during the TrF movement cycle (Figure 3). Tokuriki and Aoki [40] noted the same asymmetrical phasic activation pattern for splenius relative to the ipsilateral forelimbs during canter, measured using intramuscular EMG. They summarised that the splenius is bilaterally activated during the late-swing phase of the TrF, just prior to impact [40]. This agrees with the activity onset detected here, in which the muscle remained active during the diagonal support phase of TrF and LdH. At this point in the stride cycle, sagittal pitching of the trunk and neck segments are largely "in phase", resulting in a "nose down"—or clockwise—pitching angle [7,29,30], which occurs during 50% of the stride cycle and corresponds to the activity duration of the splenius observed here, supporting previous suggestions that the splenius is bilaterally activated to counteract the downward movement of the head and neck [7]. In the remaining 50% of the canter stride, which includes the suspension phase and the single limb support phases of the LdF and TrH, sagittal pitching of the trunk and neck segments are "out of phase" and the neck segment is elevated in a "nose up" or counterclockwise position [7,29,30]. During this time, Gellman et al. [29] reported that active muscular work is required to reverse downward angular rotation and raise the head and neck, after which the nuchal ligament passively provides most of the mechanical work required to elevate the head and neck through the release of elastic strain energy. Our findings support this claim, as splenius activation was not observed during the single support and suspension phases. However, splenius activity observed during LdF stance may represent the active muscular contribution for reversing the neck segment rotation [29], particularly during the high decelerating forces experienced by this limb [5,15], which together may contribute to vertical lifting of the COM for the upcoming suspension phase [30]. Further studies are required to investigate the relationship between splenius activity and head and neck kinematics at canter, but our findings provide objective support for the splenius making an active contribution to the characteristic body pitching mechanisms that occur during this gait [7,29,30].

4.2. Electromyographic and Kinematic Differences between Leading and Trailing Hindlimbs

Kinematic findings from the hindlimbs corroborate a previous report of greater LdH protraction and greater TrH retraction during canter on a treadmill [4]. These were associated with significantly greater LdH hip joint flexion during swing and significantly greater TrH hip joint extension during stance. Additionally, Back et al. [4] reported significantly greater peak MTPJ extension in TrH and peak tarsal flexion in LdH during stance, which was also observed here but did not reach statistical significance when analysed using SPM. In contrast to Back et al. [4], who observed significantly greater TrH stifle flexion only during early stance, our evaluation of continuous joint angle data revealed significantly more flexion of the TrH stifle throughout stance and the majority of swing. Again, discrepancies for variables reaching significance may be due to methodological differences between studies, as described above. In particular, the use of SPM in this study allows comparison between continuous angle–time waveforms to statistically compare, for the first time, the limb movements across the entire canter stride cycle, whereas previous kinematic investigations of canter compared discrete kinematic variables between limbs [4,16]. Furthermore, to reduce inter- and intra-subject variability, we normalised joint angle–time data to the standing position, which was not performed in the other comparative studies [4,16] and may account for some discrepancies.

The significantly greater and delayed peak protraction velocity of TrH during swing is probably related to the peak retraction angle occurring significantly later, necessitating faster protraction during late swing to enable correct limb positioning for impact. During early stance, the MTPJ extended more rapidly in the TrH than the LdH, suggesting that the TrH is more rapidly loaded [18] and/or generates propulsive forces more rapidly than the LdH [5]. This significant peak in TrH MTPJ extension velocity was followed by significant peaks in extension velocity of the hip and stifle joints that were not present in the LdH and occurred at approximately mid-stance, which coincided with significantly greater TrH hip joint extension and stifle joint flexion. Taken together, these findings suggest that the proximal joints of the TrH actively damp vertical loading, as has been observed as a compensatory strategy in lame horses [41]. Integration of GRF and kinematic data is required to confirm this, but our kinematic results from the hindlimbs corroborate the propulsive and supporting functions of the TrH and LdH, respectively [4,5,15].

A main burst of activation from late swing to approximately mid-stance was observed for the middle gluteal and biceps femoris muscles during canter, which agrees with previous equine EMG studies [23,42–44]. Muscle activity during the first half of stance is related to limb loading and the generation of positive work, primarily by the hip joint [45], which is stabilized by contraction of the middle gluteal and hamstring muscles [46]. Quiescent activity during late stance phase and the majority of swing phase, appears to reflect a passive contribution of the gluteal and biceps to hip flexion and limb protraction, supporting the highly economical locomotor strategy of horses, which has been described for faster gaits, such as canter [47]. We observed significantly greater ARV and significantly longer activity duration for the TrH gluteal compared to LdH. This finding may be related to the generation of greater muscular force for stabilizing the more extended TrH hip joint during stance [46] and to produce the large propulsive forces required to generate a strong push-off for the rapid reversal of COM movement during stance [5]. Like forelimb movement and triceps activity, earlier—albeit non-significant—onset of gluteus activity in the TrH coincided with the significantly earlier initiation of hip extension and greater limb retraction velocity in late swing. This suggests an active muscular contribution to earlier reversal of this limb's direction of movement.

In contrast to the gluteal, significant between-limb differences were not observed for biceps activity, except for a significantly delayed activation offset in the LdH. St. George et al. [28] reported significantly greater ARV for the LdH biceps when appropriate sEMG signal processing and analysis procedures were employed. The same recommended procedures were employed here, but our findings did not reach statistical significance for ARV. Mean difference values between limbs were similar between studies at approximately 20% (17.5% vs. 21.5% reported by [28]), but we observed greater SD values, which may account for non-significant findings for ARV in this different group of horses. Still, the differing roles of the LdH and TrH are shown by the significantly greater TrH gluteal activity that stabilises the more extended hip joint and generates the highest propulsive forces across all limbs at canter [5,15]. In the LdH, greater—albeit non-significant—biceps activity may reflect its role for stabilising the hip, stifle, and hock joints against the greater decelerative and vertical forces experienced by this limb [5].

4.3. Practical Applications for Equestrian Training

The canter is an essential gait for equestrian competition and training, particularly for dressage and jumping disciplines, which aim to develop an equine athlete that exhibits straightness, balance, and symmetry of gait [4,10,48,49]. However, it is widely accepted within the equestrian and scientific community that horses display a motor asymmetry that can manifest as a preference to use one canter lead over the other [48,49]. As such, attempts to correct the "sidedness" or motor asymmetry of a horse is central to most equestrian training programmes [48–50]. In the scientific literature, there is contention surrounding whether motor asymmetry is inherent, the result of cerebral lateralisation, and/or linked to external factors, such as asymmetrical training or rider position/laterality [49,51]. Here, we have provided objective evidence for the differing functional demands of the studied muscles when they act within the leading and trailing limbs during canter. A deficiency in muscular strength on one side of the horse's body may result in one canter lead being more physically demanding and could thus offer another factor contributing to a horse's preference to use a specific canter lead. As such, our findings provide objective evidence for training the horse equally on both canter leads to develop symmetry in muscular strength, enhance athletic performance, and mitigate the risk of overuse injuries. In addition, an understanding of the differing neuromuscular demands between leading and trailing limbs during canter may allow trainers to better identify muscular imbalances and to implement exercises to improve muscular symmetry during canter. These exercises may include, but are not limited to, lateral movements [49,51] and/or working the horse at various speeds and inclines, each of which have been shown to elicit modifications in muscular activation or workload [26,42,43,52,53].

4.4. Study Limitations

Kinematic and sEMG data were collected unilaterally from the right side of the horses, so movement and muscle activity of the leading and trailing limbs could not be compared within the same stride. Furthermore, the measurement of one hind limb meant that impact of either the LdH or TrH was used for stride splitting depending on the canter lead, which may confound comparisons of temporal stride characteristics between leading and trailing limbs. This method did, however, allow direct comparison of movement and muscle activity when the same limb functioned as the leading or trailing limb as in previous studies of asymmetrical gaits [4,16,26]. In addition, we studied a relatively equal distribution of 67 left- and 64 right-lead canter strides, which permitted direct comparisons between limbs. When researchers acquire bilateral kinematic and sEMG data during canter, they should consider the potential for sEMG asymmetry due to electrode placement and underlying tissue differences between left- and right-side muscles [54], which our study design mitigated.

Canter speed, which was not standardised, is known to affect muscle activity and kinematics [55]. However, speed did not differ between left- and right-lead canters, and standard deviation values for this variable were relatively low compared to other studies of ridden, overground canter [6,9,16]. Horses were ridden by their normal rider, so the rider's influence was not standardised. Interestingly, Tokuriki and Aoki [40,44,56] reported that the rider did not influence the phasic activation patterns of intramuscular EMG signals from biceps femoris, triceps brachii, and splenius during canter when compared to unridden conditions. In addition, the joint angle–time diagrams and kinematic findings reported here were similar to a study of unridden horses that standardised canter speed using a treadmill [4]. As such, we suggest that our findings are externally valid within the context of ridden horse training and performance. Finally, future work with larger numbers of horses is required to study differences in leading and trailing limbs within the wider population.

5. Conclusions

This study combined sEMG and motion capture to conduct the first comparative study of muscle activation and movement within the leading and trailing fore- and hindlimbs during ridden, overground canter. We observed significantly greater protraction in the LdF and LdH through respectively greater elbow and hip flexion during swing phase when compared to the trailing limbs, but these differences were not associated with significant differences in triceps activity between LdF and TrF. In the trailing limbs, we observed significantly greater retraction than the leading limbs during stance, driven by significantly greater TrF elbow and TrH hip joint extension. In the hindlimbs, this difference was associated with significantly greater gluteal ARV and activity duration in the TrH, which reflects the requirement for greater muscular force to stabilize the more extended TrH hip joint during stance and to produce large propulsive forces. We also observed a significant phasic shift for earlier splenius activation within the LdF stride cycle, which reflected bilateral activation to counteract the downward movement of the head and neck during TrF and LdH diagonal support. Our findings provide novel insight into the underlying alterations in muscle activation that facilitate the differing biomechanical functions of the leading and trailing, fore- and hind limbs, as well as the splenius' active contribution to the characteristic body pitching mechanisms in cantering horses. These findings have real world applications for equestrians, as they provide objective justification for exercising the horse equally on both canter leads to promote balanced muscular development and to mitigate the risk of overuse injury.

Author Contributions: Conceptualization, L.B.S.G., S.J.H., J.R., S.H.R., H.M.C. and J.K.S.; methodology, L.B.S.G., S.J.H., J.R., H.M.C., S.H.R. and J.K.S.; software, L.B.S.G.; validation, L.B.S.G., S.J.H., J.R., H.M.C., S.H.R. and J.K.S.; formal analysis, L.B.S.G. and J.K.S.; investigation, L.B.S.G. and S.J.H.; resources, L.B.S.G. and S.J.H.; data curation, L.B.S.G., S.J.H., J.R. and J.K.S.; writing—original draft preparation, L.B.S.G.; writing—review and editing, L.B.S.G., S.J.H., S.H.R., H.M.C., J.R. and J.K.S.; visualization, L.B.S.G.; supervision, S.J.H.; project administration, L.B.S.G. and S.J.H. All authors have read and agreed to the published version of the manuscript.

Funding: This research received no external funding.

Institutional Review Board Statement: The animal study protocol was approved by the University of Central Lancashire's Animal Projects Committee (RE/13/04/SH).

Informed Consent Statement: Written informed consent was obtained from all horse owners and riders involved in the study.

Data Availability Statement: The data presented in this study are openly available in UCLanData at https://doi.org/10.17030/uclan.data.00000371 (accessed on 9 May 2023), reference number 371.

Acknowledgments: The authors would like to thank the horse owners and riders for their involvement in this study and D. Holt for her help with data collection.

Conflicts of Interest: Co-author S.H.R. is employed at Delsys Inc., the manufacturer of the EMG sensors used in this study. The remaining authors declare no conflict of interest.

References

1. Hildebrand, M. Analysis of asymmetrical gaits. *J. Mammal.* **1977**, *58*, 131–156. [CrossRef]
2. Leach, D. Recommended terminology for researchers in locomotion and biomechanics of quadrupedal animals. *Cells Tissues Organs* **1993**, *146*, 130–136. [CrossRef] [PubMed]
3. Leach, D.; Ormrod, K.; Clayton, H. Standardised terminology for the description and analysis of equine locomotion. *Equine Vet. J.* **1984**, *16*, 522–528. [CrossRef] [PubMed]
4. Back, W.; Schamhardt, H.; Barneveld, A. Kinematic comparison of the leading and trailing fore- and hindlimbs at the canter. *Equine Vet. J.* **1997**, *29*, 80–83. [CrossRef]
5. Merkens, H.W.; Schamhardt, H.C.; Van Osch, G.; Hartman, W. Ground reaction force patterns of Dutch Warmbloods at the canter. *Am. J. Vet. Res.* **1993**, *54*, 670.
6. Clayton, H. The extended canter: A comparison of some kinematic variables in horses trained for dressage and for racing. *Cells Tissues Organs* **1993**, *146*, 183–187. [CrossRef]

7. Faber, M.; Johnston, C.; Schamhardt, H.; Van Weeren, P.; Roepstorff, L.; Barneveld, A. Three-dimensional kinematics of the equine spine during canter. *Equine Vet. J.* **2001**, *33*, 145–149. [CrossRef]
8. Burns, T.E.; Clayton, H.M. Comparison of the temporal kinematics of the canter pirouette and collected canter. *Equine Vet. J.* **1997**, *29*, 58–61. [CrossRef]
9. Clayton, H.M. Comparison of the collected, working, medium and extended canters. *Equine Vet. J.* **1994**, *26*, 16–19. [CrossRef]
10. Deuel, N.R.; Park, J.-J. The gait patterns of Olympic dressage horses. *J. Appl. Biomech.* **1990**, *6*, 198–226. [CrossRef]
11. Clayton, H.M. Time-motion analysis of show jumping competitions. *J. Equine Vet. Sci.* **1996**, *16*, 262–266. [CrossRef]
12. St George, L.; Hobbs, S.J.; Sinclair, J.; Richards, J.; Roddam, H. Does equestrian knowledge and experience influence selection and training practices for showjumping horses? *Comp. Exerc. Physiol.* **2019**, *15*, 123–135. [CrossRef]
13. Hellsten, E.T.; Viklund, Å.; Koenen, E.; Ricard, A.; Bruns, E.; Philipsson, J. Review of genetic parameters estimated at stallion and young horse performance tests and their correlations with later results in dressage and show-jumping competition. *Livest. Sci.* **2006**, *103*, 1–12. [CrossRef]
14. Wallin, L.; Strandberg, E.; Philipsson, J. Genetic correlations between field test results of Swedish Warmblood Riding Horses as 4-year-olds and lifetime performance results in dressage and show jumping. *Livest. Prod. Sci.* **2003**, *82*, 61–71. [CrossRef]
15. Niki, Y.; Ueda, Y.; Masumitsu, H. A force plate study in equine biomechanics 3. The vertical and fore-aft components of floor reaction forces and motion of equine limbs at canter. *Bull. Equine Res. Inst.* **1984**, *1984*, 8–18.
16. Crevier-Denoix, N.; Falala, S.; Holden-Douilly, L.; Camus, M.; Martino, J.; Ravary-Plumioen, B.; Vergari, C.; Desquilbet, L.; Denoix, J.M.; Chateau, H. Comparative kinematic analysis of the leading and trailing forelimbs of horses cantering on a turf and a synthetic surface. *Equine Vet. J.* **2013**, *45*, 54–61. [CrossRef]
17. Witte, T.; Knill, K.; Wilson, A. Determination of peak vertical ground reaction force from duty factor in the horse (*Equus caballus*). *J. Exp. Biol.* **2004**, *207*, 3639–3648. [CrossRef]
18. McGuigan, M.P.; Wilson, A.M. The effect of gait and digital flexor muscle activation on limb compliance in the forelimb of the horse *Equus caballus*. *J. Exp. Biol.* **2003**, *206*, 1325–1336. [CrossRef]
19. Harrison, S.M.; Whitton, R.C.; King, M.; Haussler, K.K.; Kawcak, C.E.; Stover, S.M.; Pandy, M.G. Forelimb muscle activity during equine locomotion. *J. Exp. Biol.* **2012**, *215*, 2980–2991. [CrossRef]
20. Jansen, M.; Van Raaij, J.; Van den Bogert, A.; Schamhardt, H.; Hartman, W. Quantitative analysis of computer-averaged electromyographic profiles of intrinsic limb muscles in ponies at the walk. *Am. J. Vet. Res.* **1992**, *53*, 2343–2349.
21. Zsoldos, R.; Kotschwar, A.; Kotschwar, A.; Groesel, M.; Licka, T.; Peham, C. Electromyography activity of the equine splenius muscle and neck kinematics during walk and trot on the treadmill. *Equine Vet. J.* **2010**, *42*, 455–461. [CrossRef] [PubMed]
22. Zsoldos, R.; Kotschwar, A.; Kotschwar, A.; Rodriguez, C.; Peham, C.; Licka, T. Activity of the equine rectus abdominis and oblique external abdominal muscles measured by surface EMG during walk and trot on the treadmill. *Equine Vet. J.* **2010**, *42*, 523–529. [CrossRef] [PubMed]
23. Robert, C.; Valette, J.; Degueurce, C.; Denoix, J. Correlation between surface electromyography and kinematics of the hindlimb of horses at trot on a treadmill. *Cells Tissues Organs* **1999**, *165*, 113–122. [CrossRef] [PubMed]
24. Licka, T.; Frey, A.; Peham, C. Electromyographic activity of the longissimus dorsi muscles in horses when walking on a treadmill. *Vet. J.* **2009**, *180*, 71–76. [CrossRef]
25. Licka, T.F.; Peham, C.; Frey, A. Electromyographic activity of the longissimus dorsi muscles in horses during trotting on a treadmill. *Am. J. Vet. Res.* **2004**, *65*, 155–158. [CrossRef] [PubMed]
26. Hodson-Tole, E. Effects of treadmill inclination and speed on forelimb muscle activity and kinematics in the horse. *Equine Comp. Exerc. Physiol.* **2006**, *3*, 61–72. [CrossRef]
27. Kienapfel, K.; Preuschoft, H.; Wulf, A.; Wagner, H. The biomechanical construction of the horse's body and activity patterns of three important muscles of the trunk in the walk, trot and canter. *J. Anim. Physiol. Anim. Nutr.* **2018**, *102*, e818–e827. [CrossRef]
28. St George, L.; Roy, S.; Richards, J.; Sinclair, J.; Hobbs, S.J. Surface EMG signal normalisation and filtering improves sensitivity of equine gait analysis. *Comp. Exerc. Physiol.* **2019**, *15*, 173–185. [CrossRef]
29. Gellman, K.S.; Bertram, J. The equine nuchal ligament 2: Passive dynamic energy exchange in locomotion. *Vet. Comp. Orthop. Traumatol.* **2002**, *15*, 07–14.
30. Dunbar, D.C.; Macpherson, J.M.; Simmons, R.W.; Zarcades, A. Stabilization and mobility of the head, neck and trunk in horses during overground locomotion: Comparisons with humans and other primates. *J. Exp. Biol.* **2008**, *211*, 3889–3907. [CrossRef]
31. St George, L.; Clayton, H.M.; Sinclair, J.; Richards, J.; Roy, S.H.; Hobbs, S.J. Muscle Function and Kinematics during Submaximal Equine Jumping: What Can Objective Outcomes Tell Us about Athletic Performance Indicators? *Animals* **2021**, *11*, 414. [CrossRef] [PubMed]
32. De Luca, C.J. The use of surface electromyography in biomechanics. *J. Appl. Biomech.* **1997**, *13*, 135–163. [CrossRef]
33. Hermens, H.J.; Freriks, B.; Disselhorst-Klug, C.; Rau, G. Development of recommendations for SEMG sensors and sensor placement procedures. *J. Electromyogr. Kinesiol.* **2000**, *10*, 361–374. [CrossRef] [PubMed]
34. Hobbs, S.J.; Richards, J.; Clayton, H.M. The effect of centre of mass location on sagittal plane moments around the centre of mass in trotting horses. *J. Biomech.* **2014**, *47*, 1278–1286. [CrossRef] [PubMed]
35. Holt, D.; St George, L.; Clayton, H.; Hobbs, S.J. A simple method for equine kinematic gait event detection. *Equine Vet. J.* **2017**, *49*, 688–691. [CrossRef]

36. Back, W.; Schamhardt, H.; Savelberg, H.; Van den Bogert, A.; Bruin, G.; Hartman, W.; Barneveld, A. How the horse moves: 1. Significance of graphical representations of equine forelimb kinematics. *Equine Vet. J.* **1995**, *27*, 31–38. [CrossRef]
37. Back, W.; Schamhardt, H.; Savelberg, H.; Van Den Bogert, A.; Bruin, G.; Hartman, W.; Barneveld, A. How the horse moves: 2. Significance of graphical representations of equine hind limb kinematics. *Equine Vet. J.* **1995**, *27*, 39–45. [CrossRef]
38. St George, L.; Hobbs, S.J.; Richards, J.; Sinclair, J.; Holt, D.; Roy, S. The effect of cut-off frequency when high-pass filtering equine sEMG signals during locomotion. *J. Electromyogr. Kinesiol.* **2018**, *43*, 28–40. [CrossRef]
39. Witte, T.; Hirst, C.; Wilson, A. Effect of speed on stride parameters in racehorses at gallop in field conditions. *J. Exp. Biol.* **2006**, *209*, 4389–4397. [CrossRef]
40. Tokuriki, M.; Aoki, O. Neck muscles activity in horses during locomotion with and without a rider. In *Equine Exercise Physiology 3*; Persson, S., Lindholm, A., Jeffcott, L., Eds.; ICEEP Publications: Davis, CA, USA, 1991; pp. 146–150.
41. Buchner, H.; Savelberg, H.; Schamhardt, H.; Barneveld, A. Limb movement adaptations in horses with experimentally induced fore-or hindlimb lameness. *Equine Vet. J.* **1996**, *28*, 63–70. [CrossRef]
42. Robert, C.; Valette, J.; Denoix, J. The effects of treadmill inclination and speed on the activity of two hindlimb muscles in the trotting horse. *Equine Vet. J.* **2000**, *32*, 312–317. [CrossRef]
43. Robert, C.; Valette, J.P.; Pourcelot, P.; Audigie, F.; Denoix, J.M. Effects of trotting speed on muscle activity and kinematics in saddlehorses. *Equine Vet. J.* **2002**, *34*, 295–301. [CrossRef]
44. Tokuriki, M.; Aoki, O. Electromyographic activity of the hindlimb muscles during the walk, trot and canter. *Equine Vet. J.* **1995**, *27*, 152–155. [CrossRef]
45. Dutto, D.J.; Hoyt, D.F.; Clayton, H.M.; Cogger, E.A.; Wickler, S.J. Joint work and power for both the forelimb and hindlimb during trotting in the horse. *J. Exp. Biol.* **2006**, *209*, 3990–3999. [CrossRef] [PubMed]
46. Denoix, J.M. *Biomechanics and Physical Training of the Horse*; Taylor & Francis: Boca Raton, FL, USA, 2014.
47. Biewener, A.A. Muscle-tendon stresses and elastic energy storage during locomotion in the horse. *Comp. Biochem. Physiol. Part B Biochem. Mol. Biol.* **1998**, *120*, 73–87. [CrossRef]
48. Wells, A.; Blache, D. Horses do not exhibit motor bias when their balance is challenged. *Animal* **2008**, *2*, 1645–1650. [CrossRef] [PubMed]
49. Byström, A.; Clayton, H.; Hernlund, E.; Rhodin, M.; Egenvall, A. Equestrian and biomechanical perspectives on laterality in the horse. *Comp. Exerc. Physiol.* **2020**, *16*, 35–45. [CrossRef]
50. Eisersiö, M.; Roepstorff, L.; Rhodin, M.; Egenvall, A. A snapshot of the training schedule for 8 professional riders riding dressage. *Comp. Exerc. Physiol.* **2015**, *11*, 35–45. [CrossRef]
51. Krueger, K.; Schwarz, S.; Marr, I.; Farmer, K. Laterality in horse training: Psychological and physical balance and coordination and strength rather than straightness. *Animals* **2022**, *12*, 1042. [CrossRef]
52. Robert, C.; Valette, J.; Denoix, J.M. The effects of treadmill inclination and speed on the activity of three trunk muscles in the trotting horse. *Equine Vet. J.* **2001**, *33*, 466–472. [CrossRef]
53. Crook, T.; Wilson, A.; Hodson-Tole, E. The effect of treadmill speed and gradient on equine hindlimb muscle activity. *Equine Vet. J.* **2010**, *42*, 412–416. [CrossRef] [PubMed]
54. Miller, R.A.; Thaut, M.H.; McIntosh, G.C.; Rice, R.R. Components of EMG symmetry and variability in parkinsonian and healthy elderly gait. *Electroencephalogr. Clin. Neurophysiol. Electromyogr. Mot. Control* **1996**, *101*, 1–7. [CrossRef] [PubMed]
55. Hof, A.; Elzinga, H.; Grimmius, W.; Halbertsma, J. Speed dependence of averaged EMG profiles in walking. *Gait. Posture* **2002**, *16*, 78–86. [CrossRef] [PubMed]
56. Tokuriki, M.; Aoki, O.; Niki, Y.; Kurakawa, Y.; Hataya, M.; Kita, T. Electromyographic activity of cubital joint muscles in horses during locomotion. *Am. J. Vet. Res.* **1989**, *50*, 950–957. [PubMed]

animals

MDPI

Article

Efficient Development of Gait Classification Models for Five-Gaited Horses Based on Mobile Phone Sensors

Haraldur B. Davíðsson [1,2], Torben Rees [3], Marta Rut Ólafsdóttir [2] and Hafsteinn Einarsson [1,*]

1 Department of Computer Science, University of Iceland, 101 Reykjavík, Iceland
2 Horseday ehf., 102 Reykjavík, Iceland
3 TöltSense Ltd., Newton Abbot TQ12 5ND, UK
* Correspondence: hafsteinne@hi.is

Simple Summary: This study explored the use of mobile phone sensors to accurately classify the gaits of five-gaited horses. The data were collected from horses and riders using a mobile phone in the rider's pocket and an existing multi-sensor gait classification system. A machine learning model was then trained to classify the gaits using input from the phone's accelerometer and gyroscope, achieving an accuracy of 94.4%. This research demonstrates that mobile phones can be used to gather data on horse gaits, reducing the cost of large-scale studies. This efficient method for acquiring labelled data will be invaluable for ongoing research into horse riding activities.

Abstract: Automated gait classification has traditionally been studied using horse-mounted sensors. However, smartphone-based sensors are more accessible, but the performance of gait classification models using data from such sensors has not been widely known or accessible. In this study, we performed horse gait classification using deep learning models and data from mobile phone sensors located in the rider's pocket. We gathered data from 17 horses and 14 riders. The data were gathered simultaneously from movement sensors in a mobile phone located in the rider's pocket and a gait classification system based on four wearable sensors attached to the horse's limbs. With this efficient approach to acquire labelled data, we trained a Bi-LSTM model for gait classification. The only input to the model was a 50 Hz signal from the phone's accelerometer and gyroscope that was rotated to the horse's frame of reference. We demonstrate that sensor data from mobile phones can be used to classify the five gaits of the Icelandic horse with up to 94.4% accuracy. The result suggests that horse riding activities can be studied at a large scale using mobile phones to gather data on gaits. While our study showed that mobile phone sensors could be effective for gait classification, there are still some limitations that need to be addressed in future research. For example, further studies could explore the effects of different riding styles or equipment on gait classification accuracy or investigate ways to minimize the influence of factors such as phone placement. By addressing these questions, we can continue to improve our understanding of horse gait and its role in horse riding activities.

Keywords: horse; smartphone sensors; inertial measurement unit; gait classification; machine learning

1. Introduction

Mobile devices have become an accepted part of our everyday lives, and with the rapid pace of technological progress, their applications are constantly evolving. With sophisticated built-in motion sensors, users expect their devices to be able to perform human activity recognition. However, the devices are not only limited to the classification of human activities, since they can also be used for animal activity classification. Gait classification has been implemented in commercial smartphone apps such as Equilab (https://equilab.horse, accessed on 1 May 2022), which can recognize four gaits (walk, trot, canter, and tölt). The work of this paper was performed in collaboration with Horseday ehf., who are working on an app that can perform equine gait classification for five-gaited Icelandic horses, i.e., it can recognize flying pace in addition to the four other gaits.

Published work on equine gait classification dates back to the landmark work by Hildebrand in 1965 [1]. In that work, he described a standard for the task, using variables derived from limb movements and step placement. Since then, specially designed motion sensor systems for horses have been used to collect data for gait events and classification. Such data have been used to predict the timing of hoof contact [2,3], to monitor lameness [4], to analyse equestrian show jumping and dressage training movements [5], and to detect indications of fatigue during training [6]. Furthermore, machine learning models using data from horse-mounted sensors for gait classification have been tested [7], and the accuracy of the gait classification models on such sensor data reached 97% in a recent study by Bragança et al. [8]. Furthermore, mobile phone sensors have been shown to have a good agreement with validated specialist IMUs when both devices are attached to the horse [9].

Moreover, Bragança et al. [8] showed that a long short-term memory (LSTM) model [10] that received the raw sensor data as the input performed only slightly worse than the model using Hildebrand's variables. Similarly, convolutional networks have been used to classify raw accelerometer data from sensors strapped to the horses [11]. Although the models reach good accuracy using inputs from horse-mounted sensors, they still require the rider to explicitly attach sensors to the horse's limbs and body. This inconvenience leads us to the question of what accuracy can be reached using wearable human sensors carried in the rider's pocket. Studies on three-gaited horses (walk, trot, canter) show that gait classification can be performed using their sensor recordings [12,13]. However, it is not clear to what extent this would apply to the five-gaited Icelandic horse using smartphone sensors.

In this paper, we studied the accuracy of gait classification for all five gaits of the Icelandic horse using models trained on data from mobile phones in the rider's pocket. We specifically studied the Icelandic horse, which can perform two additional gaits, tölt and flying pace, on top of the three standard ones, walk, canter, and trot, due to a gene mutation [14]. We used the TöltSense (https://toltsense.com, accessed on 1 May 2022) system (TS) to label the training data. In previous studies, gait labelling was performed by recording the horse with a camera in a controlled environment and labelling the gait by watching the recording [8] or by timing gait switches using a stopwatch [13]. The TS automates the gait labelling process, which makes data acquisition significantly more accessible. The system further makes the labelling process objective and feasible in a diverse and natural environment.

Our study aims to answer the following research question: What accuracy of gait classification for all five gaits of the Icelandic horse can be reached using models trained on data from mobile phones in the rider's pocket? Our two objectives were to evaluate the accuracy of gait classification using the TS system and to evaluate the gait classification accuracy of models trained using the rotated sensor signals from mobile phones and TS gait labels. Our hypothesis was that models trained using TS labels and the rotated sensor signals from mobile phones will perform well in gait classification of Icelandic horses.

2. Materials and Methods

For both the mobile phone sensor model and TöltSense validation studies, the local Ethics Committee (The Icelandic Food and Veterinary Authority and the Ethics Review Board at the Royal College of Veterinary Surgeons) waived the need for a formal review and approval. It was concluded that the study is outwith the European Directive 2010/63/EU as it does not meet the threshold for causing any pain, distress, suffering or lasting harm. All the methods in each individual study were carried out in accordance with the approved guidelines and regulations. Informed consent was obtained from the owner of the animals and riders in a written manner when needed. Informed consent for publication was obtained from the rider in Figure 1.

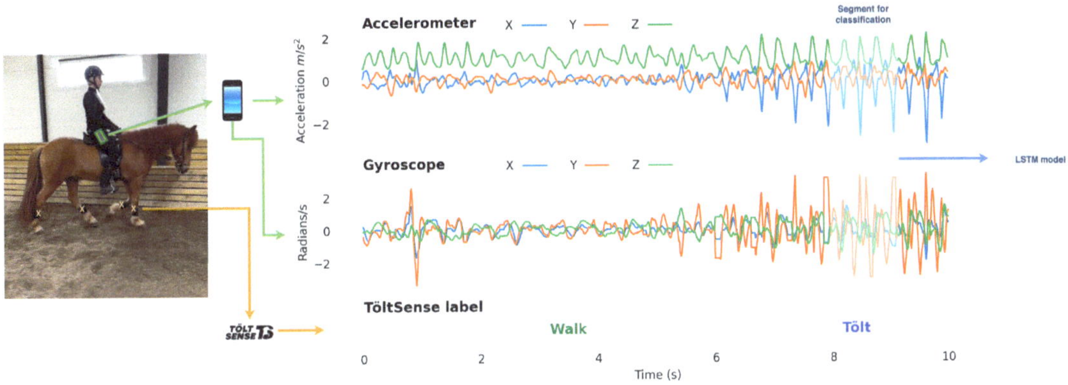

Figure 1. Data labelling with the TS application. The left panel shows the location of the sensors. The TöltSense sensors are strapped to the lateral aspect of the metacarpal/metatarsal bone, and the phone is placed in the rider's pocket. The right panel shows the data from the mobile sensor after rotation to a given frame of reference (world-frame) and the gait labels as a horse switches from walk to tölt. The X and Y curves correspond to variations in the acceleration and gyroscope signal in the horizontal plane, and the Z curve corresponds to variations on the vertical axis. The sign of the signal on a given axis corresponds to the direction of the signal on that axis. The highlighted segment shows an example of the input we used for the Bi-LSTM model.

2.1. The TöltSense System

To acquire labels for our training set, we used the TöltSense system (TS). The TS is a training tool designed to classify and analyse the quality of Icelandic horse gaits and provide feedback to the rider in real-time. The system is composed of motion sensors and a mobile app to report analysis results to the user. The four wireless motion sensors were attached to the horse's lower limbs, and they were kept synchronized to within 8ms of each other. The cross-platform mobile app processes the signals and generates gait labels (see Figure 1) with up to 99.7% accuracy (see the Results Section). The TS is not based on machine learning, but on the definitions of the gaits [15] by the International Federation of Icelandic Horse Associations (FEIF). The TS is based on the principle that a handcrafted algorithm can determine gaits if the hoof-on and hoof-off timings are measured with sufficient accuracy.

2.2. Dataset and Labelling—TöltSense Validation

Eight Icelandic horses of varying levels of training and ability were ridden and filmed while wearing the TS equipment at a horse farm in the U.K. Some of the sessions were captured during warm-up for an oval track competition in an indoor arena. The rest were captured during a training day on an oval track.

At the beginning of each session, the press of the TS app's "START" button was recorded (see Figure 2). This button press initiated the creation of a log file of gait classifications and timestamps, and recording it provided a reference point to line up the video with the TS log. Each video was trimmed to start exactly when the "START" button was pressed so that the times in the video would correspond to the times in the app log.

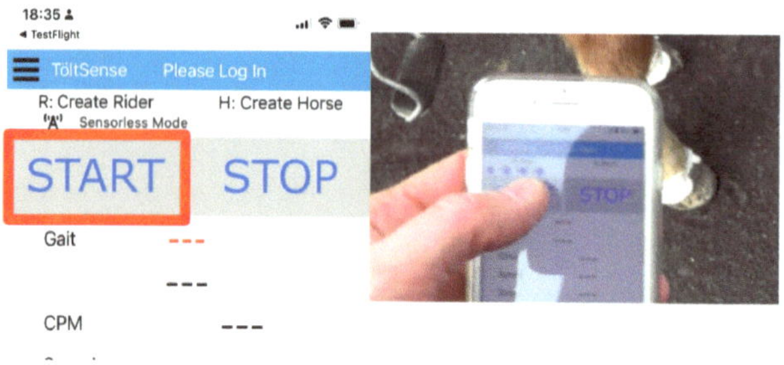

Figure 2. Töltsense interface and an example frame from a video of how the starting event was filmed with the press of the START button.

A panel of 4 qualified Icelandic sport judges independently suggested gait labels while watching the videos, using a custom-made web application (see Figure 3). For each video, a continuous observation window of 4–5 min was defined so as to include as many transitions and gaits as possible and to avoid judges having to watch unnecessary footage. At no point were the classifications of the TS revealed to the judges.

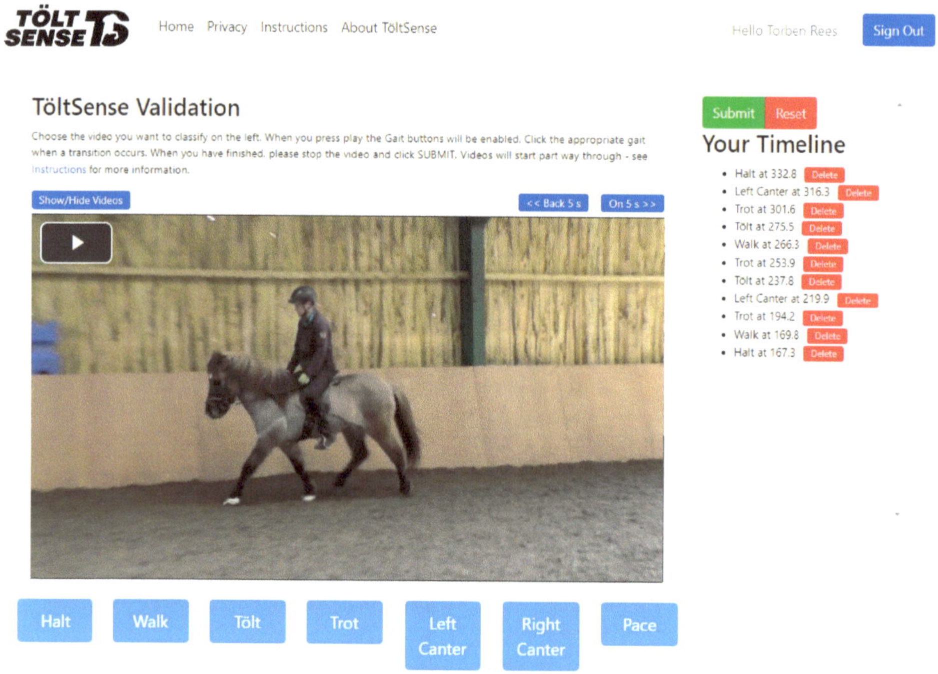

Figure 3. The web application used by the judges to assign gait labels to video segments.

A gait was determined every 250 ms by choosing the most-common label suggested during the given time interval. Such a majority vote was applied throughout the observation window, and a new data point was created whenever the majority gait changed. This processing step resulted in a series that defined the gait at any given moment during the observation window. We refer to this time series as aggregate judge classifications. An illustration of this time series is shown for a single example in Figure 4, and the speed of one horse with TS gait labels is shown in Figure 5. The values in the time series correspond to the gaits according to Table 1.

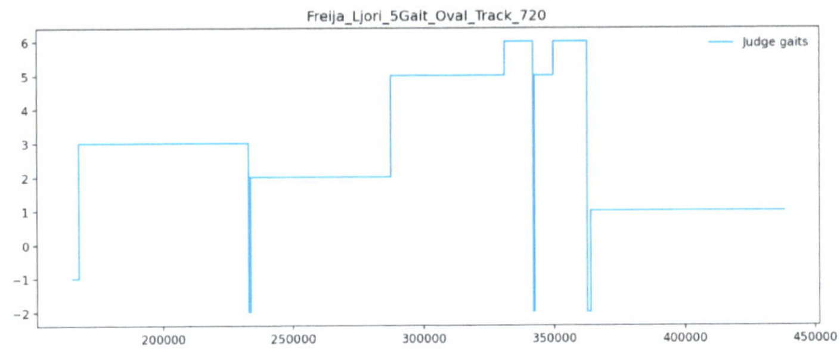

Figure 4. Plot of aggregate judge classifications against time, showing initial unclassified period (−1) and three periods of dispute (−2). The y-axis corresponds to the chosen label as defined in Table 1.

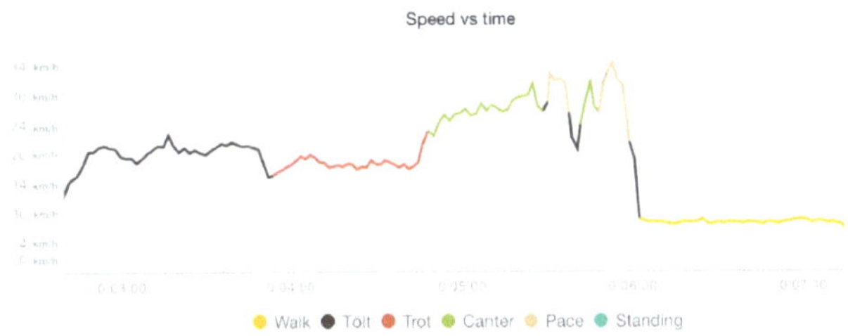

Figure 5. Plot of speed vs. time colour coded by gait from the TöltSense session overview screen.

Table 1. Gait labels used by judges. The table shows the gait labels from the TöltSense system that the judges used to label the video segments.

TöltSense Label	Number
No majority/disputed	−2
Not classified	−1
Halt	0
Walk	1
Trot	2
Tölt	3
Left Canter	4
Right Canter	5
Pace	6

The category "No majority/disputed" was required because there were occasions where the judges did not agree on the gait. Mostly, these were brief periods around gait transitions. However, Icelandic horses often display movements that are "between gaits" (e.g., pacey tölt, or 4-beat trot), and in these cases, it is not clear which gait is being shown. If qualified observers do not agree on the gait, there is no ground truth to compare the TS against, so periods labelled as −2 were excluded from the assessment. "Not classified" appears once at the very start of each session before any classification has been given; such periods were also excluded. The other labels are self-explanatory, but note that the left and right canter are included as separate gaits because it is important to demonstrate that the TS can distinguish between them.

The TS calculates the gait label every time a hoof-on event is registered from any leg. Hence, the gait labels are produced at a variable rate from about 4 Hz to 10 Hz, depending on the horse's activity. A sliding window of 1 s length with a step of 0.5 s was used to produce a timeline for analysis. For each window, all gait labels falling within that window were collected, and the most-frequent gait label was taken and paired with the timestamp from the middle of the window. The timestamp of the first sample in the log was subtracted from all windows, which resulted in a timeline of gaits starting at 0 s and progressing forward at 0.5 s intervals for the whole session.

With the two time series acquired, the series from the TS should be regarded as the "predicted value" set, and the series aggregated from the judges is the "true value" set. For each video, an observation window was defined, where we have both a TS prediction and the ground truth labels generated by judges. We took the timestamp from the predicted value and retrieved the ground truth value at that given time to make a prediction–truth pair, or "test case".

As mentioned above, when aggregate judge classifications resulted in −2 or −1, the test case was discarded. In addition, it was appropriate to discard test cases that were very close to transitions (as defined by the TöltSense or judges). In other words, leeway should be allowed for both the TS and judges when it comes to identifying and registering the moment of a transition. There are several reasons for this. First, there was always a delay between the horse making the transition, the judge recognising the transition has occurred, and then, again, a delay before the gait button is clicked in the web application. The TS may already have correctly recorded the transition when the judge clicks the button, so a false negative will be produced. Second, in cases of momentary loss or the change of gait (for example, a few steps of trotty tölt in the middle of a section of trot going straight back to trot), a judge is unlikely to react fast enough to register the gait change. If he/she does, it is likely to be registered late.

On the other hand, the TS is very likely to register the momentary gait change, and so, again, a false positive or false negative may be produced. There are also cases where the human eye (and hand) is quicker to register the gait change than the TS. The main example is the transition to walk, where the stride frequency is low, and it takes longer for the TS to build a buffer of steps to analyse as opposed to when going into a fast tölt, for example. In such cases, the judges may log a transition before the TS does, which results in a false negative. For these reasons, we applied a 1 s exclusion period for transitions (as identified by either the TS or the judges) as a fair degree of leeway. Any test cases falling within these exclusion periods were removed from the analysis.

2.3. Dataset and Labelling—Gait Classification with a Mobile Phone

The mobile phone sensor data were collected and labelled between May and August 2021 using the TöltSense (TS, https://toltsense.com/, accessed on 1 May 2022) system (see Figure 1). The data were collected on a horse farm in southern England and across various horse farms and training centres in Iceland. Seventeen different Icelandic horses and fourteen different riders were used for the measurements, and the phone was placed in a pocket on the rider's clothing, chosen by the rider. The phone location varied between riders with the phone placed in pockets on either trousers or jackets. The horses were ridden on different surfaces outdoors, on a track, sandy arena, or a trail. In this manner, 5.8 h of labelled data were collected, which corresponded to thousands of short segments for each gait.

The sensors from the TS system were attached to the lateral aspect of the metacarpal or metatarsal bone and set to a sampling frequency of 125 Hz, an acceleration range of ±16 g, and an angular velocity of 2000 deg/s. The TS system was responsible for synchronization between sensors and data processing, as well as capturing the phone sensor data into a log file and appending a gait label to each sample. It performs limb stride parameter calculations by detecting hoof-on/-off times using a built-in algorithm. The results of these calculations are then used to generate the gait labels. The TS system outputs 10 different labels, as can be seen in Table 2. The gait labels were the only data used from the TS system in this study, and they were generated whenever a hoof struck the ground, which was up to ten times a second for a fast tölt, i.e., four times per stride with up to 2.5 strides per second.

Table 2. Mapping from the TöltSense labels to the ones used in this study.

TöltSense Label	Label
Standing	Not Used
Walk	Walk
Trot	Trot
Tölt	Tölt
L Canter	Canter
R Canter	Canter
L Cross Canter	Canter
R Cross Canter	Canter
Flying Pace	Flying Pace

The phone models used for this study were different models of Samsung phones and iPhones. The data logged from the iPhones were sampled at a 50 Hz rate, whereas the data from the Samsungs were sampled at a higher rate, ranging from 100–1200 Hz, depending on the model. The data consisted of measurements from the accelerometer and gyroscope, which were subsequently rotated to a given frame of reference. One rotation was to the world-frame using a quaternion generated by the phone. We note that rotating the movement signal to the world-frame is standard practice and has been suggested by earlier studies on equine gait analysis [9,16]. Furthermore, such a rotation makes the signal more interpretable since it isolates acceleration in the vertical axis to a single dimension in the input signal. However, the world-frame does not give a clear indication of how the signal is varying in the lateral dimensions with respect to the horse. For that reason, we also studied a rotation to the horse's frame of reference. We used the 1 Hz GPS signal to acquire the horse's running direction in the x-y plane as an angle in the range $[0, 360)$ by comparing two consecutive longitude and latitude measurements. To determine the direction, we used a smoothed version of the horse's direction in the x-y plane, where we averaged the degree in which it was moving over a 1 s window. To compute a circular average, we unwrapped the signal by changing elements that had an absolute difference from their predecessor of more than 180 degrees to their period-complementary value. After averaging, we wrapped the signal again to obtain a direction in the range $[0, 360)$. The direction and speed were obtained using the Android/iOS location APIs.

For the sake of clarity, we note that the model receives six dimensions as the input, acceleration around the x-, y-, and z-axis and angular velocity along the same axes in the given frame of reference. We also explored the variations of the input signal, by adding speed as a dimension in the input signal or only including data from the accelerometer or gyroscope.

2.4. Pre-Processing of Signals from Mobile Phone Sensors

The data were pre-processed using common libraries for Python: NumPy, Pandas, and PyTorch. The rides that were sampled at more than 50 Hz were downsampled to 50 Hz. It may be noted that previous results indicate that downsampling to 50 Hz does not have a large impact on gait classification performance [11] or vertical movement symmetry measures in trot [17].

We split the data into a training set and a test set to measure generalization performance. The test set contained data from four horses that were not observed in the training set and a rider/horse combination that was not in the training set (see Table 3). We split the data into segments, as is illustrated with the blue rectangle in Figure 1. When generating the segments, we selected a segment such that it overlapped with the previous segment by 90%. We chose a fixed proportional overlap between segments instead of an absolute segment shift to reduce overfitting when studying longer intervals. For this reason, we had less training and test data for longer intervals. However, since relatively little flying pace data were present, we generated segments every 20 milliseconds for the flying pace for every window size.

As in the validation of the TS, segments were discarded that were within a 2 s period of a gait switch (here, a gait switch occurs when the Töltsense labels change) to leave out periods where the horse is in transition as such transitions might not have a reliable label. This discarding further eliminated transient labelling errors that may arise due to latency in the classification from the TS.

The ten labels from the TS system were mapped to a set of five labels representing the five gaits of the Icelandic horse (Table 2). Note that the cross canter is typically a result of rider error when transitioning to canter or flying pace (incidentally, pace horses often wear special over-reach boots to protect against strike injuries made more likely by cross canter). The two cross canters were mapped to canter, but no examples of it were actually collected in the training data. The distribution of the gaits in the training set can be seen in Figure 6.

Table 3. Overview of the horses used for the study. The total time of labelled data sums up to 5.4 h. Note that only the horses in the 2nd, 10th, and 11th row are five-gaited.

Horse No.	Location	Rides	Walk	Trot	Tölt	Canter	Flying Pace	Total Time
1	England	1	1026 s	212 s	376 s	190 s	0 s	30 min
2	England	2	1488 s	98 s	253 s	39 s	85 s	33 min
3	England	2	767 s	427 s	973 s	154 s	0 s	39 min
4	Iceland	3	470 s	416 s	935 s	42 s	0 s	31 min
5	Iceland	2	394 s	121 s	710 s	0 s	0 s	20 min
6	Iceland	4	1394 s	628 s	2275 s	88 s	0 s	73 min
7	Iceland	2	1319 s	712 s	1161 s	257 s	0 s	57 min
8	Iceland	1	354 s	192 s	496 s	63 s	0 s	18 min
9	Iceland	1	157 s	120 s	212 s	32 s	0 s	8 min
10	Iceland	2	0 s	0 s	0 s	0 s	28 s	0.5 min
11	Iceland	1	0 s	0 s	0 s	0 s	27 s	0.5 min
12	England	1	155 s	55 s	67 s	40 s	0 s	5 min
13	England	1	144 s	0 s	338 s	0 s	0 s	8 min
14	England	1	141 s	90 s	144 s	102 s	0 s	8 min
15	England	1	124 s	61 s	100 s	14 s	0 s	5 min
16	England	1	117 s	41 s	80 s	24 s	0 s	4 min
17	England	1	134 s	80 s	134 s	38 s	0 s	6 min

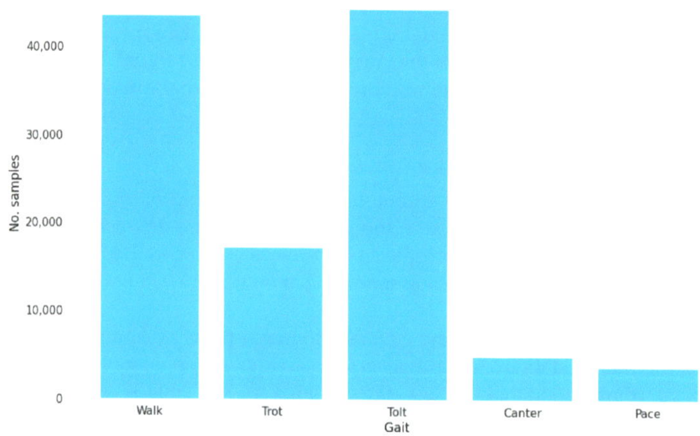

Figure 6. The distribution of horse gaits in the dataset for 1.5 s segments.

The training set was split into a training and validation with an 85/15 split, and the samples were shuffled for training. The leave-one-outtest set contained rides from Horse Nos. 1, 2, 8, 9, and 11 while the rest were used for training. Rides from Subject No. 2

were used in both sets, but the rides had different riders. However, the rides contained a different phone model and a different rider.

2.5. The Gait Classification Model

The main model used for gait classification in this study was a recurrent neural network (RNN), namely, a long short-term memory (LSTM), an architecture widely used for time series classification and regression tasks [10]. Other similar RNN architectures were also tested such as a gated recurrent unit (GRU, [18]) and a bidirectional LSTM [19]. A 1-dimensional convolutional neural network was also tested.

The LSTM model contained a single LSTM layer with 200 units; the Bi-LSTM model had 400 units; the GRU model had 200 units. For the 1-dimensional CNN model, we had four layers with a kernel size of 3. The layer dilation rates were 12, 8, 4, and 1; the number of inputs was n_i, 16, 32, and 64, where n_i is the number of input features used; the number of outputs was 16, 32, 64, and 128. In all models, the final layer added was a 128-dimensional linear layer (see Figure 7 for the LSTM model). The models were trained for 20 epochs with a batch size of 64 using the ADAM optimizer [20] and early stopping monitoring the loss of the validation set. All models were trained using cross-entropy as the loss function.

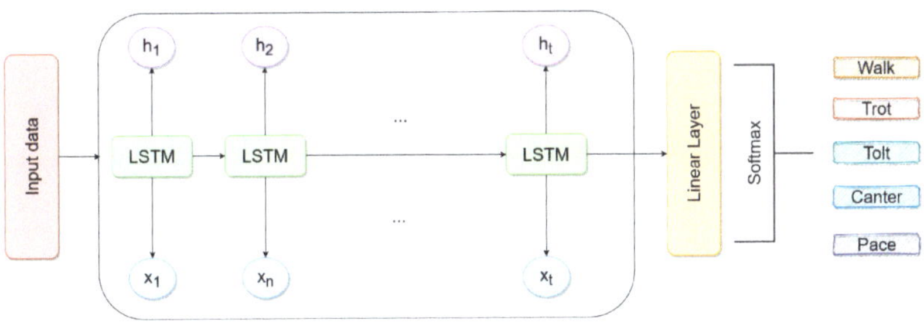

Figure 7. The model architecture used in this study.

The model's input was the output of the mobile sensors rotated to a given frame of reference where one axis (z) represents the vertical dimension and the others (x and y) represent the horizontal dimensions. In the world-frame, the horizontal axes correspond to the south–north and east–west directions. In the horse-frame, they correspond to the front–back and left–right directions. We also studied the effect of adding speed as an additional input feature, where the speed was calculated based on the GPS coordinates. The acceleration signal had three dimensions; the gyroscope signal had three dimensions; the speed signal had one dimension.

2.6. Smoothing Classifier Output

The model prediction only took in a segment of mobile sensor data and output a label. Due to the training approach, the model might make mistakes, which can be easily corrected on sequential data. As an example, because the model is not given its output for the last segment, it can claim that a horse is performing tölt and then brief walking for 100 milliseconds and then tölt again. Intuitively, horses do not perform such a switch from one gait to another and back within a 100-millisecond time period.

For this reason, two post-processing methods were used for smoothing the classifier output that could be applied to the leave-one-outtest datasets since they were in sequential order. The former method makes use of the linear layer of the network, which outputs a probability vector of the labels. The vector output of the softmax layer is updated with respect to the vectors preceding it in time using the exponential weight decay defined as:

$$z_0 = \boldsymbol{h}_0, \text{ and } z_t = \frac{z_{t-1} + \boldsymbol{h}_t}{2}. \quad (1)$$

The vector $\boldsymbol{h}$ denotes the output from the LSTM and z the refined vector after using exponential decay. This method ameliorates the problem to some extent, but does not fix it completely. To further refine the result, we applied a majority vote window of size 7, which we slid over the gaits as determined by the z_t vectors (for an illustration, see Figure 8). Concretely, we define

$$g_t = \arg\max z_t \quad (2)$$

as the gait chosen at time t through the largest component of z_t. We then define g'_t as the most common gait in the set

$$\{g_{t-3}, g_{t-2}, g_{t-1}, g_t, g_{t+1}, g_{t+2}, g_{t+3}\}$$

where ties are broken by using g_t. The sequence g'_t represents the output of our method after the two post-processing steps.

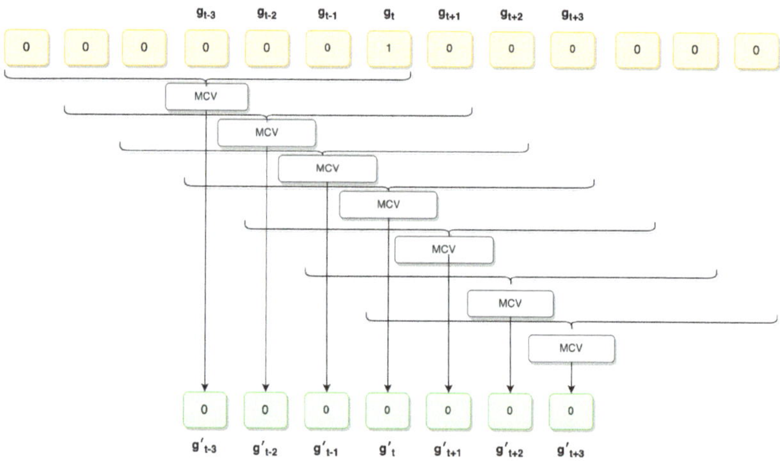

Figure 8. Sliding window majority vote. Here, g_t represents the chosen gait after the first pre-processing step and g'_t represents the chosen gait after the majority vote. MCV is an abbreviation for "Most-Common Value", and the curly brackets represent the window on which the most-common value is selected.

By applying the post-processing step, the prediction depends not only on past predictions, but also on future predictions, smoothing the signal.

2.7. Performance Measures

To measure the performance of the model across all gaits, we used the micro-averaged classification accuracy defined as

$$\frac{\text{number of correctly classified examples}}{\text{total number of examples}}, \quad (3)$$

which corresponds to the sum of the diagonal in a confusion matrix divided by the sum of all entries. For the accuracy of particular gaits, we report the one-vs.-all accuracy, i.e., where the classification is viewed as a binary classification problem with the gait in one class and all other gaits in the other class. We further report the macro-averaged gait classification accuracy where we averaged single gait classification accuracies over the gaits.

3. Results

3.1. Validation of TöltSense Labels

A total of 4421 one-second windows were generated from the TS logs, which included 179 gait transitions. Excluding cases that were subsequently marked as −2 or −1 and without exclusion periods, 4371 valid test cases were generated. Factoring in transition exclusion periods reduces the number of valid test cases (see the table below). The accuracy of the TS predictions was calculated simply as the total number of correct predictions divided by the total number of valid test cases.

In Table 4, we show how the calculated accuracy varied when we altered the exclusion period for both judge-identified and TS-identified transitions.

Table 4. Gait classification accuracy for different sizes of exclusion windows.

TS Excl (ms)	Judge Excl (ms)	Test Cases	Accuracy
2000	2000	3358	99.73%
1000	1000	3757	98.86%
1000	0	3909	97.95%
0	1000	3990	96.62%
0	0	4371	93.89%

The exclusion period was varied from 0 s to 2 s, and it was found that the longer the period, the greater the accuracy was. Without any exclusion periods, the micro-averaged accuracy was 93.89%, and with 2 s for each, the micro-averaged accuracy was 99.73%. The gait distribution is shown in Figure 9, and the confusion matrix for the case where both the TS and judge exclusion period was 1000ms is shown in Figure 10. The confusion matrix without any exclusion periods is shown in Figure 11.

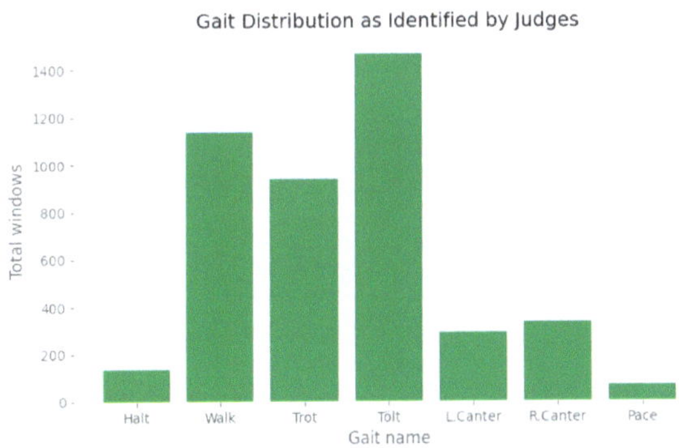

Figure 9. Distribution of gaits as identified by the judges. We note that pace is under-represented.

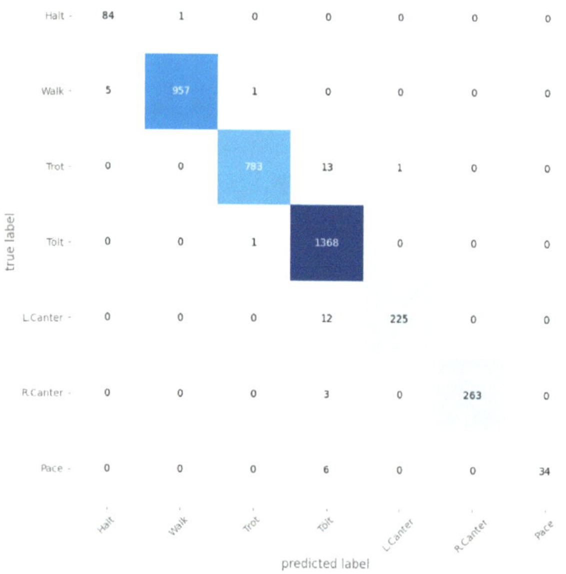

Figure 10. A confusion matrix for the case where both the TS and judge exclusion period was 1000 ms.

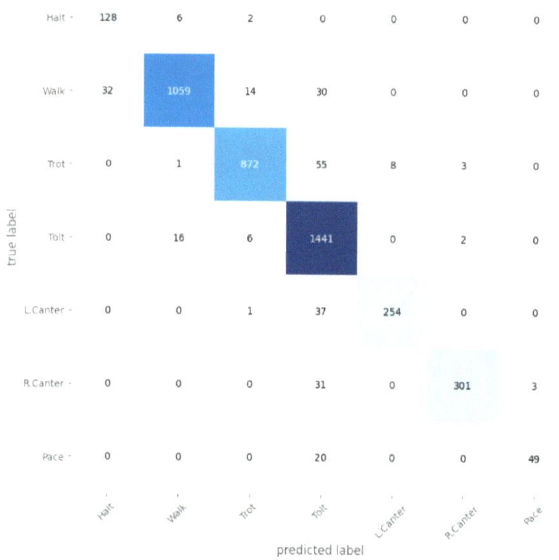

Figure 11. A confusion matrix for the case where both the TS and Judge exclusion period was 0 ms.

3.2. *Comparing Sequence Models on Mobile Phone Sensor Data*

The results of the mobile phone sensor study were based on data collected from 17 horses (see the Methods Section). When comparing sequence models, cross-validation was used where each horse was left out. For other experiments, we used a separate test set. Four of the horses were left out from the training data to measure the test performance.

Since only a few horses were able to perform flying pace, we had one horse both in the training and test data, but the rider was different in each set.

We compared several models in the gait classification task using cross-validation, where each horse was left out separately. The micro-averaged classification accuracy, averaged over the horses, is shown in Table 5. All models had accuracy scores exceeding 90%, with the Bi-LSTM model reaching the highest at 94.4%.

For each horse, detailed results based on the Bi-LSTM model are shown in Table 6. We observed the highest accuracy for walking at 97%. Canter was at 94%, flying pace at 93%, tölt at 89%, and trot at 82%. However, for four horses, the micro-averaged accuracy was worse (see the Discussion Section). The model performed well, as we hypothesized. Specifically, the model did not confuse the gaits of the Icelandic horse, tölt and flying pace.

Table 5. The average micro-averaged gait classification accuracy was computed for each horse using cross-validation, where the horse was left out for evaluation. The cross-validation was repeated five times for each model, and the results were averaged.

Model	Macro avg.
Bi-LSTM	94.4
GRU	91.2
LSTM	93.3
1D CNN	93.9

Table 6. We performed cross-validation where each horse was left out. For each horse, we ran the evaluation with five different initializations of the Bi-LSTM model and report the micro average for each gait. The macro average over all the gaits is 0.91. The amount of training data for each horse can be found in Table 3.

Horse ID.	Walk	Trot	Tölt	Canter	Flying Pace	Micro avg.
1	1.0	1.0	1.0	1.0	-	1.0
2	0.98	0.72	0.82	1.0	0.87	0.95
3	1.0	0.97	0.99	1.0	-	0.99
4	0.83	0.82	0.96	0.61	-	0.89
5	0.99	0.68	0.94	-	-	0.94
6	0.99	0.97	0.99	0.69	-	0.98
7	1.0	0.88	0.92	0.99	-	0.95
8	0.95	0.92	1.0	1.0	-	0.97
9	0.93	0.88	1.0	1.0	-	0.96
10	-	-	-	-	0.95	0.95
11	-	-	-	-	0.9	0.9
12	0.98	0.44	0.74	0.96	-	0.87
13	0.97	0.0	0.98	-	-	0.97
14	1.0	1.0	1.0	1.0	-	1.0
15	1.0	0.57	0.61	1.0	-	0.82
16	0.97	0.66	0.5	1.0	-	0.74
17	1.0	0.95	0.93	0.99	-	0.94
Macro avg.	0.97	0.82	0.89	0.94	0.93	0.94

3.3. Using the Horse's Frame of Reference Improves Classification Performance

Using the world-frame as a frame of reference isolates vertical variations in acceleration to a single axis. However, rotations to the horse-frame can further isolate variations in acceleration along the left–right axis and the front–back axis. We thus hypothesized that rotation to the horse-frame could lead to better classification performance. We trained an LSTM network with 200 units on 1.5 s-long segments of accelerometer and gyroscope measurements from 17 horses (see Table 3 for information about the horses). The distribution of the collected segments is shown in Figure 6. The dataset was quite imbalanced, but with the data acquisition approach, we managed to collect thousands of segments for each gait.

We evaluated the model on data left out from five rides, and it reached an average accuracy of 96.1% when training on the signal rotated to the horse's frame of reference (see Figure 12 for the best run) compared to an average accuracy of 93.9% for a signal rotated to the world-frame (see Figure 13 for the best run).

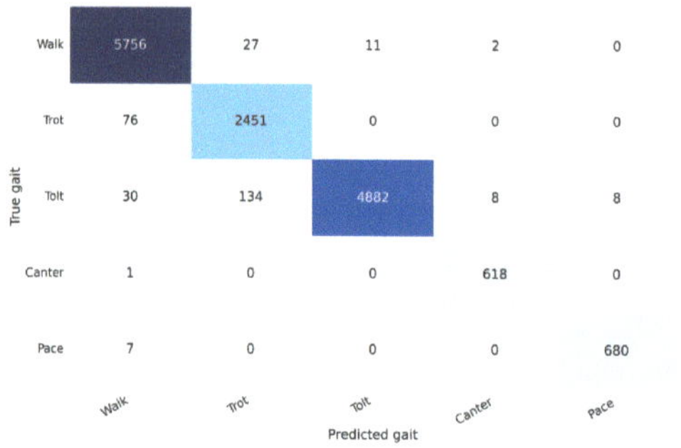

Figure 12. Confusion matrix for the gait classification model on the test set with 98.0% accuracy (best out of 9 random seeds with average accuracy at 96.1% and median accuracy at 95.8%). We use an input interval of length 1.5 s, where the input signal is aligned to the horse's frame of reference.

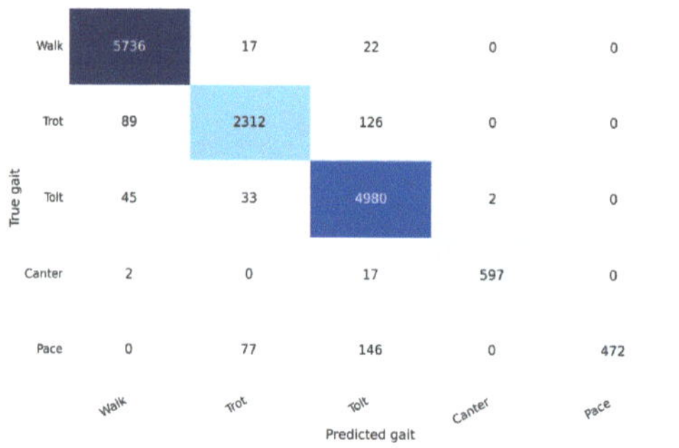

Figure 13. Confusion matrix for the gait classification model on the test set with 96.1% accuracy (best out of 9 random seeds with average accuracy at 93.9% and median accuracy at 92.7%). We use an input interval of length 1.5 s, where the input signal is aligned to the world-frame.

3.4. The Model Is Robust to Choice of Interval Length

Achieving a good performance with short intervals or less data can make predictions more responsive in an interactive environment since the model needs less time to react to gait changes. For recurrent models such as LSTMs, a shorter input can further reduce the computational cost of the inference task, which is ideal for mobile devices. For an LSTM model, the performance does not seem to depend strongly on the interval length in the range of 0.5–4 s (see Figure 14). The maximum accuracy on the test set was achieved for a 3 s interval, but the mean accuracy was highest for a 4 s interval. For an interval of length 1.5 s, the accuracy of the model averaged around 96% over nine evaluations on the test set where the model was trained each time using a different random seed. It may be noted that the variation in the test accuracy also increased with longer intervals. This can to some extent be attributed to the decreased size of the training and test sets for longer interval lengths, which leads to larger relative deviations in measures of performance on the test set.

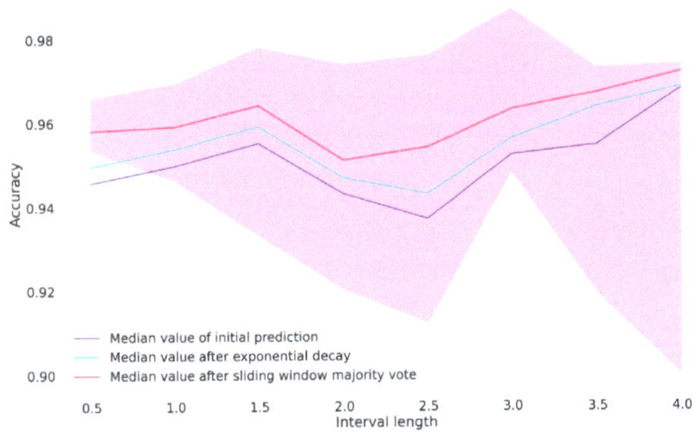

Figure 14. Accuracy over all gaits for each interval length (in seconds) using a rotation to the horse's frame of reference. The blue and red lines show the result of post-processing the classification result to achieve a higher accuracy score. The shaded area is bounded by the highest and lowest reported accuracy for each interval after post-processing. The accuracy is averaged over 9 evaluations on the test set, where the model was trained using a different random seed each time.

3.5. Performance Comparison for Input Signal Variations

We further studied the effect of varying sampling rates and what signals we trained the model on for 1.5-s intervals when the signals had been rotated to the horse's frame of reference. These variations reflect that not all mobile devices have a gyroscope and an accelerometer and the sampling rates vary significantly. In addition, we studied the effect that the speed had on the classification performance. The speed was derived from the GPS data on the phone's placement and not from the accelerometer. Table 7 shows the result.

Table 7. Classification accuracy on the test set for different signal combinations and rates for 1.5 s segments and a rotation to the horse-frame with the best performance for each rate in bold. The numbers reported are the median micro-averaged accuracy over 9 random seeds (a different random seed was used each time the model was trained and evaluated on the test set). **G** stands for Gyroscope only, **A** for Accelerometer only and **G+A** for Gyroscope and Accelerometer.

	without Speed			with Speed		
Rate	G	A	G+A	G	A	G+A
10 Hz	80.8	**96.9**	92.2	76.7	95.7	91.1
15 Hz	91.4	**97.4**	96.8	92.4	96.1	96.0
25 Hz	92.3	**97.8**	97.1	92.5	97.1	96.6
50 Hz	92.6	96.8	96.4	90.7	**97.3**	95.8

The result suggests that acceleration is the most-important input signal for gait classification. From the evaluation, we cannot conclude that the addition of gyroscope signals or speed consistently improved the model accuracy. Since acceleration reflects variations in speed, the speed signal might not be providing additional information that the model can benefit from. Furthermore, the speed signal might not be available indoors or in situations where the GPS is not reliable.

Regarding sampling rates, we did not observe a large drop in performance when they were lowered with only acceleration as the input. However, we saw a big difference in performance for 10 Hz and 15 Hz when the input from the gyroscope was used. The performance also did not clearly increase with a higher sampling rate, since we observed the best performance for 25 Hz, but not for 50 Hz.

4. Discussion

In this article, we presented the gait classification performance of the first phone-based classifier that recognizes all five gaits of the Icelandic horse, including flying pace. We showed that the gait classification for five-gaited horses can reach 94.4% accuracy with the model receiving only raw mobile sensor data from the accelerometer and gyroscope rotated to the horse-frame based on measurements from the magnetometer and a GPS signal. That is, specific feature engineering was not required. Instead of labelling the data by hand, we used a novel efficient approach to label the data by simultaneously collecting data from smartphones and the TS gait labelling system. That system generates a gait label based on four IMU sensors attached to a horse's limbs, and thus, the gait label is based on a signal for the limb movements. The kind of information that the TS can generate would normally require an expert eye on the ground or an in-depth frame-by-frame analysis of video. Such circumstances inevitably incur costs and are restrictive in terms of environment, such as being confined to a riding hall, or good lighting, or fair weather. Moreover, the volume and utility of information gathered manually is limited. By contrast, the TS is a cost-effective way to collect gait labels without any external assistance or environmental restrictions.

Through cross-validation, the method achieved accuracy scores above or equal to 0.9 for all gaits except trot (0.82) and tölt (0.89). In that regard, the most-common confusion in the model was between tölt and trot. It is conceivable that more training data from different horses and riders would improve the performance on trot since the performance on the training set was better than on the test set, which can indicate mild overfitting.

Tölt is characterized by a four-beat gait in which the horse lifts its hooves off the ground in a diagonal sequence. It has half-suspension in both the front and hind. In contrast, trot is a two-beat gait in which the horse lifts its hooves off the ground in a diagonal sequence, but with a moment of suspension. Tölt is considered to be the gait between trot and flying pace. We note that tölt can be ridden at different variations, speeds, and quality [15], some of which can be hard to differentiate from trot. Experienced human observers might even disagree on trotty tölt and tölty trot, especially at higher speeds, where they might be harder to tell apart [21]. Furthermore, trot can be ridden using three main riding techniques: sitting, rising, and a two-point seat where the rider stands in the stirrups. These techniques influence how the rider moves along with the horse, and they can also influence the horse's motion pattern [22]. We speculate that different riding techniques could make the mobile sensor movements more similar to other gaits. Together, these differences might explain the confusion in the model. To improve the performance of models relying on mobile phone sensors, it could be worthwhile to study whether different combinations of riding styles and gaits can be distinguished in mobile sensor recordings.

On the test set, the model reached a median classification accuracy of 96.9% with sampling rates down to 10 Hz. We observed a higher accuracy for 25 Hz signals than 50 Hz signals when comparing signal combinations. In principle, performance can increase by lowering the sampling rate since it translates to shorter input sequences for the model. A recurrent neural network such as an LSTM model might handle shorter inputs better [23,24]. However, lowering the sampling rate too much can cause the signal to contain less information about the underlying gait, which possibly explains the performance drop for the 15 Hz and 10 Hz signals. When exploring signal combinations, we also observed that speed did not lead to improved accuracy, in agreement with prior work [8].

To ensure the reliability of our measurements with respect to TS labels, we further validated TS accuracy in a separate study. We demonstrated a very high level of agreement between the TS and qualified sport judges when classifying the gait of Icelandic horses. The use of exclusion periods around transitions can take the agreement to over 99%, but the agreement was around 94% even without any exclusion. We earlier framed this in terms of "accuracy" by considering the judge classifications as the ground truth. In reality, we are assessing the agreement between two different measuring approaches, and it is valid to question whether the TS is more accurate than human observers in some circumstances. There are often areas where the judges disagree about the gait. For example, a very pacey tölt coming out of canter may be classed as pace by some and tölt by others. There are also cases on the boundary between walk and tölt and between tölt and trot. It may be interesting to analyse these disagreements as a project in itself. The main shortcoming of the validation study is the lack of flying pace segments.

We acknowledge that this study is limited to Icelandic horses. However, the methods we have applied to collect the data can be used to collect data for a large population of different horse breeds in diverse environments using various wearable sensors. More test data would further allow us to better measure the generalization performance. That would be especially beneficial for flying pace, the gait for which we had the fewest measurements [25]. To improve the results further, we note that it is known that sensor placement can affect model performance [9,26], and we hypothesize that phone placement could have an effect, which would explain the worse classification performance for some horse–rider pairs. We speculate that our results could be improved by making sure that factors such as the phone's placement, phone model, riding surface, and clothing (loose vs. tight) are standardized. To mitigate the phone's placement problem, a model could be trained that takes the placement into account, which could improve overall performance. Furthermore, to improve the user experience of an app, a model could be trained to automatically infer the phone's placement (and possibly even the type of riding surface) such that a user would not need to assign it himself/herself. Further improvements could be achieved with better mobile phone sensors. For example, we used a 1Hz GPS signal to estimate direction, but a higher sampling rate could allow for more detailed estimates of direction and other important parameters. For example, Pfau et al. managed to estimate essential stride parameters using a 10 Hz GPS signal [27]. Another improvement could be achieved by using several mobile sensors, such as jointly from a smartwatch and a smartphone. Estimating speed has been shown to be better with more than a single horse-mounted sensor [28], and it thus is reasonable to ask whether several human-attached sensors improve gait classification performance.

Recordings based on mobile phones open up a variety of possibilities in horse-related activity tasks. For example, it makes it feasible to study horse behaviour at a large scale through volunteer participation. Such data can be used to classify horses, define phenotypes, and possibly relate their behaviour to genomic data. Furthermore, data obtained from mobile phone sensors have been used for lameness detection [9,29], but such studies could benefit from the labelling approach we used here. Sensors attached to a horse have been used to identify lameness [30–32], and commercial products have been developed for that task (see, for example, https://equisense.com/ accessed on 1 May 2022 and https://equinosis.com/ accessed on 1 May 2022).

Traditionally, the human eye has been considered the gold standard for gait classification. Bragança et al. [8] claimed based on their results that human visual and subjective assessment is not optimal. Furthermore, results on lameness detection using human observers have reported low intraobserver agreement [33,34]. Therefore, when models can exceed human performance for tasks such as lameness detection, then they will possibly be better suited for data labelling. Similar to our labelling approach, data could be captured simultaneously from mobile phone sensors attached to the horse and a label from a well-performing model (we acknowledge that commercial products can be difficult to trust due to too rarely disclosed accuracies). That dataset can then be used to train a model for lameness detection. Alternatively, there is also the possibility of applying unsupervised approaches such as anomaly detection methods to detect unusual recordings at a large scale.

5. Conclusions

In this paper, we investigated the feasibility of using mobile phone sensors for gait classification in Icelandic horses, a breed known for its ability to perform five gaits: walk, trot, canter, tölt, and flying pace. We used the TöltSense (TS) system to label our training data and evaluated the accuracy of different machine learning models on these data. Our results showed that it is possible to achieve high accuracy in gait classification using mobile phone sensors, with the best-performing model reaching an accuracy of 94.4%.

These findings have significant implications for the field of gait classification. Mobile phones are widely available and portable devices that are often carried by individuals, making them a convenient and accessible option for gait classification. Our results suggest that mobile phone sensors can be used as a reliable alternative to sensors attached to the animal, offering a more practical and convenient solution for gait classification in certain contexts.

However, it is important to note that the accuracy of gait classification can be influenced by various factors, such as the environment in which the data are collected and the quality of the sensors. Further research is needed to fully understand the limitations and potential of mobile phone sensors for gait classification in different contexts and with different types of animals.

In conclusion, our study demonstrated the feasibility of using mobile phone sensors for gait classification in Icelandic horses, offering a convenient and accessible alternative to traditional methods. These findings have the potential to broaden the scope of gait classification research and to facilitate the development of mobile-phone-based applications for gait classification.

Author Contributions: Conceptualization, T.R., M.R.Ó. and H.E.; methodology, H.B.D., T.R. and H.E.; software, H.B.D., T.R. and H.E.; validation, H.B.D., T.R. and H.E.; data curation, M.R.Ó. and T.R.; writing—original draft preparation, H.B.D., T.R. and H.E.; writing—review and editing, H.B.D., T.R. and H.E.; supervision, H.E. and T.R.; project administration, H.E. and T.R.; funding acquisition, H.E. All authors have read and agreed to the published version of the manuscript.

Funding: This research was funded by the Icelandic directorate of labour, the University of Iceland, and Horseday ehf.

Institutional Review Board Statement: Ethical review and approval were waived for this study. It was concluded that it is outwith the European Directive 2010/63/EU as it does not meet the threshold for causing any pain, distress, suffering or lasting harm.

Informed Consent Statement: Informed consent was obtained from all subjects involved in the study.

Data Availability Statement: The datasets used and analysed during the current study are available from Horseday ehf. upon reasonable request.

Acknowledgments: We would like to thank Thilo Pfau for helpful comments on the manuscript. We would also like to thank Ann Winter, Nanco Lekkerkerker, Rebecca Hughes, and Harriet Vincent for labelling in the TöltSense validation study. We would further like to thank the Icelandic Directorate of Labour, the University of Iceland, and Horseday for funding H.B.D. in the summer of 2021.

Conflicts of Interest: H.E. declares no conflict of interest. H.B.D.'s work in the summer of 2021 was partially funded by Horseday ehf., and he has been employed by Horseday ehf. since the fall of 2021. M.R.Ó. is a shareholder of Horseday ehf., and T.R. is the owner of Toltsense Ltd.

Abbreviations

The following abbreviations are used in this manuscript:

TS	TöltSense
RNN	Recurrent neural network
LSTM	Long short-term memory
GPS	Global positioning system
GRU	Gated recurrent unit
CNN	Convolutional neural network

References

1. Hildebrand, M. Symmetrical Gaits of Horses. *Science* **1965**, *150*, 7001–708. [CrossRef]
2. Olsen, E.; Haubro Andersen, P.; Pfau, T. Accuracy and Precision of Equine Gait Event Detection during Walking with Limb and Trunk Mounted Inertial Sensors. *Sensors* **2012**, *12*, 8145–8156.
3. Holt, D.; George, L.B.S.; Clayton, H.M.; Hobbs, S.J. A simple method for equine kinematic gait event detection. *Equine Vet. J.* **2017**, *49*, 688–691. [CrossRef] [PubMed]
4. Bosch, S.; Serra Bragança, F.; Marin-Perianu, M.; Marin-Perianu, R.; Van der Zwaag, B.J.; Voskamp, J.; Back, W.; Van Weeren, R.; Havinga, P. EquiMoves: A Wireless Networked Inertial Measurement System for Objective Examination of Horse Gait. *Sensors* **2018**, *18*, 850.
5. Eerdekens, A.; Deruyck, M.; Fontaine, J.; Damiaans, B.; Martens, L.; De Poorter, E.; Govaere, J.; Plets, D.; Joseph, W. Horse Jumping and Dressage Training Activity Detection Using Accelerometer Data. *Animals* **2021**, *11*, 2904. [CrossRef]
6. Pasquiet, B.; Biau, S.; Trébot, Q.; Debril, J.F.; Durand, F.; Fradet, L. Detection of Horse Locomotion Modifications Due to Training with Inertial Measurement Units: A Proof-of-Concept. *Sensors* **2022**, *22*, 4981. [CrossRef]
7. Robilliard, J.J.; Pfau, T.; Wilson, A.M. Gait characterisation and classification in horses. *J. Exp. Biol.* **2007**, *210*, 187–197.
8. Serra Bragança, F.M.; Broomé, S.; Rhodin, M.; Björnsdóttir, S.; Gunnarsson, V.; Voskamp, J.P.; Persson-Sjodin, E.; Back, W.; Lindgren, G.; Novoa-Bravo, M.; et al. Improving gait classification in horses by using inertial measurement unit (IMU) generated data and machine learning. *Sci. Rep.* **2020**, *10*, 17785.
9. Pfau, T.; Weller, R. Comparison of a standalone consumer grade smartphone with a specialist inertial measurement unit for quantification of movement symmetry in the trotting horse. *Equine Vet. J.* **2017**, *49*, 124–129. [CrossRef]
10. Hochreiter, S.; Schmidhuber, J. Long Short-Term Memory. *Neural Comput.* **1997**, *9*, 1735–1780. [CrossRef]
11. Eerdekens, A.; Deruyck, M.; Fontaine, J.; Martens, L.; De Poorter, E. Automatic equine activity detection by convolutional neural networks using accelerometer data. *Comput. Electron. Agric.* **2020**, *168*, 105139. [CrossRef]
12. Casella, E.; Khamesi, A.; Silvestri, S. A framework for the recognition of horse gaits through wearable devices. *Pervasive Mob. Comput.* **2020**, *67*, 101213. [CrossRef]
13. Maga, M.; Björnsdotter, S. Development of Equine Gait Recognition Algorithm. Master's Thesis, Lund University, Lund, Sweden, 2017.
14. Andersson, L.S.; Larhammar, M.; Memic, F.; Wootz, H.; Schwochow, D.; Rubin, C.J.; Patra, K.; Arnason, T.; Wellbring, L.; Hjälm, G.; et al. Mutations in DMRT3 affect locomotion in horses and spinal circuit function in mice. *Nature* **2012**, *488*, 642–646. [CrossRef] [PubMed]
15. Kristjánsson, Þ.; Reynisson, G.; Bárðarson, S.; Ævarsson, S. The Gaits of the Icelandic Horse, Basic Definitions. 2014. Available online: https://www.lhhestar.is/static/files/gangtegundir_2017p_engl.pdf (accessed on 1 October 2021).
16. Pfau, T.; Witte, T.H.; Wilson, A.M. A method for deriving displacement data during cyclical movement using an inertial sensor. *J. Exp. Biol.* **2005**, *208*, 2503–2514.
17. Pfau, T.; Reilly, P. How low can we go? Influence of sample rate on equine pelvic displacement calculated from inertial sensor data. *Equine Vet. J.* **2021**, *53*, 1075–1081. [CrossRef]
18. Chung, J.; Gulcehre, C.; Cho, K.; Bengio, Y. Empirical evaluation of gated recurrent neural networks on sequence modeling. *arXiv* **2014**, arXiv:1412.3555.
19. Graves, A.; Schmidhuber, J. Framewise phoneme classification with bidirectional LSTM and other neural network architectures. *Neural Netw.* **2005**, *18*, 602–610. [CrossRef]
20. Kingma, D.P.; Ba, J. Adam: A Method for Stochastic Optimization. In Proceedings of the 3rd International Conference on Learning Representations, ICLR 2015, San Diego, CA, USA, 7–9 May 2015.
21. Zips, S.; Peham, C.; Scheidl, M.; Licka, T.; Girtler, D. Motion pattern of the toelt of Icelandic horses at different speeds. *Equine Vet. J.* **2001**, *33*, 109–111. [CrossRef]
22. Persson-Sjodin, E.; Hernlund, E.; Pfau, T.; Haubro Andersen, P.; Rhodin, M. Influence of seating styles on head and pelvic vertical movement symmetry in horses ridden at trot. *PLoS ONE* **2018**, *13*, e0195341. [CrossRef]
23. Li, S.; Li, W.; Cook, C.; Zhu, C.; Gao, Y. Independently recurrent neural network (indrnn): Building a longer and deeper rnn. In Proceedings of the IEEE Conference on Computer Vision and Pattern Recognition, Salt Lake City, UT, USA, 18–23 June 2018; pp. 5457–5466.
24. Khandelwal, U.; He, H.; Qi, P.; Jurafsky, D. Sharp Nearby, Fuzzy Far Away: How Neural Language Models Use Context. In Proceedings of the Proceedings of the 56th Annual Meeting of the Association for Computational Linguistics (Volume 1: Long Papers), Melbourne, Australia, 15–20 July 2018; pp. 284–294.
25. Kaur, H.; Pannu, H.S.; Malhi, A.K. A Systematic Review on Imbalanced Data Challenges in Machine Learning: Applications and Solutions. *ACM Comput. Surv.* **2019**, *52*, 79:1–79:36.
26. Serra Braganca, F.; Rhodin, M.; Wiestner, T.; Hernlund, E.; Pfau, T.; Van Weeren, P.; Weishaupt, M.A. Quantification of the effect of instrumentation error in objective gait assessment in the horse on hindlimb symmetry parameters. *Equine Vet. J.* **2018**, *50*, 370–376. [CrossRef]
27. Pfau, T.; Bruce, O.; Edwards, W.B.; Leguillette, R. Stride frequency derived from GPS speed fluctuations in galloping horses. *J. Biomech.* **2022**, *145*, 111364. [CrossRef] [PubMed]

28. Darbandi, H.; Serra Bragança, F.; van der Zwaag, B.J.; Voskamp, J.; Gmel, A.I.; Haraldsdóttir, E.H.; Havinga, P. Using different combinations of body-mounted imu sensors to estimate speed of horses—A machine learning approach. *Sensors* **2021**, *21*, 798. [CrossRef] [PubMed]
29. Marunova, E.; Dod, L.; Witte, S.; Pfau, T. Smartphone-Based Pelvic Movement Asymmetry Measures for Clinical Decision Making in Equine Lameness Assessment. *Animals* **2021**, *11*, 1665. [CrossRef] [PubMed]
30. Keegan, K.G.; Kramer, J.; Yonezawa, Y.; Maki, H.; Pai, P.F.; Dent, E.V.; Kellerman, T.E.; Wilson, D.A.; Reed, S.K. Assessment of repeatability of a wireless, inertial sensor–based lameness evaluation system for horses. *Am. J. Vet. Res.* **2011**, *72*, 1156–1163.
31. McCracken, M.J.; Kramer, J.; Keegan, K.G.; Lopes, M.; Wilson, D.A.; Reed, S.K.; LaCarrubba, A.; Rasch, M. Comparison of an inertial sensor system of lameness quantification with subjective lameness evaluation. *Equine Vet. J.* **2012**, *44*, 652–656.
32. Yigit, T.; Han, F.; Rankins, E.; Yi, J.; McKeever, K.; Malinowski, K. Wearable IMU-based Early Limb Lameness Detection for Horses using Multi-Layer Classifiers. In Proceedings of the 2020 IEEE 16th International Conference on Automation Science and Engineering (CASE), Hong Kong, China, 20–21 August 2020; pp. 955–960. ISSN: 2161-8089. [CrossRef]
33. Keegan, K.G. Evidence-based lameness detection and quantification. *Vet. Clin. N. Am. Equine Pract.* **2007**, *23*, 403–423. [CrossRef]
34. Arkell, M.; Archer, R.; Guitian, F.; May, S. Evidence of bias affecting the interpretation of the results of local anaesthetic nerve blocks when assessing lameness in horses. *Vet. Rec.* **2006**, *159*, 346–348. [CrossRef]

animals

MDPI

Article

Vertical Movement of Head, Withers, and Pelvis of High-Level Dressage Horses Trotting in Hand vs. Being Ridden

Hilary M. Clayton [1,*], Sarah Jane Hobbs [2], Marie Rhodin [3], Elin Hernlund [3], Mick Peterson [4], Rosalie Bos [5] and Filipe Serra Bragança [6]

1 Large Animal Clinical Sciences, Michigan State University, 736 Wilson Road, East Lansing, MI 48824, USA
2 Research Centre for Applied Sport, Physical Activity and Performance, University of Central Lancashire, Preston PR1 2HE, UK; sjhobbs1@uclan.ac.uk
3 Department of Anatomy Physiology and Biochemistry, Swedish University of Agricultural Sciences, S-750 07 Uppsala, Sweden; marie.rhodin@slu.se (M.R.); elin.hernlund@slu.se (E.H.)
4 Biosystems and Agricultural Engineering and UK Ag Equine Programs, University of Kentucky, Lexington, KY 40546, USA; mick.peterson@uky.edu
5 Sporthorse Medical Diagnostic Centre, SMDC, Hooge Wijststraat 7, NL-5384 RC Heesch, The Netherlands; bos@sporthorsemdc.co
6 Department of Clinical Sciences, Faculty of Veterinary Medicine, Utrecht University, Yalelaan 112-114, NL-3584 CM Utrecht, The Netherlands; filipe.braganca@slu.se
* Correspondence: claytonh@msu.edu

Simple Summary: Before entering high-level dressage competitions, horses are inspected for lameness while trotting in hand, but it is unclear how motion asymmetries change when horses are ridden. This study measures axial and limb asymmetries to test the hypothesis that ridden horses have greater vertical movement asymmetry of the head, withers, and pelvis than when trotting in hand. Nineteen dressage horses were evaluated trotting in hand on a firm surface and being ridden by their trainer in an arena with sand-fiber footing at collected and extended trot. Inertial measurement units (IMUs) on the head, withers, and pelvis measured data describing vertical motion and left–right asymmetry under the three trotting conditions. IMUs on the cannon bones measured left–right symmetry in limb pro-/retraction. Ridden horses had larger vertical ranges of motion of the head, withers, and pelvis, which were ascribed to the riders' effects on impulsion and engagement. Ridden horses had larger asymmetries in head and withers MaxDiff and pelvic MinDiff in collected trot. These were thought to reflect left–right differences in muscular strength that affected the ability to raise the forehand and lower the haunches.

Abstract: Prior to international competitions, dressage horses are evaluated for fitness to compete while trotting in hand on a firm surface. This study compares the kinematics of experienced dressage horses trotting under fitness-to-compete conditions vs. performing collected and extended trot when ridden on a sand-fiber arena surface. The hypotheses are that the vertical range of motion (ROM) and left–right asymmetries in minimal and maximal heights of axial body segments at ridden trot exceed those when trotting in hand. Inertial measurement units (IMUs) attached mid-dorsally to the head, withers, and pelvis of 19 actively competing dressage horses measured the vertical ROM and left–right asymmetries in minimal (MinDiff) and maximal (MaxDiff) heights of the midline sensors. The vertical ROM was greater for both types of ridden trot, reflecting greater impulsion in response to the riders' aids. Head MinDiff/MaxDiff and withers MaxDiff were significantly higher under both ridden conditions. Pelvis MinDiff was significantly the largest for collected trot. Compared with trot in hand, left–right differences in limb protraction were larger for extended and collected trot in the forelimbs but only for extended trot in the hind limbs. The rider's influence increases the horse's impulsion and vertical ROM, which may exacerbate inherent asymmetries in muscular strength when lowering the haunches and elevating the withers.

Keywords: head asymmetry; withers asymmetry; pelvic asymmetry; limb pro-/retraction; collected trot; extended trot; fit to compete

1. Introduction

Equestrian sports are based on locomotor skills that require varying combinations of speed, endurance, and power. Locomotion is a result of ground reaction forces (GRFs) generated when the hooves press against the ground. The resultant GRF can be represented by three perpendicular components, each having a different effect on the horse's center of mass (CoM): the vertical component pushes the body upwards, the longitudinal component controls craniocaudal accelerations, and the transverse component is necessary for turning. In a lame horse, the generation of vertical GRF and impulse during the stance phase of the lame limb are reduced compared with the compensating limb [1–4]. This results in asymmetrical vertical excursions of the CoM and axial body segments on the two diagonals [1–4].

Inertial measurement units (IMUs) measure accelerations from which displacements are calculated. When attached to specific body segments, they offer an accurate method of determining segmental displacements and rotations. In relation to the study reported here, IMUs characterize body motion [5] and detect left–right asymmetries in the vertical motion of axial body segments and the longitudinal motion of the limb segments [2,6]. These asymmetries are consequences of differences in GRFs generated by the left and right limbs. Forelimb asymmetries mostly affect the poll and withers, while hind limb asymmetries have more effect on the pelvis. The ability of IMUs to detect asymmetries that fall below the threshold of detection of the human eye is particularly useful in the diagnosis of lameness in clinical practice [7].

Interestingly, the use of IMUs has revealed high prevalence of movement asymmetries in various populations of horses that are in active training and are described as "sound" by their owners [3,8–11]. Similar asymmetries have been reported in horses showing limb length discrepancy [12], trotting around a circle [6], or being ridden at a rising trot [13]. Limited information is available regarding the effect of a rider, per se, on gait symmetry at the trot and, thus, differences in horses' kinematics at the in-hand evaluation compared with the performance in the competition arena.

A question that needs to be addressed in horses with asymmetrical movements of the axial body segments is whether the horse is lame/in pain or whether other confounding influences are involved. One possible confounder is motor laterality originating in the cerebral cortex and resulting in asymmetrical muscular strength or use of the contralateral limb pairs. There is, as yet, insufficient evidence to support or refute an effect of motor laterality on gait symmetry in trotting horses. One study found that 12 of 13 values that were above the commonly used asymmetry limits for PMinDiff were towards the right side, but no other parameter had the same skewed distribution [14]. A different study of 65 young warmblood horses did not find convincing evidence that vertical movement asymmetry was associated with the horses' perceived laterality patterns [15].

The study reported here addresses gait asymmetry in high-level, actively competing dressage horses under two practical conditions that occur during international dressage competitions (CDI): trot in hand and ridden trot at slow (collected) and fast (extended) speeds. Trot in hand is part of a mandatory, subjective evaluation of the horse's health and soundness. It is usually performed on a track at least 30 m long with a firm, level, clean, and non-slippery surface. Horses are led from the left side on a loose rein wearing a bridle or halter. The horse walks away from the inspector for a short distance, trots to the end of the track, turns by walking in a clockwise direction, and trots back to the starting point. A decision is made that the horse is accepted (fit to compete), not accepted (unfit to compete), or questionable, in which case the horse is moved to a holding box for further evaluation. Since there is no appeal against the ground jury's decision, it is important for the inspection to be fair and honest.

The dressage test is performed on an arena surface that is predominantly sand, to which the addition of other materials is allowed. The prescribed test movements are judged and scored subjectively. Criteria evaluated by judges include left–right symmetry in spatiotemporal variables and spinal movements, and one of the responsibilities of the chief judge is to stop the performance if the horse appears to be lame. The extent to which the horse's own kinematic pattern and the presence of a rider affect locomotor asymmetries is highly relevant in this context. Lower-level competitions do not have a fitness-to-compete evaluation, which puts the onus on the judge to recognize and assess the importance of locomotor asymmetries.

This study evaluates the vertical ROM (range of motion) and movement symmetry in axial body segments and pro-/retraction of the limbs in a group of experienced dressage horses under conditions simulating the CDI fitness-to-compete inspection and the competition performance. The objectives are to measure and compare locomotor asymmetries under the two conditions and, in particular, to evaluate the effects due to the presence of a rider, the trotting speed of the horse, and the type of footing. The hypotheses are that the vertical ROM of the axial body segments, the asymmetries in minimal and maximal heights of axial body segments, and the asymmetries in limb pro-/retraction at trot are greater when horses are ridden compared with trotting in hand.

2. Materials and Methods

2.1. Horses and Riders

The subjects were 19 dressage horses (mean $\pm$ SD; height: 166.7 $\pm$ 7.4 cm; age: 10.7 $\pm$ 3.2 years; sex: 5 stallions, 11 geldings, and 3 mares) ridden by their regular riders. Inclusion criteria were that horses were assessed as sound by their trainers and two clinicians, horses and riders were able to perform at Prix St. George level or higher, and they were actively competing in high-level dressage competitions. Prior to acceptance into the study, two experienced lameness clinicians (M.R. and E.H.) performed a clinical examination consisting of visual inspection and palpation of the musculoskeletal system.

2.2. Study Design and Data Collection

Data were collected by using 15 wireless ProMove-mini IMUs (Inertia Technology B.V., Enschede, The Netherlands), each of which weighed 20 g. The sensors have two aligned accelerometers that provide a single fused signal with high precision and range, a gyroscope that measures angular velocity in a range of $\pm 2000^{\circ}/s$, and a compass to measure magnetic field intensity. The IMUs are actively time-synchronized within a precision of 100 ns and a sampling frequency of 200 Hz, which is ample for trotting data [16]. They transmit over a distance up to 30 m to the Inertia Gateway, which coordinates the individual nodes and streams data through the gateway to a laptop computer running Equimoves software (version 0.0.211001). Additionally, each sensor has an on-board SD card with 2 Gb memory, which stores data if the horse moves outside of the wireless transmission range. Stored data are retrieved on completion of the data collection. For further details, see Bosch et al. [17]. The IMUs were also synchronized with 3 video cameras.

IMU nodes were attached to the poll, withers, lumbar spine region just behind the saddle, left and right tuber coxae, pelvis above and between the tubera sacrale, the cannon region of each limb, and the four hooves. The head sensor was mounted on the crown piece of the bridle by using hook and loop tape. At the withers, lumbosacral region, pelvis, and tuber coxae, sensors were attached to the skin with animal polster and double-sided tape. A lightweight protection boot with a sensor pocket on its lateral aspect was attached to the cannon region of each limb. Hoof sensors were attached on the lateral aspect of the hooves and wrapped with duct tape (Figure 1).

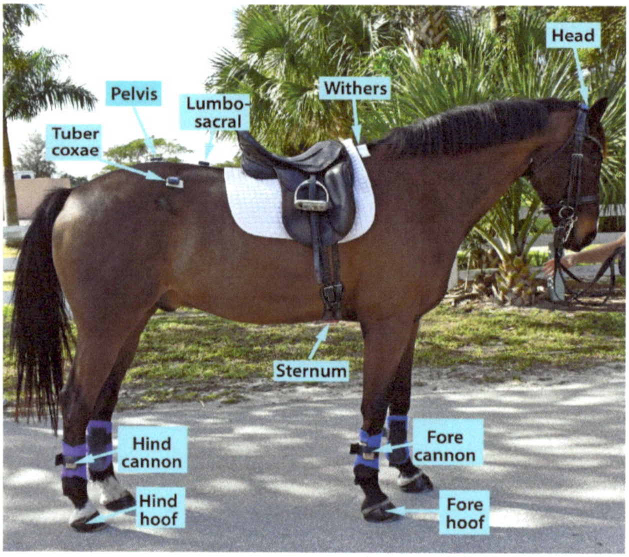

Figure 1. IMU locations. Sensors on the limbs are attached bilaterally. Photo courtesy of Dr. Hilary M. Clayton.

The in-hand evaluation involved walking and trotting the horses approximately 30 m in a straight line over a firm surface. Since horses were evaluated at different venues, the surfaces were not identical and consisted of packed clay, packed gravel, or asphalt. Video recordings made from the cranial, caudal, and lateral views were synchronized with data from the IMUs.

Each horse wore its usual tack for the ridden part of the study. They were ridden in arenas with similar but not identical footing based on sand with added geotextiles/fibers. Horses warmed up in the arena at the rider's discretion and then performed a dressage test written for the study. It included all dressage gaits performed in straight lines and, when appropriate, on left and right circles, and lateral movements. Two 5 min rest intervals were included. The riders familiarized themselves with the test beforehand, and during testing, it was read to them through ear buds.

2.3. Data Processing and Analysis

Data from the sensors were analyzed with EquiMoves software, which converted the recorded vertical accelerations into vertical displacements. Stride segmentation was based on angular velocity data from a gyroscope [17], and stride durations were measured. The cannon-mounted IMUs detected hoof-on and hoof-off events, which marked the transitions between swing and stance phases for each limb [17]. Speed could not be measured because the roof of the covered arenas interfered with satellite communication.

The dorsal midline sensors follow a sinusoidal path with two cycles per stride (Figure 2). The following variables were extracted from the raw data:

- Stride duration: Time elapsing between successive occurrences of the same event in successive strides.
- HROMz, WROMz, and PROMz: Vertical range of motion (ROMz) calculated as the difference between the minimal and maximal heights of the head (H), withers (W), and pelvis (P) sensors during each diagonal stance phase.
- HMinDiff, WMinDiff, and PMinDiff: Absolute difference between the two minima of the heights of the head (H), withers (W), and pelvis (P) sensors during the stride.
- HMaxDiff, WMaxDiff, and PMaxDiff: Absolute difference between the two maxima of the heights of the head (H), withers (W), and pelvis (P) sensors during the stride.
- ProMaxDiff: Difference in maximal protraction between contralateral limbs in late swing. Measured as the absolute difference between left and right cannon segment angles relative to the vertical at maximal protraction when the distal cannon bone is maximally dorsal to its proximal end.
- RetMaxDiff: Difference in maximal retraction between contralateral limbs shortly after lift-off. Measured as the absolute difference between the left and right cannon segment angles relative to the vertical at maximal retraction when the distal cannon segment is maximally palmar/plantar to its proximal end.

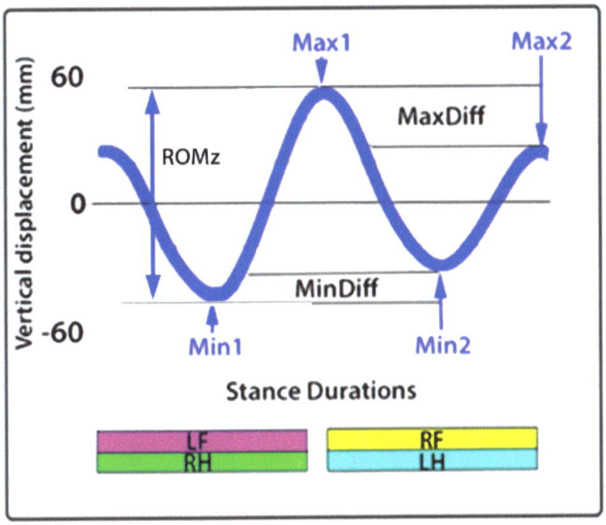

Figure 2. Sinusoidal pattern of the vertical motion of a dorsal midline sensor during one stride at trot showing the two minima, two maxima, and measurement of MinDiff, MaxDiff, and ROMz. The bars at the bottom indicate stance phase durations of the diagonal limb pairs. LF: left fore; RF: right fore; LH: left hind; RH: right hind.

2.4. Statistical Analysis

Descriptive statistics were performed, and boxplots, showing means, inter-quartile ranges, and individual data points, were created to demonstrate stride duration, ROM, upper-body symmetry parameters, and symmetry in maximum cannon protraction and retraction for the three trot conditions (extended, collected, and in hand).

All variables except stride duration were square root-transformed to achieve a normal distribution of model residuals. By using R-studio (version 3.6.3) and the package lme4 (version 1.1), linear mixed models were obtained for all variables with horse as a random effect and trot conditions (in hand, extended, and collected) as fixed effects. For pairwise comparisons, *p*-values of ≤ 0.05 were regarded as significant.

3. Results

All horses completed all phases of the data collection required for this study. The following description refers only to statistically different findings ($p \leq 0.05$).

3.1. Stride Duration

Stride duration (LSmean) was significantly longer in collected trot (0.85 s) compared with trot in hand (0.78 s) and extended trot (0.78 s), which did not differ from each other (Figure 3).

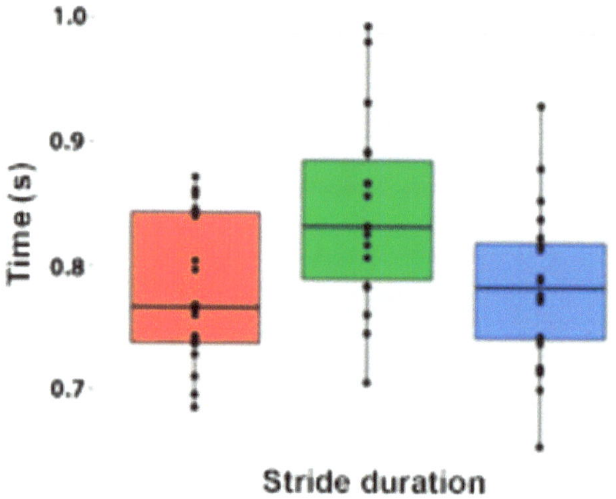

Figure 3. Boxplot showing arithmetic means, inter-quartile ranges, and individual data points for stride duration during extended (orange), collected (green), and in-hand (blue) trot.

3.2. Vertical Range of Motion

Differences between the vertical ROM in the three types of trot followed the same pattern for the head, withers, and pelvis, with trot in hand having a significantly smaller vertical ROM than both ridden conditions, which did not differ from each other (Table 1, Figure 4).

Table 1. Linear mixed model output with pairwise comparison for vertical ranges of motion among trot conditions. Values are LSmeans with 95% confidence intervals for ROM (mm). For each sensor location (head, withers, and pelvis), LSmean values with different superscripts differ significantly ($p < 0.05$).

Sensor Location	Condition	LSmean	Lower C.I.	Upper C.I.
Head	Extended trot	123.4 ^{b}	107.8	140.1
	Collected trot	129.3 ^{b}	113.3	146.4
	Trot in hand	82.4 ^{a}	70.2	95.5
Withers	Extended trot	90.3 ^{b}	79.7	101.5
	Collected trot	97.5 ^{b}	86.5	109.1
	Trot in hand	79.3 ^{a}	69.6	89.5
Pelvis	Extended trot	102.3 ^{b}	89.6	115.9
	Collected trot	106.9 ^{b}	93.9	120.8
	Trot in hand	86.2 ^{a}	74.8	98.4

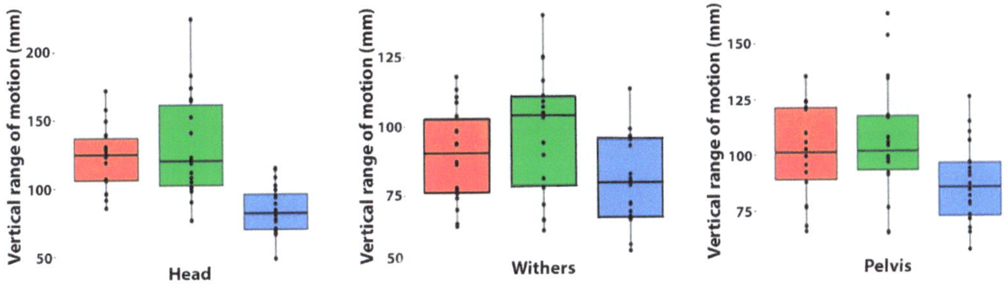

Figure 4. Boxplots showing arithmetic means, inter-quartile ranges, and individual data points for vertical range of motion of the head (**left**), withers (**center**), and pelvis (**right**) for extended trot (orange), collected trot (green), and in-hand trot (blue).

3.3. MinDiff

MinDiff values for the head, withers, and pelvis are shown in Table 2 and Figure 5. HMinDiff was larger for both types of ridden trot than trot in hand. WMinDiff had low values that did not differ among trot conditions. PMinDiff was higher for collected trot than trot in hand.

Table 2. LSmean values from mixed model analysis with 95% confidence intervals for mean absolute values of MinDiff and MaxDiff of head, withers, and pelvis (mm). For each sensor location, LSMean values of MinDiff or MaxDiff with different superscripts differ significantly ($p < 0.05$).

		MinDiff			MaxDiff		
		LSmean	Lower C.I.	Upper C.I.	LSmean	Lower C.I.	Upper C.I.
Head	Extended trot	17.3 [b]	12.4	23.1	12.8 [b]	8.2	17.9
	Collected trot	17.5 [b]	12.6	23.3	16.9 [b]	11.9	22.8
	Trot in hand	10.3 [a]	6.7	14.6	5.8 [a]	3.2	9.1
Withers	Extended trot	4.7 [a]	2.7	6.8	7.5 [b]	5.0	10.4
	Collected trot	6.4 [a]	4.4	8.8	8.6 [b]	6.0	11.8
	Trot in hand	5.2 [a]	3.4	7.3	4.9 [a]	3.0	7.2
Pelvis	Extended trot	8.51 [a,b]	5.2	12.7	5.7 [a]	3.3	8.6
	Collected trot	10.5 [b]	6.7	15.0	5.8 [a]	3.5	8.8
	Trot in hand	5.9 [a]	3.3	9.2	5.9 [a]	3.6	8.8

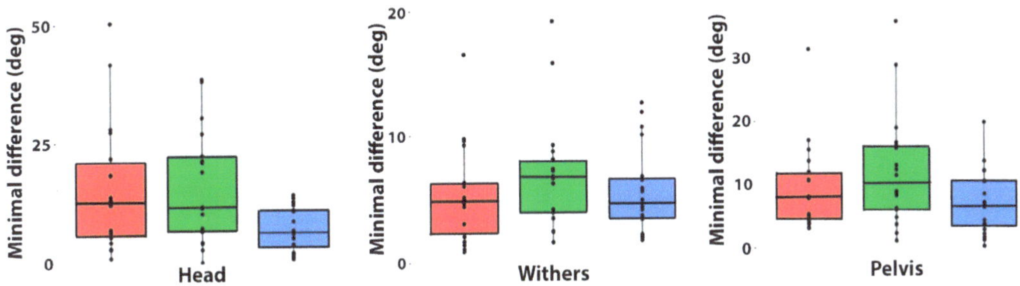

Figure 5. Boxplots showing absolute left–right differences in minimal values for height of the head (**left**), withers (**center**), and pelvis (**right**) for extended trot (orange), collected trot (green), and in-hand trot (blue).

3.4. MaxDiff

MaxDiff values for the head, withers, and pelvis are shown in Table 2 and Figure 6. HMaxDiff and WMaxDiff were higher in both types of ridden trot compared with trot in hand, but there were no differences between extended and collected trot. There were no significant differences in PMaxDiff among trot conditions.

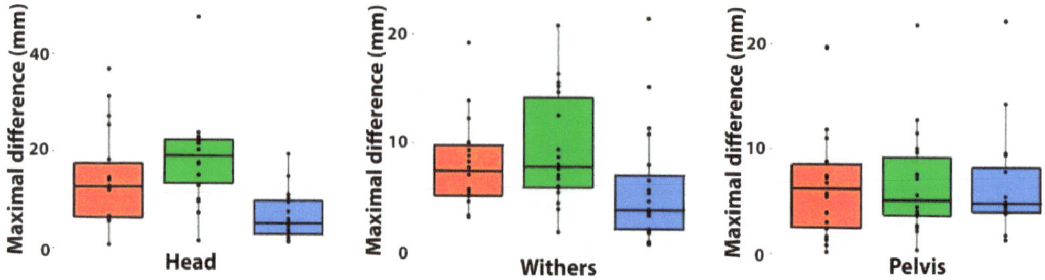

Figure 6. Boxplots showing absolute left–right differences in maximal values for the height of the head (**left**), withers (**center**), and pelvis (**right**) for extended trot (orange), collected trot (green), and in-hand trot (blue).

3.5. Limb Protraction and Retraction

Fore ProMaxDiff for the left and right limbs in late swing (Table 3, Figure 7) did not differ between collected and extended trot, but both ridden conditions had a larger asymmetry in the forelimb protraction angle than trot in hand. Fore RetMaxDiff did not differ among trot conditions. In the hind limbs, ProMaxDiff was higher in extended trot than collected trot or trot in hand, which did not differ from each other. HindRetMaxDiff did not differ among the three trot conditions (Table 3, Figures 8 and 9).

Table 3. LSmean from mixed model analysis with 95% confidence intervals for mean absolute values of ProMaxDiff and RetMaxDiff of the fore- and hind limbs. For forelimbs and hind limbs, LSmean values of ProDiff or RetDiff with different superscripts differ significantly ($p < 0.05$).

		ProMaxDiff (deg)			RetMaxDiff (deg)		
		LSmean	Lower C.I.	Upper C.I.	LSmean	Lower C.I.	Upper C.I.
Fore	Extended trot	2.9 [b]	1.9	4.0	5.0 [a]	2.8	7.9
	Collected trot	2.3 [b]	1.5	3.3	0.7 [a]	3.9	0.81
	Trot in hand	0.7[a]	0.3	1.3	1.7 [a]	0.6	3.4
Hind	Extended trot	2.3 [b]	1.4	3.4	1.7 [a]	1.0	2.5
	Collected trot	2.1 [a]	1.3	3.2	1.5 [a]	0.9	2.3
	Trot in hand	1.5 [a]	0.8	2.4	1.0 [a]	0.5	1.6

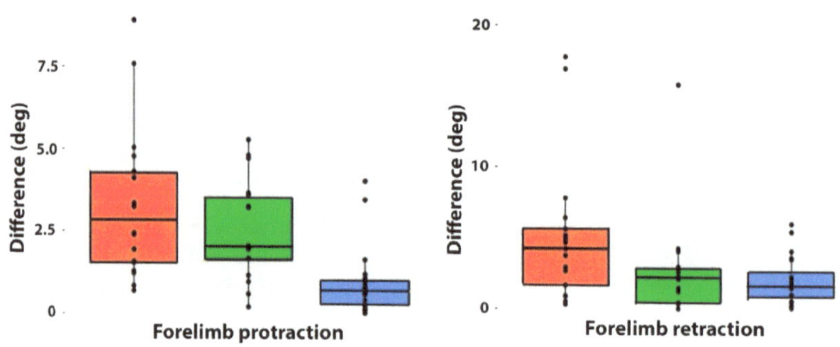

Figure 7. *Cont.*

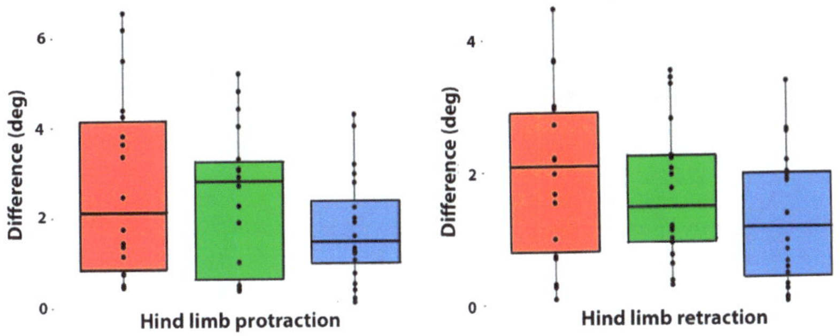

Figure 7. Boxplots showing arithmetic means, inter-quartile ranges, and individual data points for absolute left–right differences in contralateral limb maximal protraction (**left graphs**) and contralateral limb maximal retraction (**right graphs**) in the forelimbs (**top row**) and hind limbs (**bottom row**) for extended trot (orange), collected trot (green), and in-hand trot (blue).

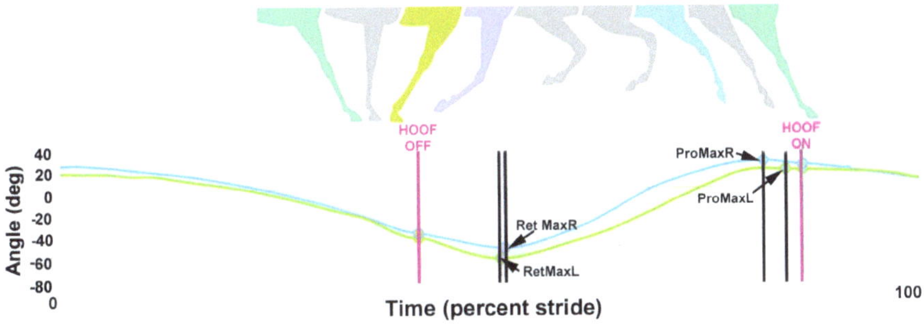

Figure 8. An example from one horse of the magnitude and timing of maximal protraction and retraction in the left (green) and right (blue) forelimbs. Illustration courtesy of Rosalie Bos.

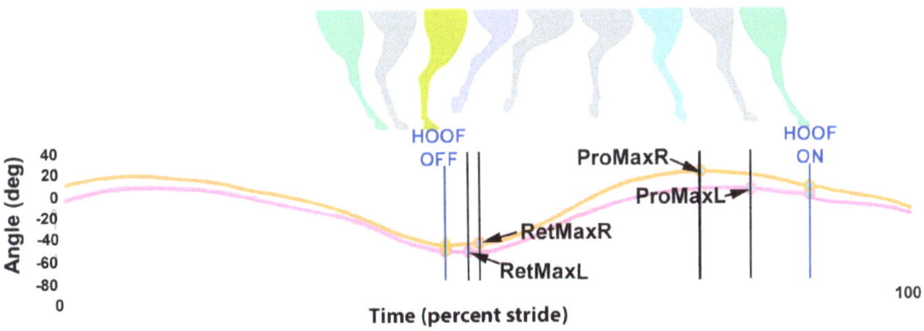

Figure 9. An example from one horse of the magnitude and timing of maximal protraction and retraction in the left (pink) and right (orange) hind limbs. Illustration courtesy of Rosalie Bos.

4. Discussion

This study compared stride variables of actively competing dressage horses trotting in hand on a firm surface and being ridden at collected and extended trot on a soft arena surface. This mimics the situations during the fitness-to-compete evaluation and the dressage test performance, respectively, at CDI competitions. The fit-to-compete examination involves visual evaluation by members of the ground jury in consultation with an FEI official veterinarian. The horse should appear healthy and free from marked gait abnormality or lameness at the trot. Horses that are judged to be lame are excluded from the competition.

Issues influencing the visual examination include the limited temporal and spatial resolution of the human eye [18], the lack of agreement even between experienced lameness clinicians [19], the possibility of expectation bias in which an individual's judgement is influenced by past events, and a perception among competitors that subjectivity may influence the outcome. The possibility of using an objective method to detect gait asymmetries indicative of lameness has been raised.

Asymmetry is a hallmark of lameness but is also a feature of normal gait in people [20] and likely also in animals. Small but consistent asymmetries in the GRFs generated by the left and right legs result in asymmetrical vertical oscillations of the CoM [21]. Small differences between the left and right sides of the body in spatiotemporal variables describing the magnitude or timing of the movements or forces may be regarded as functional rather than pathological asymmetries [8,11]. The human eye may not have sufficient temporal or spatial resolution to detect subtler differences, which is one of the benefits of using IMUs. With regard to lameness detection, the trained human eye has shown better consistency within than between individuals, but IMUs perform better in detecting subtle asymmetries and are more consistent than humans.

Non-pathological gait asymmetries become important when evaluating horses on an individual basis, as in a pre-purchase examination, lameness evaluation, or determination of fitness to compete. Contralateral asymmetries in the vertical trajectory of axial body segments can be detected by IMUs attached to the head, withers, and pelvis. A more difficult problem is knowing whether the asymmetries are simply individual variations of normality or manifestations of pathology. In other words, the challenge lies in defining the limits of normality and determining whether there is overlap between the degree of asymmetry under normal and pathological conditions. Considerable information has been gathered from studies of horses of different ages, breeds, sport disciplines, and levels of training [8,14,15,22–29], confirming that the limits of asymmetry vary among different populations of horses. Therefore, specific limits of asymmetry would need to be established for each sport before objective gait symmetry measurements could be used to determine fitness to compete.

The established method of in-hand fit-to-compete inspections is being challenged in some countries. It has been suggested, for example, that horses could be evaluated while being ridden during competition warm-up. In addition to the challenges inherent in evaluating horses in hand, asymmetry during a ridden evaluation is affected by the rider–horse weight ratio [30], the rider's posture [31], the rider's asymmetry pattern [32], the fit of the saddle [33], whether the rider is posting or sitting in the saddle [13], and the influence of the rider's aids on the horse's performance as presented in the results shown here. Evaluation of the horse in hand avoids the many confounding factors associated with the tack and the rider.

The use of two different surfaces was an integral part of the study design. The footing for the fitness-to-compete evaluation is firmer than the competition footing, which implies higher concussive forces during impact, higher peak loading forces at midstance, and greater rotational shear resistance during breakover [1,34]. On a firm surface, the hoof is decelerated abruptly after contact, which exacerbates discomfort, for example, in horses with bone or joint problems, such as arthritis. During push-off, the toe cannot penetrate a firm surface, resulting in high tensile forces in the distal check ligament and deep digital flexor tendon, which exert pressure on the navicular bone and its bursa. Thus, the fit-to-compete evaluation on a firm surface is likely to exaggerate gait asymmetries associated with lameness and facilitate the detection of mildly lame horses prior to the start of competition. In contrast, the footing in the competition arena is formulated to dampen impact accelerations more gradually and provide appropriate shear resistance to allow for toe penetration while still providing stability during push-off [34]. A softer surface tends to increase stride duration and between-measurement variation [35], but only collected trot showed a longer stride duration in the study reported here. This is consistent with a previous study showing that collected trot has a longer stride duration than extended trot [36], so this is regarded as a gait-related change. The fact that we found no differences in symmetry parameters between hard and soft surfaces agrees with Marunova et al. [37], who reported no difference in head or pelvic symmetry parameters in horses trotting on hard vs. soft surfaces.

Ideally, dressage horses change speed within a gait by increasing stride length while maintaining a consistent stride duration/rate. A visible change in the stride rate is penalized. A previous study in a comparable group of horses ridden in a sand arena had significantly longer stride duration in collected trot (0.78 ms) than extended trot (0.72 ms), which was associated with large reductions in stance duration in both fore- and hind limbs during the extensions [36]. Those values are somewhat shorter than the 0.85 ms and 0.78 ms reported here and may be related to the differences between a sand surface versus a composite surface.

With regard to the rider's influence on the horse's movement, effects can be categorized as gravitational and inertial changes due to the rider's weight and movements vs. trained responses to the rider's aids. When a rider sits passively, peak vertical GRF increases in both the fore- and hind limbs of the horse [38]. The presence of a rider can change the vertical motion symmetry of the horse's head and pelvis, but the effects vary among individual horses [30]. Several studies have evaluated how rider weight, expressed relative to the weight of the horse, affects the horse's movement. When very heavy riders performed rising trot, locomotor asymmetry increased to the extent that the horses appeared temporarily lame [30]. Rising trot, per se, induces locomotor asymmetry, because when the rider pushes against the stirrups during the rising phase, it creates downward momentum, which counteracts hind limb push-off and simulates push-off lameness in the hind limb the rider sits on [13]. In the study reported here, all riders were of an appropriate size and weight for their horses, and they rode in sitting trot throughout. In CDI competitions, all trot work is performed sitting, so assuming the riders' weight distribution is symmetrical, the rider's weight has an equal effect on the two diagonals [14].

Asymmetries in muscular strength are associated with asymmetrical GRF generation on the left and right sides of the body in people with no self-reported injuries or pain. And they result in consistent asymmetry in CoM vertical oscillations [21]. One leg is described as having a propulsive function characterized by generating more hip power at push-off, while the other leg plays a greater role in support associated with power absorption at the knee [20]. If laterality plays a similar role in horses, it may offer an explanation for some non-pathological asymmetries in the movements of the axial body segments.

Head movements are more susceptible to external influences and distractions than those of the withers or pelvis [39]. In sound horses, asymmetries related to distractions are somewhat random and can be removed mathematically by a signal decomposition method [40]. Another factor with the potential to influence head height variables is neck position. Unridden horses choose to walk with the neck almost horizontal, but in trot, the neck is raised, and the head is carried about 20 cm higher than at walk [41]. The elevation of the neck relieves tension from the nuchal ligament and other elastic structures in the dorsal neck, so the head oscillation pattern becomes more dependent on active muscular contractions involving mainly the splenius and cervical trapezius [42]. This effect is amplified in highly trained dressage horses, which adopt an even higher head and neck posture, implying greater reliance on muscular support and the possibility of contralateral, strength-related asymmetries being responsible for the larger HMinDiff and HMaxDiff in ridden horses.

Several studies have applied limits of symmetry based on having one or multiple asymmetry parameters >6 mm for HMinDiff or HMaxDiff or >3 mm for PMinDiff or PMaxDiff, with the SD less than the mean value. Vertical motion exceeding these values has been reported in 83% of Standardbred foals and 45% of Swedish warmblood foals [25]. Asymmetries are even more prevalent in Standardbred yearlings, with 93% exceeding these limits during in-hand trials and 94% during track trials. Interestingly, 20% of horses switched sides between in-hand and track trials. There was no group-level effect between in-hand and track trials, but there was considerable individual variation [25]. The high prevalence of vertical motion asymmetries in such young horses suggests that they are non-pathological. Based on these limits, a large number of experienced performance horses have been classified as asymmetrical. As an example, one or more values fell outside the limits of symmetry in horses trotting in a straight line on hard/soft surfaces, in 67/74% of dressage horses, 67/75% of eventers, and 72/66% of show jumpers [14].

The fact that the horses' axial body segments showed a larger range of vertical motion with a rider supports the first part of the experimental hypothesis that vertical excursions are greater in ridden horses compared with unridden horses. The higher ROMz values for horses ridden at sitting trot imply greater energy expenditure to project the combined bodyweights of horse and rider more vertically, which is contrary to the natural tendency of the neuromotor control system to conserve energy, as shown by the lower values for ROMz when trotting in hand. The sport of dressage rewards competitors for moving with energy and impulsion, which implies the generation of large vertical GRFs to propel the horse's CoM into a higher trajectory during the suspension phases [43]. The larger vertical excursions of the head, withers, and pelvis in ridden horses are interpreted as an effect of the rider's aids encouraging the horse to move with greater impulsion.

The emphasis on having large dorsoventral displacement of the CoM during trotting [44], favors the selection of dressage horses with the ability to project their body into lofty suspensions. Horses with larger overall vertical excursions of the CoM are likely to show larger absolute differences in height between the left and right minima and maxima of the axial body segments than horses with a smaller range of vertical motion. Sport-specific requirements for energy efficiency vs. extravagant movements are reflected in the different threshold levels reported for lameness detection in horses competing in different sports when evaluated by using the same measurement system [23,45]. To compensate for differences in the height of the withers of dressage horses, the evaluation of relative rather than absolute threshold differences is used to normalize for inherent height-related differences in ROMz and its effects on the minima and maxima. This procedure is offered as an option in some gait evaluation systems.

As dressage training progresses, the roles of the fore- and hind limbs become more specialized, with the hind limbs providing more propulsion, while the forelimbs control speed and the direction of movement. Fore- and hind limbs also play different roles in the postural changes associated with developing self-carriage, which is characterized by rotating the body in a nose-up direction around the CoM through a combination of lengthening the forelimbs to raise the withers and shortening the hind limbs to lower the pelvis [46]. As a result of their different mechanical responsibilities, forelimb asymmetries affected primarily MaxDiff, and hind limb asymmetries affected primarily MinDiff. These increases in asymmetries in the minimal and maximal heights of the midline markers in ridden horses support the second part of the experimental hypothesis.

During trotting, the hind hoof typically lifts off slightly earlier than the diagonal forehoof, and the CoM moves ahead of the still-grounded forehoof in terminal stance [47].

This allows the forelimb to exert extra push-off force to elevate the forehand into the suspension phase [46]. The horse's ability to raise the withers is a characteristic of self-carriage, with maximal withers height occurring around the time of forehoof lift-off into the suspension phase [46]. The fact that WMaxDiff was larger for both ridden conditions may reflect differences in neural drive or strength of the extensor musculature between the left and right forelimbs when the rider creates more uphill carriage. This type of asymmetry can simulate forelimb push-off lameness [48].

The pelvis, on the other hand, showed asymmetry in PMinDiff, which was greater in collected trot vs. trot in hand. The role of the hind limbs in collection is to lower the haunches by accepting weight with the joints in a more flexed position. This is controlled by eccentric contractions of the extensor musculature, primarily the gluteals and hamstrings. Of the three conditions evaluated, collected trot would be expected to show the greatest lowering of the haunches and require the greatest eccentric muscular strength. In lame horses, an increase in PMinDiff would be ascribed to a weight-bearing type of lameness, since the lowering of the pelvis is correlated with peak vertical GRF [48]. In dressage horses, asymmetrical neural drive or strength in the gluteal and hamstring muscles could simulate a weight-bearing hind limb lameness. It has been reported that when horses are ridden by a dressage rider [39] or are ridden with greater collection [37], hind limb asymmetry/lameness increases.

Normal human gait has been reported to show clear asymmetries in spatiotemporal variables during swing, including foot position, which are regarded as a normal expression of laterality so long as they do not exceed 8-10% [49]. Asymmetries in plantar-flexor electromyographic activity have also been related to limb dominance, and it is possible that they are similarly related to the effects of laterality in horses. Asymmetries in limb pro- and retraction have been associated with lameness [3,50,51]. For example, in forelimb lameness, the lame limb tends to be less protracted and, in general, to have a more vertical orientation throughout stance, which allows it to support the body in an elevated position. The body is then lowered during the stance phase of the compensating limb, which has higher vertical GRF and rotates through a greater range of angular motion during stance [52].

Dressage riders encourage their horses to perform with greater cadence and expression of the forelimbs, which includes showing greater forelimb protraction in the swing phase. Some horses have a visible difference between the left and right forelimbs in their positions of maximal protraction which would be recognized as higher ForeProDiff for the ridden conditions as reported here. Asymmetrical contributions of the forelimb musculature to limb elevation and protraction may be responsible for the larger asymmetry in horses being ridden to show greater expression compared with those trotting in hand. The hypothesis regarding larger asymmetries in limb pro-/retraction in ridden horses was supported by larger differences in forelimb protraction when horses were ridden at collected and extended trot and for hind limb protraction in extended trot only. The data indicating there were no significant differences among the conditions in the maximal retraction angles of the fore- or hind limbs do not support our hypothesis.

There is considerable variability in assessments of gait symmetry or lameness among owners, veterinarians, and objective measurement systems [11]. Subjective evaluation is inconsistent, even between experts [11,12], and it seems likely that fitness-to-compete assessments may be equally inconsistent. The human eye does not recognize asymmetry until the difference reaches at least 25% [18], whereas IMUs detect subtle differences below the detection threshold of the human eye [7]. The inherent objectivity and accuracy of evaluation using IMUs at the fitness-to-compete evaluation would be fair to competitors and provide an equal playing field if appropriate threshold values that are specific to this population of horses could be established [23,45]. However, it is important that the IMUs are precisely placed over the underlying anatomical landmarks and correctly oriented [53–55], especially when sensors are applied by different individuals.

Markerless tracking has shown results comparable to IMUs for the classification of asymmetries under field conditions [56,57]. Thus, data collection at the fit-to-compete evaluation could be collected with minimal adaptation of the current procedure and without concerns about the precision of marker attachment. However, defining acceptable limits of asymmetry for trot in hand presents the same problems as marker-based evaluations. In both cases, the large variability and presence of numerous outliers is a significant issue when screening individuals.

Limitations to the study include the relatively small number of participants; a much larger pool of mature, experienced competitors would be needed to establish the limits of asymmetry in this population. Horses were evaluated on different surfaces for in-hand and ridden data collection, and data were collected at different venues to mimic competition conditions, so these were not regarded as limitations. All horses were specialized in the same sport and were of similar ages and levels of training, which is required for a single-sport evaluation, but the results should not be generalized to other equine populations.

5. Conclusions

The mechanical effects of the rider's weight interact with trained responses to the rider's aids to change the dressage horse's posture and alter the functional responsibilities of the fore- and hind limbs. The higher ROMz of all axial body segments when horses were being ridden compared with trotting in hand resulted from experienced dressage horses developing greater impulsion in response to the rider's aids. Increases in WMaxDiff, PMinDiff, and Fore ProMaxDiff were ascribed to the riders' influence on impulsion, collection, and forelimb expression, respectively, with the contralateral limbs responding to different degrees, perhaps as a consequence of asymmetrical muscular strength. The differences presented here constitute a step towards establishing normative asymmetry values for a population of trained dressage horses. This is relevant to discussions about the use of objective tests or ridden evaluations to determine whether a horse is fit to compete.

Author Contributions: Conceptualization, F.S.B. and R.B.; methodology, H.M.C., S.J.H., M.R., E.H., M.P., R.B. and F.S.B.; software, F.S.B.; validation F.S.B. and R.B.; formal analysis, H.M.C., S.J.H., M.R., E.H., M.P., R.B. and F.S.B.; investigation, H.M.C., S.J.H., M.R., E.H., M.P., R.B. and F.S.B.; resources, H.M.C.; data curation, H.M.C., S.J.H., M.R., E.H., M.P., R.B. and F.S.B.; writing—original draft preparation, R.B. and H.M.C.; writing—review and editing, S.J.H., M.R., E.H., M.P. and F.S.B.; project administration, S.J.H., M.P. and F.S.B. All authors have read and agreed to the published version of the manuscript.

Funding: This research received no external funding.

Institutional Review Board Statement: This study was conducted in accordance with the Declaration of Helsinki and was approved by the Institutional Review Board of UNIVERSITY OF KENTUCKY (Ethics number 2019-3150) and the Ethics Committee of UNIVERSITY OF CENTAL LANCASHIRE (STEMH 961). Written informed consent was provided by the riders prior to commencing the study. Written informed consent was obtained from the owner of the animals (or an authorized agent for the owner).

Informed Consent Statement: Informed consent was obtained from all subjects involved in the study and from the owner or owner's representative for each of the participating horses and judges.

Data Availability Statement: Data and templates related to this study can be accessed at: https://uclandata.uclan.ac.uk/id/eprint/502 (accessed on 9 January 2025).

Acknowledgments: The authors thank the riders who volunteered their time and expertise for this study.

Conflicts of Interest: The authors declare no conflicts of interest.

References

1. Serra Bragança, F.M.; Rhodin, M.; van Weeren, P.R. On the Brink of Daily Clinical Application of Objective Gait Analysis: What Evidence Do We Have So Far from Studies Using an Induced Lameness Model? *Vet. J.* **2018**, *234*, 11–23. [CrossRef]
2. Serra Bragança, F.M.; Roepstorff, C.; Rhodin, M.; Pfau, T.; van Weeren, P.R.; Roepstorff, L. Quantitative Lameness Assessment in the Horse Based on Upper Body Movement Symmetry: The Effect of Different Filtering Techniques on the Quantification of Motion Symmetry. *Biomed. Signal Process. Control* **2020**, *57*, 101674. [CrossRef]
3. Marshall, J.F.; Lund, D.G.; Voute, L.C. Use of a Wireless, Inertial Sensor-Based System to Objectively Evaluate Flexion Tests in the Horse. *Equine Vet. J.* **2012**, *44*, 8–11. [CrossRef] [PubMed]
4. Weishaupt, M.A.; Wiestner, T.; Hogg, H.P.; Jordan, P.; Auer, J.A. Compensatory Load Redistribution of Horses with Induced Weight-Bearing Forelimb Lameness Trotting on a Treadmill. *Vet. J.* **2006**, *171*, 135–146. [CrossRef]
5. Warner, S.M.; Koch, T.O.; Pfau, T. Inertial Sensors for Assessment of Back Movement in Horses during Locomotion over Ground. *Equine Vet. J.* **2010**, *42*, 417–424. [CrossRef] [PubMed]
6. Pfau, T.; Stubbs, N.C.; Kaiser, L.J.; Brown, L.E.A.; Clayton, H.M. Effect of Trotting Speed and Circle Radius on Movement Symmetry in Horses during Lunging on a Soft Surface. *Am. J. Vet. Res.* **2012**, *73*, 1890–1899. [CrossRef]
7. McCracken, M.J.; Kramer, J.; Keegan, K.G.; Lopes, M.; Wilson, D.A.; Reed, S.K.; LaCarrubba, A.; Rasch, M. Comparison of an Inertial Sensor System of Lameness Quantification with Subjective Lameness Evaluation. *Equine Vet. J.* **2012**, *44*, 652–656. [CrossRef]
8. Rhodin, M.; Egenvall, A.; Andersen, P.H.; Pfau, T. Head and Pelvic Movement Asymmetries at Trot in Riding Horses in Training and Perceived as Free from Lameness by the Owner. *PLoS ONE* **2017**, *12*, e0176253. [CrossRef]
9. Donnell, J.R.; Frisbie, D.D.; King, M.R.; Goodrich, L.R.; Haussler, K.K. Comparison of Subjective Lameness Evaluation, Force Platforms and an Inertial-Sensor System to Identify Mild Lameness in an Equine Osteoarthritis Model. *Vet. J.* **2015**, *206*, 136–142. [CrossRef]
10. Keegan, K.G.; Wilson, D.A.; Kramer, J.; Reed, S.K.; Yonezawa, Y.; Maki, H.; Pai, P.F.; Lopes, M.A.F. Comparison of a Body-Mounted Inertial Sensor System–Based Method with Subjective Evaluation for Detection of Lameness in Horses. *Am. J. Vet. Res.* **2013**, *74*, 17–24. [CrossRef]
11. Müller-Quirin, J.; Dittmann, M.T.; Roepstorff, C.; Arpagaus, S.; Latif, S.N.; Weishaupt, M.A. Riding Soundness—Comparison of Subjective With Objective Lameness Assessments of Owner-Sound Horses at Trot on a Treadmill. *J. Equine Vet. Sci.* **2020**, *95*, 103314. [CrossRef] [PubMed]
12. Hobbs, S.J.; Nauwelaerts, S.; Sinclair, J.; Clayton, H.M.; Back, W. Sagittal Plane Fore Hoof Unevenness Is Associated with Fore and Hindlimb Asymmetrical Force Vectors in the Sagittal and Frontal Planes. *PLoS ONE* **2018**, *13*, e0203134. [CrossRef]
13. Persson-Sjodin, E.; Hernlund, E.; Pfau, T.; Andersen, P.H.; Rhodin, M. Influence of Seating Styles on Head and Pelvic Vertical Movement Symmetry in Horses Ridden at Trot. *PLoS ONE* **2018**, *13*, e0195341. [CrossRef] [PubMed]
14. Zetterberg, E.; Persson-Sjodin, E.; Lundblad, J.; Hernlund, E.; Rhodin, M. Prevalence of Movement Asymmetries in High-Performing Riding Horses Perceived as Free from Lameness and Riders' Perception of Horse Sidedness. *PLoS ONE* **2024**, *19*, e0308061. [CrossRef]
15. Leclercq, A.; Lundblad, J.; Persson-Sjodin, E.; Ask, K.; Zetterberg, E.; Hernlund, E.; Andersen, P.H.; Rhodin, M. Perceived Sidedness and Correlation to Vertical Movement Asymmetries in Young Warmblood Horses. *PLoS ONE* **2023**, *18*, e0288043. [CrossRef]
16. Gmel, A.I.; Haraldsdóttir, E.H.; Serra-Bragança, F.; Lamas, L.P.; Rosa, T.V.; Stefaniuk-Szmukier, M.; Klecel, W.; Neuditschko, M.; Weishaupt, M.A. Inertial Sensor Data of Horses from Four Breeds at Walk and Trot in Hand on a Straight Line. *Data Brief* **2024**, *55*, 110764. [CrossRef]
17. Bragança, F.M.; Bosch, S.; Voskamp, J.P.; Marin-Perianu, M.; Van der Zwaag, B.J.; Vernooij, J.C.M.; van Weeren, P.R.; Back, W. Validation of Distal Limb Mounted Inertial Measurement Unit Sensors for Stride Detection in Warmblood Horses at Walk and Trot. *Equine Vet. J.* **2017**, *49*, 545–551. [CrossRef] [PubMed]
18. Parkes, R.S.V.; Weller, R.; Groth, A.M.; May, S.; Pfau, T. Evidence of the Development of "Domain-Restricted" Expertise in the Recognition of Asymmetric Motion Characteristics of Hindlimb Lameness in the Horse. *Equine Vet. J.* **2009**, *41*, 112–117. [CrossRef]
19. Fuller, C.J.; Bladon, B.M.; Driver, A.J.; Barr, A.R.S. The Intra- and Inter-Assessor Reliability of Measurement of Functional Outcome by Lameness Scoring in Horses. *Vet. J.* **2006**, *171*, 281–286. [CrossRef] [PubMed]
20. Sadeghi, H.; Allard, P.; Duhaime, M. Functional Gait Asymmetry in Able-Bodied Subjects. *Hum. Mov. Sci.* **1997**, *16*, 243–258. [CrossRef]
21. Crowe, A.; Schiereck, P.; de Boer, R.W.; Keessen, W. Characterization of Human Gait by Means of Body Center of Mass Oscillations Derived from Ground Reaction Forces. *IEEE Trans. Biomed. Eng.* **1995**, *42*, 293–303. [CrossRef] [PubMed]

22. Pfau, T.; Scott, W.M.; Sternberg Allen, T. Upper Body Movement Symmetry in Reining Quarter Horses during Trot In-Hand, on the Lunge and during Ridden Exercise. *Animals* **2022**, *12*, 596. [CrossRef] [PubMed]
23. Pfau, T.; Sepulveda Caviedes, M.F.; McCarthy, R.; Cheetham, L.; Forbes, B.; Rhodin, M. Comparison of Visual Lameness Scores to Gait Asymmetry in Racing Thoroughbreds during Trot In-hand. *Equine Vet. Educ.* **2020**, *32*, 191–198. [CrossRef]
24. Scheidegger, M.D.; Gerber, V.; Dolf, G.; Burger, D.; Flammer, S.A.; Ramseyer, A. Quantitative Gait Analysis Before and After a Cross-Country Test in a Population of Elite Eventing Horses. *J. Equine Vet. Sci.* **2022**, *117*, 104077. [CrossRef] [PubMed]
25. Zetterberg, E.; Leclercq, A.; Persson-Sjodin, E.; Lundblad, J.; Andersen, P.H.; Hernlund, E.; Rhodin, M. Prevalence of Vertical Movement Asymmetries at Trot in Standardbred and Swedish Warmblood Foals. *PLoS ONE* **2023**, *18*, e0284105. [CrossRef] [PubMed]
26. Hobbs, S.J.; Serra Braganca, F.M.; Rhodin, M.; Hernlund, E.; Peterson, M.; Clayton, H.M. Evaluating Overall Performance in High-Level Dressage Horse–Rider Combinations by Comparing Measurements from Inertial Sensors with General Impression Scores Awarded by Judges. *Animals* **2023**, *13*, 2496. [CrossRef]
27. Kallerud, A.S.; Fjordbakk, C.T.; Hendrickson, E.H.S.; Persson-Sjodin, E.; Hammarberg, M.; Rhodin, M.; Hernlund, E. Objectively Measured Movement Asymmetry in Yearling Standardbred Trotters. *Equine Vet. J.* **2021**, *53*, 590–599. [CrossRef] [PubMed]
28. Pfau, T.; Noordwijk, K.; Sepulveda Caviedes, M.F.; Persson-Sjodin, E.; Barstow, A.; Forbes, B.; Rhodin, M. Head, Withers and Pelvic Movement Asymmetry and Their Relative Timing in Trot in Racing Thoroughbreds in Training. *Equine Vet. J.* **2018**, *50*, 117–124. [CrossRef] [PubMed]
29. Rhodin, M.; Persson-Sjodin, E.; Egenvall, A.; Serra Bragança, F.M.; Pfau, T.; Roepstorff, L.; Weishaupt, M.A.; Thomsen, M.H.; van Weeren, P.R.; Hernlund, E. Vertical Movement Symmetry of the Withers in Horses with Induced Forelimb and Hindlimb Lameness at Trot. *Equine Vet. J.* **2018**, *50*, 818–824. [CrossRef]
30. Dyson, S.; Ellis, A.D.; Mackechnie-Guire, R.; Douglas, J.; Bondi, A.; Harris, P. The Influence of Rider:Horse Bodyweight Ratio and Rider-horse-saddle Fit on Equine Gait and Behaviour: A Pilot Study. *Equine Vet. Educ.* **2020**, *32*, 527–539. [CrossRef]
31. Engell, M.-T. Postural Strategies in Skilled Riders. Ph.D. Thesis, Swedish University of Agricultural Sciences, Uppsala, Sweden, 2018.
32. Gunst, S.; Dittmann, M.T.; Arpagaus, S.; Roepstorff, C.; Latif, S.N.; Klaassen, B.; Pauli, C.A.; Bauer, C.M.; Weishaupt, M.A. Influence of Functional Rider and Horse Asymmetries on Saddle Force Distribution During Stance and in Sitting Trot. *J. Equine Vet. Sci.* **2019**, *78*, 20–28. [CrossRef] [PubMed]
33. Meschan, E.M.; Peham, C.; Schobesberger, H.; Licka, T.F. The Influence of the Width of the Saddle Tree on the Forces and the Pressure Distribution under the Saddle. *Vet. J.* **2007**, *173*, 578–584. [CrossRef]
34. Hobbs, S.J.; Northrop, A.J.; Mahaffy, C.; Martin, J.H.; Clayton, H.M.; Murray, R.; Roepstorff, L.; Peterson, M. *Equine Surfaces White Paper*; Fédération Equestre Internationale: Geneva, Switzerland, 2014; 51p.
35. Hardeman, A.M.; Serra Bragança, F.M.; Swagemakers, J.H.; van Weeren, P.R.; Roepstorff, L. Variation in Gait Parameters Used for Objective Lameness Assessment in Sound Horses at the Trot on the Straight Line and the Lunge. *Equine Vet. J.* **2019**, *51*, 831–839. [CrossRef]
36. Clayton, H.M. Comparison of the Stride Kinematics of the Collected, Working, Medium and Extended Trot in Horses. *Equine Vet. J.* **1994**, *26*, 230–234. [CrossRef] [PubMed]
37. Marunova, E.; Hernlund, E.; Persson-Sjödin, E. Effect of Circle, Surface Type and Stride Duration on Vertical Head and Pelvis Movement in Riding Horses with Pre-Existing Movement Asymmetries in Trot. *PLoS ONE* **2024**, *19*, e0308996. [CrossRef] [PubMed]
38. Clayton, H.M.; Lanovaz, J.L.; Schamhardt, H.C.; Van Wessum, R. The Effects of a Rider's Mass on Ground Reaction Forces and Fetlock Kinematics at the Trot. *Equine Vet. J.* **1999**, *31*, 218–221. [CrossRef] [PubMed]
39. Licka, T.; Kapaun, M.; Peham, C. Influence of Rider on Lameness in Trotting Horses. *Equine Vet. J.* **2004**, *36*, 734–736. [CrossRef]
40. Keegan, K.G.; Pai, P.F.; Wilson, D.A.; Smith, B.K. Signal Decomposition Method of Evaluating Head Movement to Measure Induced Forelimb Lameness in Horses Trotting on a Treadmill. *Equine Vet. J.* **2001**, *33*, 446–451. [CrossRef]
41. Gellman, K.S.; Bertram, J.E.A. The Equine Nuchal Ligament 1: Structural and Material Properties. *Vet. Comp. Orthop. Traumatol.* **2002**, *15*, 1–6. [CrossRef]
42. Kienapfel, K.; Link, Y.; König, v. Borstel, U. Prevalence of Different Head-Neck Positions in Horses Shown at Dressage Competitions and Their Relation to Conflict Behaviour and Performance Marks. *PLoS ONE* **2014**, *9*, e103140. [CrossRef] [PubMed]
43. Clayton, H.M.; Schamhardt, H.C.; Hobbs, S.J. Ground Reaction Forces of Elite Dressage Horses in Collected Trot and Passage. *Vet. J.* **2017**, *221*, 30–33. [CrossRef]
44. Biau, S.; Barrey, E. Relationships between Stride Characteristics and Scores in Dressage Tests. *Pferdeheilkunde Equine Med.* **2004**, *20*, 140–144. [CrossRef]
45. Macaire, C.; Hanne-Poujade, S.; De Azevedo, E.; Denoix, J.-M.; Coudry, V.; Jacquet, S.; Bertoni, L.; Tallaj, A.; Audigié, F.; Hatrisse, C.; et al. Investigation of Thresholds for Asymmetry Indices to Represent the Visual Assessment of Single Limb Lameness by Expert Veterinarians on Horses Trotting in a Straight Line. *Animals* **2022**, *12*, 3498. [CrossRef] [PubMed]

46. Clayton, H.M.; Hobbs, S.J. An Exploration of Strategies Used by Dressage Horses to Control Moments around the Center of Mass When Performing Passage. *PeerJ* **2017**, *5*, e3866. [CrossRef] [PubMed]
47. Hobbs, S.J.; Clayton, H.M. Sagittal Plane Ground Reaction Forces, Centre of Pressure and Centre of Mass in Trotting Horses. *Vet. J.* **2013**, *198*, e14–e19. [CrossRef]
48. Pfau, T. Sensor-Based Equine Gait Analysis: More than Meets the Eye? *UK-Vet Equine* **2019**, *3*, 102–112. [CrossRef]
49. Wheelwright, E.F.; Minns, R.A.; Law, H.T.; Elton, R.A. Temporal and Spatial Parameters of Gait in Children. I: Normal Control Data. *Dev. Med. Child Neurol.* **1993**, *35*, 102–113. [CrossRef] [PubMed]
50. Munoz, A.; Cuesta, I.; Riber, C.; Gata, J.; Trigo, P.; Castejon, F.M. Trot Asymmetry in Relation to Physical Performance and Metabolism in Equine Endurance Rides. *Equine Vet. J.* **2006**, *38*, 50–54. [CrossRef]
51. Keegan, K.G.; Wilson, D.A.; Smith, B.K.; Wilson, D.J. Changes in Kinematic Variables Observed during Pressure-Induced Forelimb Lameness in Adult Horses Trotting on a Treadmill. *Am. J. Vet. Res.* **2000**, *61*, 612–619. [CrossRef]
52. Buchner, H.H.F.; Savelberg, H.H.C.M.; Schamhardt, H.C.; Barneveld, A. Limb Movement Adaptations in Horses with Experimentally Induced Fore- or Hindlimb Lameness. *Equine Vet. J.* **1996**, *28*, 63–70. [CrossRef]
53. Moorman, V.J.; Frisbie, D.D.; Kawcak, C.E.; McIlwraith, C.W. Effects of Sensor Position on Kinematic Data Obtained with an Inertial Sensor System during Gait Analysis of Trotting Horses. *J. Am. Vet. Med. Assoc.* **2017**, *250*, 548–553. [CrossRef] [PubMed]
54. Gómez Álvarez, C.B. Clinical Insights: Biomechanics and Lameness Diagnosis. *Equine Vet. J.* **2019**, *51*, 5–6. [CrossRef] [PubMed]
55. Serra Bragança, F.M.; Rhodin, M.; Wiestner, T.; Hernlund, E.; Pfau, T.; van Weeren, P.R.; Weishaupt, M.A. Quantification of the Effect of Instrumentation Error in Objective Gait Assessment in the Horse on Hindlimb Symmetry Parameters. *Equine Vet. J.* **2018**, *50*, 370–376. [CrossRef]
56. Pfau, T.; Landsbergen, K.; Davis, B.L.; Kenny, O.; Kernot, N.; Rochard, N.; Porte-Proust, M.; Sparks, H.; Takahashi, Y.; Toth, K.; et al. Comparing Inertial Measurement Units to Markerless Video Analysis for Movement Symmetry in Quarter Horses. *Sensors* **2023**, *23*, 8414. [CrossRef]
57. Kallerud, A.S.; Marques-Smith, P.; Bendiksen, H.K.; Fjordbakk, C.T. Objective Movement Asymmetry in Horses Is Comparable between Markerless Technology and Sensor-based Systems. *Equine Vet. J.* **2024**, *57*, 115–125. [CrossRef] [PubMed]

animals

MDPI

Article

Saddle Thigh Block Design Can Influence Rider and Horse Biomechanics

Rachel Murray [1,*], Mark Fisher [2], Vanessa Fairfax [3] and Russell MacKechnie-Guire [4,5]

1 Rossdales Veterinary Surgeons, Newmarket, Suffolk CB8 7NN, UK
2 Woolcroft Saddlery, Mays Lane, Wisbech PE13 5BU, UK; woolcroft2002@yahoo.co.uk
3 Fairfax Saddles, The Saddlery, Fryers Road, Bloxwich, Walsall, West Midlands WS3 2XJ, UK; vanessa.fairfax@fairfaxsaddles.com
4 Centaur Biomechanics, Dunstaffanage House, Moreton Morrell, Warwickshire CV35 9BD, UK; russell.mackechnie-guire@hartpury.ac.uk
5 Department of Clinical Science and Services, The Royal Veterinary College, Hawkshead Lane, Brookman's Park, Hatfield AL9 7TA, UK
* Correspondence: rachel.murray@rossdales.com

Simple Summary: There is increasing interest in the effect of saddle design on horse kinematics, but little evidence of the influence on rider–saddle interaction and how this affects horse movement patterns. We aimed to investigate the effect of changing the design of the saddle's thigh block on the interaction between the rider and saddle and the effect this has on rider movement and horse movement. To do this, we used a seat pressure mat between the rider and the saddle and tracking technology to analyse horse and rider movement. Elite level sports horses, ridden by elite level riders, were trotted in well-fitting dressage saddles that were identical, except for the thigh block design. During straight-line locomotion when in sitting trot, results showed that a thigh block with a more deformable face (thigh block F) resulted in a greater contact area and more pressure between the rider's seat and the saddle as well as a more upright rider position when the horse's limbs were on the ground. An association between thigh block design, horse spinal movement, and forelimb flexion was also seen. These findings illustrated the importance of optimizing rider–saddle–horse interaction.

Abstract: The association between rider–saddle interaction and horse kinematics has been little studied. It was hypothesized that differences in a thigh block design would influence (a) rider–saddle interface pressures, (b) rider kinematics, and (c) equine limb/spinal kinematics. Eighteen elite sport horses/riders were trotted using correctly fitted dressage saddles with thigh blocks S (vertical face) and F (deformable face). Contact area, mean, and peak pressure between rider and saddle were determined using an on-saddle pressure mat. Spherical markers allowed for the measurement of horse/rider kinematics using two-dimensional video analysis. The kinematics of the equine thoracolumbosacral spine were obtained using skin-mounted inertial measuring units. Results were compared between thigh blocks (paired t-test $p \leq 0.05$). With F, the contact area, mean, and peak pressure between rider and saddle were significantly higher ($p = 0.0001$), and the rider trunk anterior tilt was reduced, indicating altered rider–saddle interaction. The horse thoracic axial rotation and flexion/extension were reduced ($p = 0.01$–0.03), caudal thoracic and lumbar lateral bend was increased ($p = 0.02$–0.04), and carpal flexion increased ($p = 0.01$–0.05) with F compared to S. During straight-line locomotion when in sitting trot, thigh block F was associated with altered rider–saddle interaction and rider and equine kinematics, leading to a more consistent rider–saddle interface, a more upright rider trunk during stance, an increased horse thoracic stability and lumbar lateral bend, and forelimb flexion, supporting the importance of optimising rider–saddle–horse interaction.

Keywords: kinematics; dressage; equine; pressure

1. Introduction

There have been significant advances in the understanding of the effect that saddle fit and design has on equine locomotion [1–7], but there has been less study of the influence of the saddle–rider interaction on rider kinematics and equine locomotion [8]. The saddle provides an interface between the rider and horse, aligning the rider's centre of mass (CoM) with the horse's CoM. A rider's ability to perform a pelvic tilt has been reported to influence horse–rider synchronisation [9], and increased pelvic mobility and control resulted in fewer conflict behaviours [10]. Therefore, it is possible that a saddle design restricting the function of the rider could impact the interaction with the horse and potentially influence the horse to adopt a locomotor pattern to compensate [11].

In trot, there are two flexion/extension cycles per stride, and the horse's diagonal limbs are synchronised, resulting in large vertical and longitudinal accelerations [12]. The rider's axial body segments (pelvis, trunk, head) accommodate the translational and rotational movements of the horse's trunk, which allows the arms and legs to function independently, applying precise aids to the horse [13]. For each stride cycle, during the first half of the diagonal stance phase, the axial segments alter, with the rider's pelvis rotating anteriorly whilst the trunk rotates posteriorly, resulting in lordosis of the rider's lumbar spine. The hip joint is flexed and abducted, and the rider's thigh is flexed and adducted. During the second half of the horse diagonal stance phase, the segmental rotations are reversed [14].

The rider's pelvis is the platform that supports the upper and lower segments and allows for effective weight distribution through the rider's seat, applying subtle cues to the horse. The features of the rider-facing side of the saddle in relation to the rider segments are important considerations, as restrictions of any of the rider segments may compromise the effectiveness of the rider's seat and affect the mobility and ability of the rider to effectively absorb the dynamic forces that occur during locomotion. Whilst the rider may still be able to direct the horse to perform the required tasks, the rider's effectiveness or synchronicity with the horse may be compromised, which could impact the horse's movement; thus, it is important to evaluate the effect that the rider's compensatory strategies may have on the horse [15].

One of the features of the rider-facing side of the saddle is the knee block. Knee blocks are non-deformable, and their function is to support the rider's knee, as the knee is resisted from travelling forwards during locomotion. Over the past decade, knee block size has increased, with the knee block evolving to support the thigh and being referred to as thigh blocks. Various thigh block designs are available in terms of shape, size, height, and position. A rider may influence a thigh block selection, with some riders preferring a larger thigh block, as it will provide additional support whilst riding, whereas others may feel that a larger thigh block is restrictive. Although thigh blocks are a prominent feature on the saddle, little is known about their effect on the rider and, consequently, the horse.

Therefore, it is possible that restriction of rider movement by a thigh block during the stride cycle might alter the rider's movement patterns, the effectiveness of the seat, and their ability to move synchronously with the horse, which, in turn, has the potential to affect equine locomotion. The aim of this study was to investigate the effect that thigh block shape and design has on the kinematics of elite horses and riders during straight line locomotion when performing the sitting trot. It is hypothesised that the contact area and the magnitude of pressures between the rider's seat and saddle, rider trunk and leg kinematics, and horse thoracolumbar and limb kinematics would differ between two different thigh block designs positioned on a standardised saddle: thigh block S (a conventional, vertical-faced solid block) and thigh block F (a block with a multi-layered deformable face).

2. Materials and Methods

Ethics and welfare committee approval was attained from the Royal Veterinary College and the Animal Health Trust committees (URN 2018 1785-2 and 14-2016, respectively). Before the study, riders provided informed consent using a standardized form. Riders and horses could be withdrawn at any stage in the study.

2.1. Horses

Eighteen elite sports horses (12 dressage and 6 event horses; thirteen geldings, four mares, and one stallion) were included in the study. They had a mean (± standard deviation) wither height of 1.65 ± 0.09 m, body mass of 595 ± 27 kg, and were aged 11 ± 1 years. Horses underwent regular therapy and veterinary assessments as part of their management programme and were assessed prior to the study. This assessment included veterinary visual observations when walking and trotting in a straight line and a physiotherapy examination by an Association of Chartered Physiotherapists in Animal Therapy chartered physiotherapist. On the day of data collection, the horses' gait asymmetry was quantified using a validated sensor system [16]. Horses were included in the study if they had no lameness or orthopaedic problems and were deemed fit to perform upon the veterinary and physiotherapy examination.

2.2. Riders

Two male and two female FEI Grand Prix Dressage and one male and one female FEI ranked five-star event riders were recruited with an average (±standard deviation) height 1.78 ± 0.06 m and body mass 71 ± 10 kg. All riders were healthy and uninjured.

2.3. Saddles, Girths and Bridles

Horses were ridden in their usual dressage saddle, girth, and bridle, which were under regular assessment and maintenance. On the day of the study, static and dynamic saddle fit to both rider and horse were assessed independently by five Society of Master Saddlers Qualified Saddle Fitters. The same model of dressage saddle, as described by Murray et al., 2017 [5], was used, with the only variation being the thigh block design. Thigh block S was a moulded block, 260 mm long, featuring a vertical face covered in leather with no additional padding. Thigh block F was 260 mm long; however, the rider-facing aspect of the thigh block was concave and layered with three closed-cell foams of varying densities to form a deformable face. For both the thigh block S and thigh block F conditions, saddle seat size and stirrup leather length remained the same throughout. An anatomically shaped girth not featuring any elastic was used throughout. Girth design and features have been described elsewhere [17]. All horses were ridden in an anatomically shaped snaffle bridle (Sprenger KK Ultra Snaffle Bit) with a fitted crank cavesson noseband located between the facial crest and the corner of the lips and fitted to a two-finger (index and middle finger) tightness measured between the midline of the nasal bone and noseband. All noseband tightness values were measured by the same research assistant.

2.4. Rider Kinetics—Pliance Seat Mat

A force mat was positioned on top of the saddle, quantifying the riders' seat pressures (force per unit area), (sensor size: 10 × 10 mm^2; mat dimensions: 160 mm long and 160 mm wide; sensor arrangement: 256 sensors arranged in 16 columns and 16 rows; pressure range: 2–600 kPa; and sensor resolution: 1 sensor per cm^2) (Sensor Elastisens ES Mat S2129, seat saddle mat, Pliance, Novel gmbh, Munich, Germany) (sampling rate 50 Hz) (Figure 1). To ensure that the force mat did not displace during locomotion, the force mat was positioned within a thin cover. All riders were accustomed to the experimental cover and mat prior to testing. Bluetooth technology was used to capture force mat data. Video footage was simultaneously recorded (50 Hz Panasonic, Osaka, Japan). The mat was centralized and then initialized to zero at the start of the study, between each saddle measurement set and recalibrated during the study based on the manufacturer's guidelines. Using the simultaneous video data (50 Hz) and seat pressure data, the point in the stride at which the peak pressures occurred in each thigh block type was determined. Contact area (cm^2), mean, and peak (kPa) pressure data were obtained for the sensors loaded in the region of the rider's seat bones (tubera ischii).

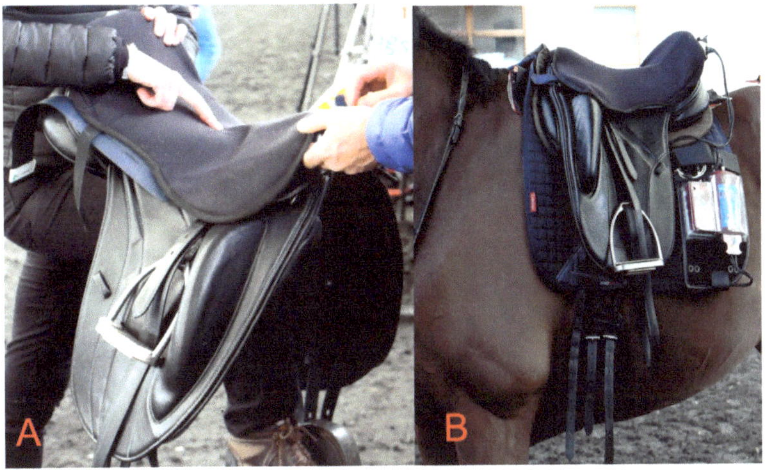

Figure 1. (**A**) Pliance force mat was positioned on top of the saddle beneath a thin cover, which was designed to prevent the force mat from displacing during locomotion. The force mat measured mean and peak pressures (kPa) with simultaneous video, and (**B**) the cables from the force mat were connected to a Pliance data logger, which was secured to the saddle pad.

2.5. Kinematics—Inertial Measurement Units

Seven inertial measurement units (IMU) (aXsens) were used, either attached to each horse's skin/hair surface using hair extension glue (Salon Pro), located over the fifth thoracic vertebra (T5) (withers); T13; and third lumbar vertebra (L3); or in custom-made pouches over the occiput (poll) and on the dorsal midline at the level of the tubera sacrale (TS), attached with double-sided tape. These were used as part of a sensor-based system (Xsens MTw Awinda), which has been validated for translational displacements derived from internal tri-axial sensor accelerations, which were then rotated into a horse-based reference frame based on the sensor orientation estimate and then double integrated into the displacement [16,18]. Data processing methods have been described elsewhere [19,20]. In brief, orientation-time signals for differential axial rotation, flexion-extension, and lateral bending values of T5, T13, L3, and TS were used to calculate differential rotational movement, as described by MacKechnie-Guire and Pfau 2021a, 2021b [2,19].

2.6. Two-Dimensional Motion Capture

Kinematic data were recorded with a high-speed video camera system, using 24 skin markers (30 mm; Quintic Consultancy, West Midlands, UK) placed on each horse using double-sided tape. Marker locations were identified by manual palpation of anatomical landmarks identifying joint centres and segment ends. Once located, white skin paint was used to mark each reference point. Markers were located on (1) dorsal extent of scapular spine, (2) greater tubercle of humerus, (3) lateral epicondyle of humerus, (4) proximal extent of the fourth metacarpal bone, (5) lateral condyle of the third metacarpal bone, (6) tuber coxae, (7) greater trochanter of the femur, (8) lateral epicondyle of the femur, (9) talus, (10) lateral condyle of the third metatarsal bone, and (11) origin of the LCL of the distal interphalangeal joint (Figure 2).

Rider kinematics in relation to the horse were quantified by applying 30 mm spherical markers on anatomical landmarks. Markers were positioned on anatomical landmarks, illustrating marker location for the rider: (1) lateral aspect of the proximal humerus, (2) lateral epicondyle of the distal humerus (3) lateral aspect of the radiocarpal joint, (4) lateral aspect of the greater trochanter of the femur, (5) lateral aspect of the proximal extent of the fibula, (6) lateral aspect of the distal extent of the fibula (Figure 2). Markers were fitted and checked between trials by the same chartered physiotherapist from the Association of Chartered Physiotherapists in Animal Therapy. To limit the effect that clothing had on marker position, riders wore fitted base layers.

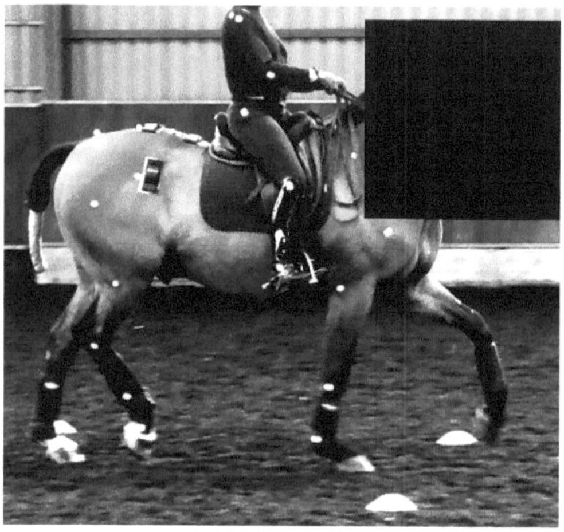

Figure 2. Illustrating marker locations for the horse and rider used for two-dimensional motion capture to compare horse and rider kinematic data between two different thigh block designs.

One high-speed camera (Quintic, Coventry, United Kingdom) was positioned at a 10 m distance from the experimental track, capturing one side of the horse and rider at 300 Hz (spatial resolution: 1300 × 400, 300 fps, at 10 m distance), with a field of view capturing two complete strides in trot. High-speed video data were recorded and downloaded to a laptop (Lenovo, Hong Kong, China) and processed using two-dimensional motion capture (Quintic Biomechanics, Quintic Consultancy, West Midlands, UK). Automatic marker tracking was used to investigate equine limb and rider kinematics.

2.7. Experimental Protocol

Horses were ridden in matching saddles (dressage monoflap saddle, 17 1/2″ seat size), with either thigh block S (a conventional vertical thigh block) or thigh block F (a multi-layered deformable-face thigh block) (Figure 3) in a randomized order (stratified randomization) with identical girth, saddle cloth, and half pad, as described by Murray et al., 2017 [5] Data were collected from half of the studied horses when they were fitted with a saddle, featuring thigh block S first followed by thigh block F second, and the remaining horses were ridden first with a saddle, featuring thigh block F first and second with thigh block S. Each horse underwent a 15 min warm up, including walk, rising/sitting trot, and canter on both left and right reins, as prescribed by the rider. After the warm-up period had been completed, the rider's seat kinetics and body kinematics were quantified along with the kinematics of the thoracolumbar spine and limbs during straight line locomotion in sitting trot.

An experimental area (50 m × 1.5 m) was created using spherical cones to define a straight line in an indoor (20 m × 60 m) arena, with electronic timing gates marking the start and end points, which were used to define speed. Data were collected from the straight-line experimental area, with the horse moving through the arena in clockwise (2 repeats) and anti-clockwise (2 repeats) directions in sitting trot, and the arena dimensions allowed for eleven repeated straight-line strides to be captured.

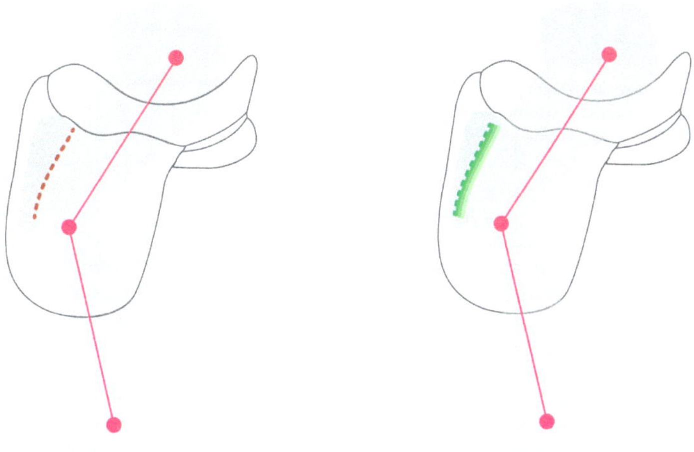

Thigh-Block S **Thigh-Block F**

Figure 3. Illustrating thigh block S, a moulded block 260 mm long featuring a vertical face covered in leather with no additional padding (red dashed lines). Thigh block F was also 260 mm long; however, the rider-facing aspect of the thigh block was concave and layered with three closed-cell foams of varying densities to form a deformable face with the most deformable layer facing the rider (three shaded green lines). Markers located on the lateral aspect of the greater trochanter of the femur, the lateral aspect of the proximal extent of the fibula, and the lateral aspect of the distal extent of the fibula.

2.8. Data Outcomes

For both conditions (thigh block S and thigh block F), kinetic (Pliance) and kinematic (IMU) data were obtained from a total of 22 ± 2 straight-line strides, and kinematic (two-dimensional video analysis) data were obtained from a total of 4 ± 1 strides (from both a clockwise/anticlockwise approach) included in the analysis. For the rider outcome parameters, mean and peak seat pressures (kPa) were quantified for 22 ± 2 straight-line strides, and the rider's trunk angle (Figure 4A), femur angle relative to the vertical (Figure 4C), and knee angle (Figure 4B) were quantified at three stride points (point of contact, midstance, and last point of contact). Outcome parameters for the IMU-derived data were flexion-extension, axial rotation, and lateral bending differential values for T5-T13, T13-L3, and L3-TS. For the two-dimensional video analysis, outcome parameters were maximum shoulder, elbow, carpal, hip, stifle, and tarsal flexion during the swing phase.

2.9. Data Analysis

Descriptive data analysis was performed to investigate the data. A Shapiro–Wilks normality test was used to determine data distribution. Paired Student's *t*-test (for parametric data) or Wilcoxon sign rank test (for nonparametric data) were performed to compare rider contact area and seat pressures, rider kinematics, and equine thoracolumbar and limb kinematics between thigh blocks S and F for each horse. All analyses were performed using statistical analysis software (Analyse-It for Microsoft Excel version 3), with a significance level of $p \leq 0.05$.

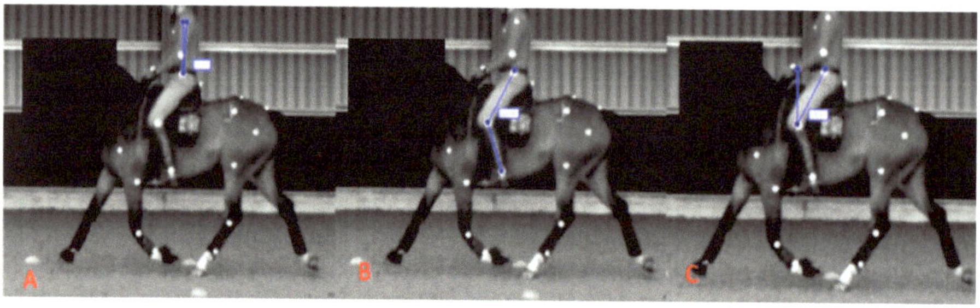

Figure 4. Illustrating the angles measured when quantifying rider kinematics: (**A**) = rider's trunk angle relative to the vertical, (**B**) = rider's knee angle, and (**C**) = rider's femur angle relative to the vertical. Rider kinematics were obtained for each stride point on both the left and right rein.

3. Results

3.1. Horse Inclusion

All horses were deemed fit to perform based on the subjective veterinary and physiotherapy assessments. No horses had hypertonicity or pain in the thoracolumbosacral epaxial musculature. From the objective movement asymmetry measures, the horses had (mean ± SD) asymmetry values (in mm): Head MinDiff 7.3 ± 5.7, Head MaxDiff −4.0 ± 2.5, Pelvis MinDiff, 2.1 ± 2.2, Pelvis MaxDiff 3.1 ± 2.6, and HHD 4.9 ± 4.3.

Rider Seat Pressures (kPa) and Contact Area (cm^2)

The maximum mean and peak pressures occurred during 75–80% of the diagonal stance phase. The differences in the seat pressure magnitude (kPa) and positioning were found between thigh blocks. Thigh block F was associated with greater mean pressures ($p \leq 0.0001$) (thigh block S, 6.2 ± 1.7 kPa; thigh block F, 7.6 ± 2.5 kPa) and peak pressures ($p \leq 0.0001$) (thigh block S, 13.5 ± 3.9 kPa; thigh block F, 15.7 ± 4.4 kPa) than thigh block S (Figure 5).

Thigh block F was associated with significantly greater total contact area between the rider's seat and saddle than thigh block S ($p = 0.0003$) (thigh block S, 401.4 ± 76.5; thigh block F 430.2 ± 65.8), with thigh block F having a 7.2% higher contact area than S. This pattern remained present when the contact area of the cranial and caudal halves of the saddle seat were compared separately with thigh block F, having a 5.5% greater contact area in the cranial half and a 9.1% higher contact area in the caudal half of the saddle (cranial: thigh block S, 211.4 ± 32.1; thigh block F, 223.0 ± 26.0. Caudal: thigh block S, 190.1 ± 53.4; thigh block F, 207.2 ± 47.2).

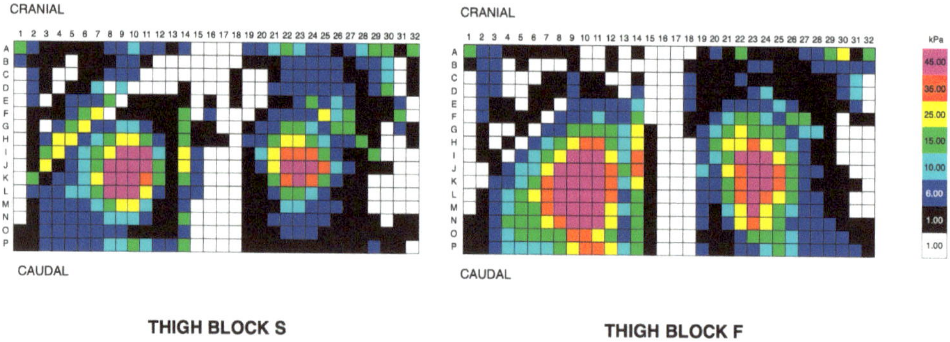

Figure 5. Pressure distribution between rider seat and saddle from one rider (dressage) using thigh block S (**left**) and thigh block F (**right**). Mean and peak pressures were greater and located further caudally with thigh block F than with thigh block S.

3.2. Rider Kinematics

Differences in rider trunk kinematics were found between thigh blocks at mid-stance. During mid-stance, the rider's trunk had less posterior tilt and was more vertical (closer to zero) with thigh block F compared to thigh block S (left rein: thigh block S, 3.4° ± 3.4°; thigh block F, 1.9° ± 2.1°; $p = 0.009$. Right rein: thigh block S, 4.2° ± 4.5°; thigh block F, 2.0° ± 2.9°; $p = 0.003$). No differences were found in the remaining rider-based parameters (All > $p = 0.06$) (Table 1).

Table 1. Rider kinematics parameters (mean ± SD) for the first point of contact, mid-stance, and last point of contact during the trot motion cycle for thigh block S and thigh block F assessed from the left (on the left rein) and right (on the right rein) sides when ridden in a straight line in identical saddles. Significant differences are shown in bold.

	Thigh Block S Left Trot Mean ± S.D	Thigh Block F Left Trot Mean ± S.D	*p* Value	Thigh Block S Right Trot Mean ± S.D	Thigh Block F Right Trot Mean ± S.D	*p* Value
			Rider's trunk angle relative to the vertical			
First Point of Ground Contact (°)	4.9 ± 4.2	4.6 ± 3.6	0.48	6.8 ± 6.4	5.7 ± 4.8	0.24
Mid-stance (°)	**3.4 ± 3.4**	**1.9 ± 2.1**	**0.009**	**4.2 ± 4.5**	**2.0 ± 2.9**	**0.003**
Last Point of Ground Contact (°)	6.1 ± 7.1	5.6 ± 6.6	0.54	5.3 ± 5.3	4.0 ± 3.9	0.06
			Rider's thigh angle relative to the vertical			
First Point of Ground Contact (°)	137.9 ± 4.3	138.4 ± 2.8	0.37	137.6 ± 1.9	136.8 ± 1.4	0.28
Mid-stance (°)	135.9 ± 3.8	135.3 ± 3.3	0.79	135.7 ± 4.1	134.5 ± 2.8	0.45
Last Point of Ground Contact (°)	138.4 ± 2.4	138.1 ± 2.5	0.59	139.6 ± 4.5	139.2 ± 3.3	0.80
			Rider's femur angle relative to the vertical			
First Point of Ground Contact (°)	23.8 ± 2.9	23.8 ± 2.7	0.50	26.9 ± 3.1	26.7 ± 3.7	0.81
Mid-stance (°)	28.4 ± 2.7	27.3 ± 4.7	0.29	27.8 ± 4.5	28.3 ± 4.6	0.64
Last Point of Ground Contact (°)	26.8 ± 3.3	26.6 ± 3.9	0.82	27.6 ± 4.7	28.3 ± 4.9	0.64

3.3. Equine Thoracolumbosacral Spinal Movement

3.3.1. T5-T13

Flexion extension (thigh block S, 9.0° ± 3.6°; thigh block F, 7.3° ± 1.7°; $p = 0.03$) and axial rotation (thigh block S, 18.3° ± 5.8°; thigh block F, 15.6° ± 3.6°; $p = 0.03$) were significantly less for thigh block F than S. No difference in lateral bending values were detected ($p \geq 0.38$).

3.3.2. T13-L3

No differences in flexion/extension were found between thigh blocks ($p \geq 0.20$), but differences were observed in axial rotation and lateral bending. Thigh block F was associated with less axial rotation (thigh block S, 14.6° ± 5.0°; thigh block F 12.4° ± 3.1°; $p = 0.02$) and greater lateral bending (thigh block S 8.6° ± 2.4°; thigh block F 9.4° ± 1.9°; $p = 0.03$) than thigh block S.

3.3.3. L3-TS

No differences between conditions were found in any differential parameters (all $p \geq 0.43$).

3.4. Limb Kinematics (Swing Phase) (°)

Maximum carpal flexion differed between conditions (smaller value = increased flexion). Thigh block F was associated with significantly greater carpal flexion than thigh block S (thigh block S, 91.4° ± 8.2°; thigh block F, 90.3° ± 8.2°; p = 0.05). No differences were found between conditions for the remaining limb kinematic parameters (all $p \geq 0.54$) (Table 2).

Table 2. Limb joint angles (mean ± SD) at peak flexion during the swing phase for horses ridden with thigh block S and thigh block F assessed from the left (on the left rein) and right (on the right rein) sides when ridden in sitting trot. Note: flexion is greater when joint angle is less.

	Thigh Block S			Thigh Block F			
	Trot Left Rein (Mean ± SD)	**Trot Right Rein (Mean ± SD)**	**Trot Pooled (Mean ± SD)**	**Trot Left Rein (Mean ± SD)**	**Trot Right Rein (Mean ± SD)**	**Trot Pooled (Mean ± SD)**	***p* Value (Left vs. Right Pooled)**
Shoulder (°)	131.8 ± 38.0	129.1 ± 32.1	130.4 ± 43.2	112.1 ± 18.8	119.3 ± 7.1	115.5 ± 14.6	0.07
Elbow (°)	100.7 ± 4.7	99.9 ± 5.1	100.3 ± 4.9	100.1 ± 4.7	98.8 ± 5.5	99.5 ± 5.5	0.19
Carpal (°)	89.8 ± 8.2	92.6 ± 8.2	91.4 ± 8.2	89.9 ± 9.0	91.5 ± 7.5	90.3 ± 8.2	**0.05**
Hip (°)	100.1 ± 10.7	99.4 ± 7.5	99.7 ± 9.1	97.6 ± 7.8	98.9 ± 7.7	98.2 ± 7.7	0.06
Stifle Flexion (°)	122.8 ± 27.6	126.9 ± 22.1	124.9 ± 24.7	120.2 ± 17.3	125.2 ± 19.3	122.7 ± 18.3	0.21
Tarsal Flexion (°)	116.2 ± 7.1	118.3 ± 7.3	117.3 ± 7.2	116.5 ± 8.2	117.6 ± 7.5	117.1± 7.8	0.33

4. Discussion

The aim of this study was to investigate the differences in rider kinematics, pressures between the rider's seat and the saddle, and horse thoracolumbosacral and limb kinematics between a dressage saddle with two different thigh block designs: a conventional vertical-faced block (thigh block S) and a multi-layered deformable block (thigh block F) when in sitting trot during straight-line locomotion. In accordance with our experimental hypothesis, different thigh block designs were associated with differences in rider and horse kinematics. Thigh block F was associated with more vertical orientations of the rider's trunk during mid-stance and greater pressures between the rider's seat and the saddle, alongside greater flexion/extension and axial rotation of the horse's cranial thoracic spine, greater axial rotation and less lateral bend in the caudal thoracic–lumbar spine, and an increase in swing phase peak carpal flexion compared to thigh block S.

Thigh blocks on saddles tend to be made from a hand-rasped block of a semi-rigid material (such as closed-cell polyethylene foam) or moulded from polyurethane foams of varying densities. This means thigh block design and shape varies radically in width, height, and length and from one model of saddle to another. How the block interfaces with the rider's thigh in motion can also be influenced by many factors such as the location of the block on the saddle, the location of the stirrup bar, the sweep of the seat, the density of the seat, as well as how the saddle is fitted and balanced on the horse. Therefore, we considered it important to ensure that all these features were identical between saddles, except for the thigh block design. In our study, these variables were controlled, and only the thigh block design was different between conditions. Thigh block S was a conventional moulded design with a vertical face against the rider's thigh, and this was compared with a unique design of a moulded block, which had a concave surface, which allowed a deformable multi-layered foam face to be incorporated against the rider's thigh (thigh block F). By only changing this one feature of the saddle, we were able to assess the effect this change had on the interface between the rider, saddle, and horse in motion.

The timing of the peak pressures beneath the rider's seat occurred during 75–80% of the diagonal stance phase of the horse stride. This part of the stride coincided with large acceleration forces, as the diagonal pair of limbs generated propulsive forces to raise the horse's trunk dorsally and cranially into suspension. During this phase of the stride, it has been reported that the rider's pelvis rotates posteriorly, the rider's trunk rotates anteriorly, and the hip joints extend and are adducted whilst the knee extends and is abducted [14].

The magnitude of mean and peak (kPa) seat pressures were greater, and the seat contact area was greater for thigh block F, which could potentially be related to the relative orientation of the rider's trunk, which had less anterior tilt throughout the horse stance phase in thigh block F. The axial segments work cohesively and are influenced by the pelvis.

Therefore, if the rider's trunk is more vertical as a function of the thigh block design, it seems reasonable to expect that the remaining segments may be altered. The findings presented here, concerning the rider-facing saddle features influencing rider kinematics, are supported by a study where saddle flaps were removed. In that study, when walking, trotting, and cantering, the rider's centre of pressure (CoP) was reduced in a medio-lateral direction and in an anteroposterior direction when performing a collected trot, extended trot, and extended canter with a flapless saddle. It was suggested that the rider's femoral segments being positioned in a more adducted position relative to the horse could provide increased stability to the rider [8]. This change in rider CoP did not alter horse stride length, however, and more detailed locomotor parameters were not reported.

We found that the flexion-extension and axial rotation values of the cranial thoracic spine (T5-T13) were decreased whilst lateral bending values were increased in the mid-thoracic and cranial lumbar spine (T13-L3) compared with thigh block S when riding in a dressage saddle with the multi-layered thigh block (thigh block F). This suggested that alterations in the rider–saddle interface could be having an impact on the horse, potentially altering the stability of the equine cranial thoracic spine. This concept was supported by a previous over-ground study quantifying back movement in horses trotting (unloaded) compared with a rider (loaded), where it was reported that axial rotation and lateral bending rotational values of the cranial thoracic (T5-T13) spine decreased whilst the kinematics of the caudal thoracic and lumber spine (T18-L3) were increased when ridden (loaded) [19,20]. It was proposed by the authors that this decrease in movement amplitude in the cranial thoracic spine may have been indicative of an attempted "stability" mechanism, in order to withstand the dynamic forces of the rider [21] (and saddle) and more efficiently transmit dynamic forces from the forelimb (and head and neck) to the cranial region of the thoracic spine. Applying this stability concept to the current study suggested that altered rider kinematics could have been having an effect on the equine locomotor apparatus, the stability of the cranial thoracic region in particular.

During the stance phase, the range of motion of the rider's trunk was more vertical when riding in thigh block F. It was proposed that the rider was able to maintain a more stable trunk position during the stance phase with thigh block F, and, as a result, this may have exerted a stabilizing effect on the horse's cranial thoracic region. In contrast, if the rider's trunk had increased its anterior–posterior trunk rotation, it was hypothesized that this could have induced instability in the horse, which could have explained the increased rotational movement of the cranial thoracic spine, as seen with thigh block S. More work is needed to confirm this concept, but this study did provide further evidence for the importance of considering the effect that the upper-side's saddle features could have on the rider–saddle interface and rider–horse interaction. It should be noted that a relatively high SD was found for the rider trunk data. This variation may have been indicative of individual rider conformation or trunk biomechanical strategies when riding. It is possible that these findings would be less applicable in less skilled riders who have less musculoskeletal strength and coordination, as suggested by findings in a previous study, where riders with less pelvic control were less synchronized with the horse [9]. In our study, we found effects of altering thigh block design on the horse and rider; thus, it is possible that altering other aspects of saddle design and, therefore, the rider–saddle interface, could also impact the rider biomechanics and potentially those of the horse. Further investigation of other features with less skilled horses/riders would be of interest.

This study did have limitations. Unfortunately, due to technical issues, data relating to the rider's pelvic kinematics were omitted from the analysis. If the study were to be repeated, quantifying rider pelvic kinematics would be useful. Some of the differences being reported here were small and, although statistically significant, may have resulted from biological variation; therefore, caution should be applied when interpreting the findings being presented. However, the only modification to the dressage saddle was the thigh block face with the deformable layers, with all the remaining upper and underside saddle features (the sweep of the seat, saddle tree, seat design/size, fit) remaining the same between thigh blocks; thus, we considered it reasonable that only small differences would be found.

We quantified the horses' back movements with the use of skin mounted IMU's, and it is appreciated that these did not directly correlate to the centre of rotation of the vertebral body, as seen in more invasive approaches [22,23], which would have had significant ethical issues. The use of IMUs to quantify back movement has been validated [18,24] for quantifying back movement during in-hand locomotion. However, it is acknowledged that no studies have validated the use of IMUs during ridden conditions. Whilst the IMUs did not contact the saddle at any point during motion and were not removed when quantifying the two experimental conditions, adding the saddle and girth may have affected the displacement of the skin and, consequently, the sensor–skin interaction. An over-ground study using IMUs positioned along the midline of the back to quantify differences in rotational movement of the back compared trotting in-hand with no saddle to horses fitted with a saddle and girth. It was reported that axial rotation in the cranial thoracic region (T5) was reduced, whereas lateral bending was increased in the mid-thoracic and lumbar regions (T13-T18 and T18-L3), the findings of which suggested that the saddle and girth could alter axial rotational values (or reduce the magnitude of skin displacement) in the cranial thoracic region [25]. Using an IMU-based approach [19,20,26,27] to compare back kinematics of horses trotting in hand and when ridden in sitting trot, similar to the aforementioned study, the axial rotation and lateral bending were reduced in the cranial thoracic region (T5-T13). However, unlike the previous in-hand study [25], axial rotation was increased in the mid-caudal segments, which may have been due to the dynamic effect of the rider. Whilst the IMUs provided a non-invasive approach to quantifying back movement, the limitations should be considered when interpreting the data presented here.

To reduce rider variables [11], only elite riders were studied, and the horses were ridden in a frame that was consistent for the level of work (with the dorsal aspect of the horse's head close to vertical); it is appreciated that the results may not be transferable to less-skilled riders and horses. Defining the horse's frame may have influenced the segmental strategy used by the riders and, consequently, the seat pressures. We chose to quantify the effect that the thigh block face had on the rider and locomotor parameters with the rider remaining seated throughout the trot cycle, which would have influenced the rider's posture. It is appreciated that different riding positions could have an effect on equine locomotion [28] and that the different riding positions may be influenced by the thigh block design. Therefore, the findings being presented here cannot be applied for all riding positions. This study quantified the immediate effects that a thigh block had on elite riders riding advanced dressage and event horses when in sitting trot during straight line locomotion. Therefore, a longitudinal study would be advantageous to determine if the differences being reported here were sustained or altered. Finally, this study only quantified horse and rider kinematics when trotting; future studies should quantify the effect that a saddle thigh block has on the rider–saddle–horse interaction when in walk and canter [29], when riding in different riding positions [28], and when used by less skilled or symmetrical riders [15].

5. Conclusions

Changing thigh block design in a dressage saddle with skilled riders was associated with altered rider kinematics, rider–saddle interactions, and equine kinematics in sitting trots in a straight line. An altered rider–saddle interface in a less restrictive thigh block was associated with greater horse thoracic stability and increased carpal flexion, supporting the importance of optimising the rider–saddle–horse interface.

Author Contributions: Conceptualization, R.M., V.F., R.M.-G. and M.F.; Methodology R.M., R.M.-G. and M.F. Formal Analysis, R.M. and R.M.-G.; Investigation, R.M.-G. and M.F.; Data Curation, R.M. and R.M.-G.; Writing—Original Draft Preparation, R.M. and R.M.-G. Writing—Review and Editing, R.M. and R.M.-G.; Visualization, R.M., V.F. and R.M.-G.; Project Administration R.M. and R.M.-G. All authors have read and agreed to the published version of the manuscript.

Funding: Data collection was funded by Fairfax Saddles. VF is a director of Fairfax saddles. VF was not involved in data collection, management, processing, or statistical analysis.

Institutional Review Board Statement: This study was approved by the Royal Veterinary College ethics and welfare committee, project number URN 2018 1785-2, and The Animal Health Trust ethics committee, project number AHT URN 14-2016.

Informed Consent Statement: Informed, written consent was obtained prior to participation in the study. At the time of the study, all riders were free from any injuries and could withdraw their participation and that of their horses from the study at any point.

Data Availability Statement: Data are restricted for confidentiality reasons, due to the calibre of horses assessed.

Acknowledgments: The authors thank the riders, owners, and research assistants for their help with data collection.

Conflicts of Interest: Vanessa Fairfax is employed by Fairfax Saddles. VF was not involved in data management, processing, or statistical analysis. None of the remaining authors of this paper have a financial or personal relationship with other people or organizations that could inappropriately influence or bias the content of the paper.

References

1. Heim, C.; Pfau, T.; Gerber, V.; Schweizer, C.; Doherr, M.; Schupbach-Regula, G.; White, S. Determination of vertebral range of motion using inertial measurement units in 27 Franches-Montagnes stallions and comparison between conditions and with a mixed population. *Equine Vet. J.* **2015**, *48*, 509–516. [CrossRef]
2. Mackechnie-Guire, R.; Mackechnie-Guire, E.; Fisher, M.; Mathie, H.; Bush, R.; Pfau, T.; Weller, R. Relationship between saddle and rider kinematics, horse locomotion and thoracolumbar pressures in sound horses. *J. Equine Vet. Sci.* **2018**, *69*, 52. [CrossRef]
3. MacKechnie-Guire, R.; MacKechnie-Guire, E.; Fairfax, V.; Fisher, D.; Fisher, M.; Pfau, T. The Effect of Tree Width on Thoracolumbar and Limb Kinematics, Saddle Pressure Distribution, and Thoracolumbar Dimensions in Sports Horses in Trot and Canter. *Animals* **2019**, *9*, 842. [CrossRef]
4. Martin, P.; Cheze, L.; Pourcelot, P.; Desquilbet, L.; Duray, L.; Chateau, H. Effects of Large Saddle Panels on the Biomechanics of the Equine Back During Rising Trot: Preliminary Results. *J. Equine Vet. Sci.* **2017**, *48*, 15–22. [CrossRef]
5. Murray, R.; Guire, R.; Fisher, M.; Fairfax, V. Reducing Peak Pressures Under the Saddle Panel at the Level of the 10th to 13th Thoracic Vertebrae May Be Associated With Improved Gait Features, Even When Saddles Are Fitted to Published Guidelines. *J. Equine Vet. Sci.* **2017**, *54*, 60–69. [CrossRef]
6. Murray, R.; Mackechnie-Guire, R.; Fisher, M.; Fairfax, V. Reducing peak pressures under the saddle at thoracic vertebrae 10-13 is associated with alteration in jump kinematics. *Comp. Exerc. Physiol.* **2018**, *14*, 239–247. [CrossRef]
7. Murray, R.; Mackechnie-Guire, R.; Fisher, M.; Fairfax, V. Could Pressure Distribution Under Race-Exercise Saddles Affect Limb Kinematics and Lumbosacral Flexion in the Galloping Racehorse? *J. Equine Vet. Sci.* **2019**, *81*, 10–27. [CrossRef]
8. Clayton, H.M.; Hampson, A.; Fraser, P.; White, A.; Egenvall, A. Comparison of rider stability in a flapless saddle versus a conventional saddle. *PLoS ONE* **2018**, *13*, e0196960. [CrossRef]
9. Walker, V.A.; Pettit, I.; Tranquille, C.A.; Spear, J.; Dyson, S.J.; Murray, R.C. Relationship between pelvic tilt control, horse-rider synchronisation, and rider position in sitting trot. *Comp. Exerc. Physiol.* **2020**, *16*, 423–432. [CrossRef]
10. Uldahl, M.; Christensen, J.W.; Clayton, H.M. Relationships between the Rider's Pelvic Mobility and Balance on a Gymnastic Ball with Equestrian Skills and Effects on Horse Welfare. *Animals* **2021**, *11*, 453. [CrossRef]
11. Peham, C.; Licka, T.; Schobesberger, H.; Meschan, E. Influence of the rider on the variability of the equine gait. *Hum. Mov. Sci.* **2004**, *23*, 663–671. [CrossRef]
12. Hobbs, S.J.; Clayton, H.M. Sagittal plane ground reaction forces, centre of pressure and centre of mass in trotting horses. *Vet. J.* **2013**, *198*, e14–e19. [CrossRef]
13. Hobbs, S.J.; St George, L.; Reed, J.; Stockley, R.; Thetford, C.; Sinclair, J.; Williams, J.; Nankervis, K.; Clayton, H.M. A scoping review of determinants of performance in dressage. *PeerJ* **2020**, *8*, e9022. [CrossRef]
14. Byström, A.; Rhodin, M.; Peinen, K.; Weishaupt, M.A.; Roepstorff, L. Basic kinematics of the saddle and rider in high-level dressage horses trotting on a treadmill. *Equine Vet. J.* **2009**, *41*, 280–284. [CrossRef]
15. MacKechnie-Guire, R.; MacKechnie-Guire, E.; Fairfax, V.; Fisher, M.; Hargreaves, S.; Pfau, T. The Effect That Induced Rider Asymmetry Has on Equine Locomotion and the Range of Motion of the Thoracolumbar Spine When Ridden in Rising Trot. *J. Equine Vet. Sci.* **2020**, *88*, 102946. [CrossRef]
16. Pfau, T.; Witte, T.H.; Wilson, A.M. A method for deriving displacement data during cyclical movement using an inertial sensor. *J. Exp. Biol.* **2005**, *208 Pt 13*, 2503–2514. [CrossRef]

17. Murray, R.; Guire, R.; Fisher, M.; Fairfax, V. Girth pressure measurements reveal high peak pressures that can be avoided using an alternative girth design that also results in increased limb protraction and flexion in the swing phase. *Vet. J.* **2013**, *198*, 92–97. [CrossRef]
18. Warner, S.M.; Koch, T.O.; Pfau, T. Inertial sensors for assessment of back movement in horses during locomotion over ground. *Equine Vet. J. Suppl.* **2010**, *42*, 417–424. [CrossRef]
19. MacKechnie-Guire, R.; Pfau, T. Differential Rotational Movement of the Thoracolumbosacral Spine in High-Level Dressage Horses Ridden in a Straight Line, in Sitting Trot and Seated Canter Compared to In-Hand Trot. *Animals* **2021**, *11*, 888. [CrossRef]
20. MacKechnie-Guire, R.; Pfau, T. Differential rotational movement and symmetry values of the thoracolumbosacral region in high-level dressage horses when trotting. *PLoS ONE* **2021**, *16*, e0251144. [CrossRef]
21. Clayton, H.; Lanovaz, J.; Schamhardt, H.; Wessum, R. The effects of a rider's mass on ground reaction forces and fetlock kinematics at the trot. *Equine Vet. J.* **1999**, *30*, 218–221. [CrossRef] [PubMed]
22. Faber, M.; Johnston, C.; Schamhardt, H.; van Weeren, R.; Roepstorff, L.; and Barneveld, A. Basic three-dimensional kinematics of the vertebral column of horses during trotting on a treadmill. *Am. J. Vet. Res.* **2001**, *62*, 757–764. [CrossRef] [PubMed]
23. Faber, M.; Johnston, C.; Schamhardv, H.; Van Weeren, P.; Roepstorff, L.; Barneveld, A. Three-dimensional kinematics of the equine spine during canter. *Equine Vet. J. Suppl.* **2001**, *33*, 145–149. [CrossRef]
24. Martin, P.; Chateau, H.; Pourcelot, P.; Duray, L.; Cheze, L. Comparison Between Inertial Sensors and Motion Capture System to Quantify Flexion-Extension Motion in the Back of a Horse. *Equine Vet. J. Suppl.* **2014**, *46*, 43. [CrossRef]
25. Deckers, I.; MacKechnie-Guire, R.; Fisher, M.; Fisher, D.; Nankervis, K. The effect of a saddle on the kinematics of the thoracolumbosacral spine at walk and trot in-hand in 11th International Conference on Equine Exercise Physiology, Uppsala, Sweden 2022. *Comp. Exerc. Physiol.* **2022**, *18* (Suppl. S1), S1–S121.
26. MacKechnie-Guire, R.; Fairfax, V.; Pfau, T. Movement symmetry values of the thoracolumbosacral region in high-level jumping horses, when trotted in-hand and ridden in a straight line with three different riding positions. *Equine Vet. J.* **2021**, *53*, 12–13.
27. MacKechnie-Guire, R.; Fairfax, V.; Pfau, T. Differential rotational movement of the thoracolumbosacral region in high-level jumping horses, when trotted in-hand and ridden in a straight line with three different riding positions. *Equine Vet. J.* **2021**, *53*, 9–10.
28. Persson-Sjodin, E.; Hernlund, E.; Pfau, T.; Haubro Andersen, P.; Rhodin, M. Influence of seating styles on head and pelvic vertical movement symmetry in horses ridden at trot. *PLoS ONE* **2018**, *13*, e0195341. [CrossRef]
29. Symes, D.; Ellis, R. A preliminary study into rider asymmetry within equitation. *Vet. J.* **2009**, *181*, 34–37. [CrossRef]

animals

MDPI

Article

Effects of Jumping Phase, Leading Limb, and Arena Surface Type on Forelimb Hoof Movement

Christina M. Rohlf [1,2,*], Tanya C. Garcia [1], Lyndsey J. Marsh [3], Elizabeth V. Acutt [4], Sarah S. le Jeune [1] and Susan M. Stover [1,2,3]

1 Department of Surgical and Radiological Sciences, University of California-Davis, Davis, CA 95616, USA; tcgarcia@ucdavis.edu (T.C.G.); sslejeune@ucdavis.edu (S.S.l.J.); smstover@ucdavis.edu (S.M.S.)

2 Biomedical Engineering Graduate Group, University of California-Davis, Davis, CA 95616, USA

3 Animal Biology Graduate Group, University of California-Davis, Davis, CA 95616, USA; ljmarsh@ucdavis.edu

4 Clinical Large Animal Diagnostic Imaging, University of Pennsylvania, Philadelphia, PA 19104, USA; evacutt@upenn.edu

* Correspondence: cmrohlf@ucdavis.edu; Tel.: +1-636-284-1015

Simple Summary: The mechanical behavior of arena surfaces has been identified as a contributor to injuries of performance horses. Evidence of excessive fetlock extension in association with stiff surfaces has propelled the installation of synthetic surfaces in performance horse arenas to reduce injury risk. However, the effect of arena surface properties on hoof slide during show jumping has not been widely studied. Therefore, this study measured the forelimb hoof motion of horses during takeoff and landing from a 1.1 m jump using a high-speed video motion capture system on five dirt and seven synthetic surfaces. Hoof slide was not significantly different between dirt and synthetic surfaces, but it was greater at takeoff than at landing and greater for the leading limb than for the trailing limb. These results indicate that horses are able to compensate for the effect of surface differences on hoof slide at a moderate jump height.

Abstract: During the stance phase of equine locomotion, ground reaction forces are exerted on the hoof, leading first to rapid deceleration ("braking") and later to acceleration ("propulsion") as the hoof leaves the ground. Excessive hoof deceleration has been identified as a risk factor for musculoskeletal injury and may be influenced by arena surface properties. Therefore, our objective was to evaluate the effect of arena surface type (dirt, synthetic) on hoof translation of the leading and trailing forelimbs during jump takeoff and landing. Solar hoof angle, displacement, velocity, and deceleration were captured using kinematic markers and high-speed video for four horses jumping over a 1.1 m oxer at 12 different arenas (5 dirt, 7 synthetic). Surface vertical impact and horizontal shear properties were measured simultaneously. The effects of surface type (dirt, synthetic), jump phase (takeoff, landing), and limb (leading, trailing) on hoof movement were assessed using ANOVA ($p < 0.05$), while the relationships of hoof movement with surface mechanical properties were examined with correlation. Slide time ($p = 0.032$), horizontal velocity of the hoof ($p < 0.001$), and deceleration ($p < 0.001$) were greater in the leading limb, suggesting a higher risk of injury to the leading limb when braking. However, surface type and jump phase did not significantly affect deceleration during braking.

Keywords: equine; show jumping; hoof slide; motion capture; arena surface; leading limb

1. Introduction

The mechanical properties of equine arena surfaces have been proposed as extrinsic risk factors for musculoskeletal injury [1]. During the stance phase of equine locomotion, ground reaction forces are exerted on the hoof, leading to first rapid deceleration ("braking") and later acceleration ("propulsion") as the hoof leaves the ground [2]. When the hoof contacts the ground, deceleration occurs first in the vertical direction [3], followed by hoof slide as the center of mass of the horse moves over the planted leg, pushing that leg forward [4]. Researchers have speculated that a shorter slide duration and greater horizontal hoof deceleration may increase musculoskeletal injury risk by imposing a large bending moment on the third metacarpal bone [5]. Shorter periods of horizontal hoof braking were also associated with greater longitudinal deceleration and high-frequency oscillations of the third metacarpal bone, which may increase the risk of damage to subchondral bone and cartilage [6]. The distance and duration of hoof slide is expected to be influenced by the surface and speed of the horse [1]. In one study, hoof deceleration was greater during trot on a sandpaper surface compared to a sand surface [7], suggesting that arena surface properties may have a significant effect on hoof deceleration.

The support, or midstance, phase follows the impact and slide phases and is characterized by relatively little hoof movement and peak vertical loads. If hoof displacement during support is large, the horse may be required to apply more muscular force to maintain speed, making the horse more susceptible to fatigue [8]. Finally, the grab, or rollover, phase occurs when the hoof rotates into the surface and lifts from the ground. The hoof is able to rotate further into surfaces with lower shear strength during grab, which may reduce strain in flexor tendons and prevent slippage [9].

Desired surface characteristics of arena surfaces, as reported by riders, significantly differ by discipline [10]. Show jumping is characterized by higher ground reaction forces [11] and higher velocities at both approach and landing than other disciplines [12,13], suggesting that a jumping surface must support higher strain rates and higher vertical and shear loads [1]. Therefore, to understand the relationship of arena surface properties and musculoskeletal injury risk of equine athletes, it is important to study hoof movement on competition surfaces during sport-specific equine locomotion.

Hoof movement during locomotion has been previously recorded with accelerometers [7,14–16] and high-speed motion capture [17,18]. The effect of limb (leading, trailing) on hoof movement during jumping has been previously reported, where the leading limb at landing exhibited a lower hoof angle, higher horizontal hoof velocity, and greater deceleration [18]. However, Hernlund et al. did not evaluate the effect of surface type or surface properties on hoof motion during jumping.

The effect of surface type on hoof movement during a gallop has been previously characterized for the hindlimb, where dirt surfaces exhibited significantly higher horizontal motion of the heel during slide than synthetic surfaces [17]. Additionally, a higher horizontal and vertical displacement of the forelimb hoof was observed on an all-waxed sand track compared to a turf track at cantering speeds [16]. By understanding the relationship between surface type, surface composition, or surface management and hoof movement, it may be possible to modify arena surfaces to optimize hoof decelerations and improve the safety of all horses that train and compete on the surface.

Therefore, our first objective was to characterize the angle, displacement, velocity, and deceleration of the forelimb hoof during jumping to evaluate the effect of limb (leading, trailing), jump phase (takeoff, landing), and surface type (dirt, synthetic). We hypothesized that horizontal hoof deceleration would be greater for the leading limb, in line with a previous study [18]. Furthermore, surfaces with greater shear forces were expected to have greater hoof deceleration; however, since shear forces were not significantly different between dirt and synthetic surface types [19] when considering a large variety of surfaces, hoof deceleration was also not expected to be different between surface types.

Our second objective was to identify relationships between hoof movement parameters and measured properties of the arena surface (compositional, manageable, shear, and vertical impact). We hypothesized that hoof horizontal motion would be negatively correlated with shear properties (i.e., adhesion, coefficient of friction, and shear force) and vertical hoof motion would be positively correlated with the vertical displacement of the surface tester and negatively correlated with other vertical impact properties such as surface stiffness and vertical deceleration at impact.

2. Materials and Methods

2.1. Study Design

A repeated measures study design was used to track solar hoof angle, position (horizontal and vertical displacements), velocity, and acceleration for four horses (one mare, three geldings; age 9.8 ± 2.1 years; weight 544 ± 66 kg) jumping three times over a 1.1 m oxer at twelve arenas in northern California (five dirt, seven synthetic). The weight of the rider and tack used for all horses was 84 kg. Horses were visually observed for orthopedic pain and discomfort by a licensed veterinarian at the beginning of each testing day (SS). No horses showed signs of lameness during the testing period. However, one horse (gelding) was unavailable for the first testing day (dirt surface) and thus only jumped on eleven of the twelve arena surfaces. These data were collected under an IACUC protocol issued by the University of California Davis (Protocol 19843-Effect of Jumping Arena Surfaces on Equine Forelimb Biomechanics; approved 3 April 2017).

Synthetic surfaces had greater than 1% fiber content by volume; none contained rubber, oil, or wax. Fibers were primarily polyester; however, polyethylene, polypropylene, and nylon fibers were also observed in some synthetic surfaces. One dirt surface had 0.6% fiber with large felt strips poorly integrated in the cushion layer. All other dirt surfaces contained 0% fiber content.

The oxer was preceded by a ground pole and two cross rails (0.56 m from ground to center) to center and standardize the approach of the horse to the measured jump (Figure 1). Horses were accustomed to the equipment by performing 3 trot trials through the jump grid without the jump poles, followed by practice jump trials which systematically added the jump elements preceding the oxer and increased the height of the oxer. Subsequently, data were collected for 3 jump trials with the complete jump grid and final oxer height (1.1 m). The takeoff and landing zones of the oxer for each surface were harrowed using a rake between each recorded jump.

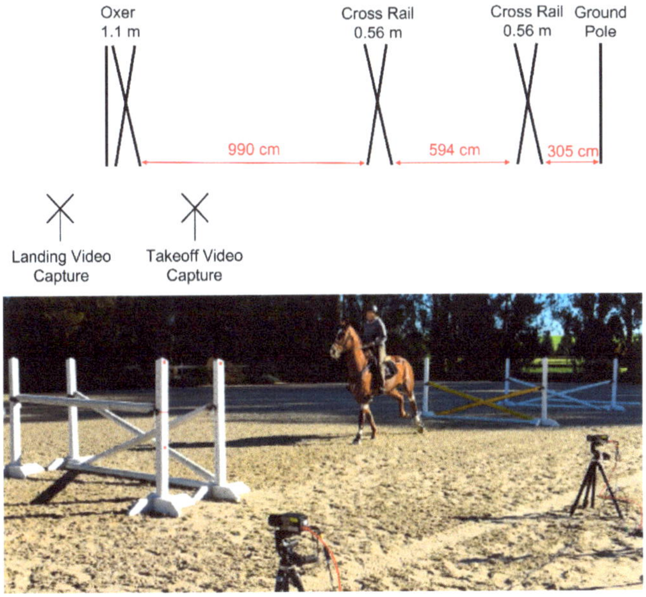

Figure 1. Scaled diagram of jumping grid (**top**) and photograph of jumping grid (**bottom**). Two high-speed cameras were used to record takeoff and landing of the final 1.1 m oxer.

2.2. Measurement of Hoof Movement

Two kinematic markers were placed on a 3D-printed extension bar and rigidly attached to the hoof wall to capture solar hoof angle, translation, and velocity while the hoof was submerged in the surface material during stance (Figure 2). The extension bar consisted of a rectangular block, which was screwed into the hoof via a patch of PMMA layered with fiberglass cloth, and a hoof wand, which was attached to the hoof block with screws prior to taking measurements. Radiographs (mediolateral projection) of the hoof, which also captured the positioning of the hoof wand, were used to translate hoof wand marker positions to virtual points at the most dorsal and palmar portions of the hoof at the solar margin ("toe" and "heel", respectively). The hoof block remained on the hoof between testing days to ensure consistent placement of the extension bar on the hoof. Two monochrome high-speed video cameras (S-PRI, AOS Technologies, Baden, Switzerland, 1280 × 1024 p, 500 fps) were centered on and calibrated in the field of view of the respective takeoff and landing zones to capture marker movement. Additionally, a wide-angle field-of-view camera (PROMON, AOS Technologies, Baden, Switzerland, 1280 × 720 p, 120 fps) and a marker on the girth were used to track true horse jump height and horizontal velocity prior to takeoff. For each jump trial, a consistent, trained observer (CR) determined whether the instrumented (left) limb was the leading or trailing forelimb at takeoff and landing. At takeoff, the instrumented forelimb was considered leading if it was the last forelimb to leave the ground; at landing, the instrumented forelimb was considered leading if it was the last forelimb to land on the ground. A second trained observer (LM) determined the video frames corresponding to hoof contact with the surface and all joint angle data were truncated to this stance phase. Marker motion was tracked throughout stance (Vicon Motus 10.0, Contemplas GMBH, Kempten, Germany).

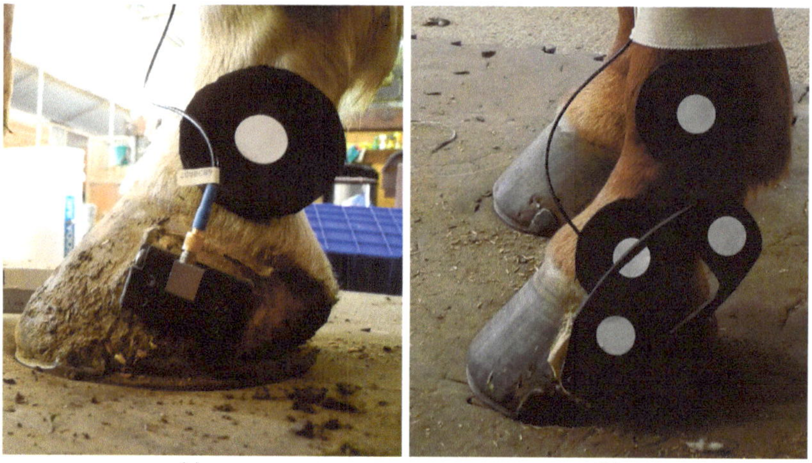

(**a**) (**b**)

Figure 2. Photograph of hoof extension bar including: (**a**) A rectangular hoof block which remained rigidly attached to the hoof wall throughout the study period; (**b**) a hoof wand with kinematic markers to track hoof rotation and translation.

The hoof angle of the solar surface of the hoof (SHA) as well as horizontal and vertical translation, velocity, and acceleration of the toe and heel were determined from marker motion using custom software (MATLAB, The MathWorks Inc., Natick, MA, USA). Solar hoof angle was defined relative to the arena surface where an angle of 0 degrees indicates that the solar surface of the hoof was parallel with the arena surface. Positive SHAs represent a hoof orientation with the dorsal wall of the hoof rotated counterclockwise with respect to the arena surface (toe down orientation); negative SHAs represent a hoof orientation with the dorsal wall of the hoof rotated clockwise with respect to the arena surface (toe up orientation) (Figure 3). Minimum, maximum, and average SHA during stance was determined for each jump trial.

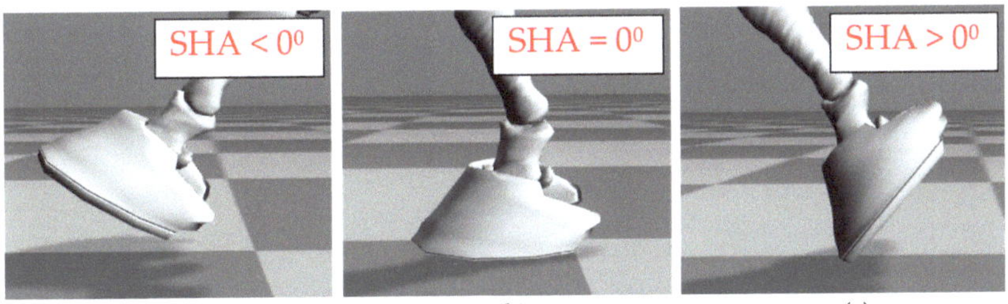

Figure 3. Definition of solar hoof angle (SHA): (**a**) Negative angles indicate that the dorsal wall of the hoof is rotated clockwise with respect to the arena surface ("toe up" orientation); (**b**) an angle of 0^0 indicates that the solar surface of the hoof is parallel to the surface; (**c**) positive angles indicate that the dorsal wall of the hoof is rotated counterclockwise with respect to the arena surface ("toe down" orientation).

Hoof translation data were also used to further divide the stance phase into three previously defined subphases [17] by a trained and consistent observer (CR): slide, support, and grab. Slide was defined as the period between the start of stance and the end of horizontal hoof motion, support was defined as the period between the end of horizontal hoof motion and start of vertical hoof motion, and grab was defined as the period between the start of vertical hoof motion and the end of stance (Figure 4). For each subphase of stance, horizontal displacement, vertical displacement, and average velocity for both the toe (dorsal extremity of the hoof in the sagittal plane) and heel (palmar extremity of the hoof in the sagittal plane) were recorded. Average deceleration during the slide phase (braking) is also reported. Displacement is defined as the difference in the position of the toe or heel between the start and end of each subphase. Horizontal displacement and horizontal velocity of the hoof are defined as positive when moving in the same direction as the center of mass of the horse. Vertical displacement and vertical velocity are defined as positive when moving farther into the arena surface.

2.3. Measurement of Arena Surface Properties

Both shear and vertical ground reaction forces were measured immediately following kinematic data collection of each horse at locations parallel to the jumping grid with surface testing equipment. Shear and vertical properties of these surfaces have been previously reported [19,20]. Shear forces and horizontal displacement were measured at 1613 Hz using a linear shear testing device with a surrogate hoof. Adhesion (a) and coefficient of friction (μ) were determined from shear tests using the Mohr–Coulomb equation ($F_{max} = F_N \times \mu + a$) in conjunction with maximum shear force (F_{max}) measured by the device and the normal force (F_N) applied to the device. Adhesion and coefficient of friction describe shear properties of the surface–hoof/horseshoe interface. Surfaces with either high adhesion or high coefficient of friction are expected to be associated with high grip and relatively low hoof slide [21]. Vertical forces, displacement, and acceleration were measured at 4545 Hz with a previously validated, portable, vertical impact device (VID) [22]. From these measured values, maximum vertical impact force and impulse were calculated from the VID force–time curve, stiffness and maximum vertical displacement were determined from VID force–displacement data, and maximum deceleration was determined from the VID acceleration data using custom software (MATLAB, The MathWorks Inc., Natick, MA, USA).

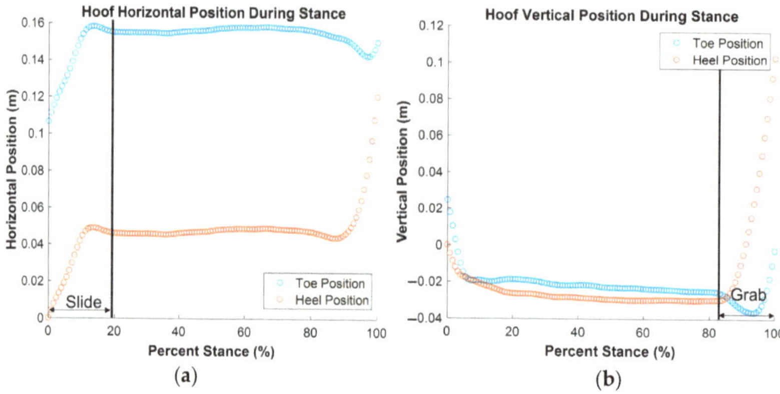

Figure 4. Subphases of stance: (**a**) Slide was defined as the region between the start of the stance phase and the end of horizontal hoof movement; (**b**) grab was defined as the region near the end of stance where the toe sank deeper into the surface. Support captured the period of the stance phase between slide and grab, where horizontal and vertical hoof displacement were minimal. Graphs depict hoof movement for a single horse at takeoff. Sample graphs depicting hoof movement at landing are presented in the Supplementary Material (Figure S1).

Cushion depth and surface temperature were also measured in conjunction with each horse, and samples (approximately 250 g) from the top two inches of the surface were collected in waterproof, airtight containers for moisture content and compositional analysis (fiber content, sand content, silt content, clay content, particle size, and fiber length) according to previously described methods [19].

2.4. Statistical Analysis

The central tendency (least squares mean/median) and variation (standard error/range) in all variables are described for normally or non-normally distributed data. The effect of jump phase (takeoff, landing), limb (leading, trailing), and arena surface material (dirt, synthetic) on SHA, displacement, velocity, and acceleration were all assessed in a single mixed-model ANOVA with horse included as a random effect and with jump height and horizontal velocity of the horse at takeoff included as covariates. Higher-level interactions between surface and phase and surface and lead were also analyzed. Normality of the ANOVA residuals was assessed using a Shapiro–Wilk test (W > 0.9). ANOVA on ranked data was used for variables with non-normally distributed residuals. The relationships of hoof motion measurements with surface composition, manageable factors, shear surface properties, and vertical impact properties were examined first using univariate regression (see Supplementary Material Tables S1–S3). For each hoof movement parameter, all related surface property variables with $p < 0.20$, as determined from the univariate regression results, were used as inputs in a multivariate stepwise regression model. Statistical significance was $p < 0.05$. SAS software (SAS Institute Inc., Cary, NC, USA) was used to perform all statistical analyses.

3. Results

3.1. Jump Characteristics

The jump height at the girth was 1.27 ± 0.07 m (mean ± standard deviation) for all horses. At takeoff, the average horizontal velocity measured at the girth increased during stance in preparation for the jump (5.32 ± 0.44 m/s before stance, 5.51 ± 0.42 m/s during stance, 5.97 ± 0.45 m/s after stance). At landing, the average horizontal velocity measured at the girth was lower than that at takeoff but also increased during stance (4.30 ± 0.48 m/s before stance, 4.39 ± 0.35 m/s during stance, 4.68 ± 0.45 m/s after stance). The resultant velocity at takeoff was directed upward, toward the jump (5.91 ± 0.43 m/s; 13.6 ± 2.8°

from horizontal) and had a higher magnitude than the resultant velocity at landing, which was, on average, directed toward the ground and away from the jump (4.70 ± 0.36 m/s; −1.83 ± 2.7° from horizontal).

3.2. Characteristics of Hoof Motion during Stance

The contact time for the hoof was significantly longer at takeoff than at landing (0.212 ± 0.006 s takeoff, 0.202 ± 0.006 s landing, $p < 0.001$), and also significantly longer when the instrumented limb was the leading limb (0.212 ± 0.006 s leading, 0.201 ± 0.006 s trailing, $p < 0.001$). Surface type (dirt, synthetic) did not have a significant effect on contact time ($p = 0.438$). However, when evaluating combined effects, the effect of leading limb on contact time was greater on dirt surfaces than on synthetic surfaces ($p = 0.028$).

Average hoof angular motion for takeoff (gray) and landing (black) is depicted in Figure 5. At the beginning of stance, the SHA was noticeably lower (more toe-up) at takeoff than at landing. The average SHA for dirt (brown) and synthetic (gray) surfaces at takeoff and landing is also shown in Figure 6. The solar hoof angle was not noticeably different between dirt and synthetic surfaces. Shaded regions represent a 95% confidence interval for the average hoof angular motion during the stance phase.

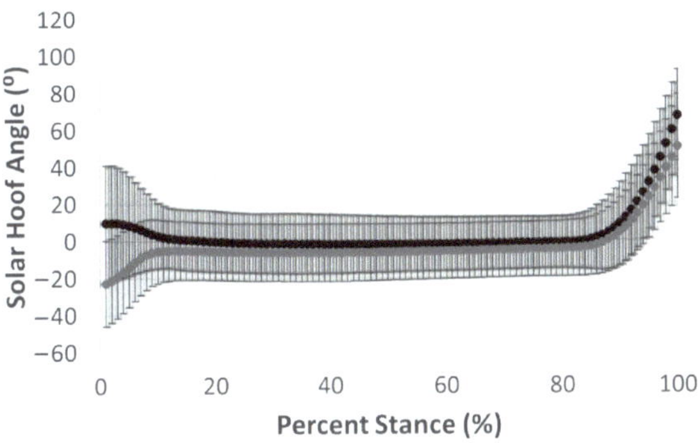

Figure 5. Average SHA normalized to percent stance at takeoff (gray) and landing (black). Bars indicate a 95% confidence interval for SHA at each percent stance.

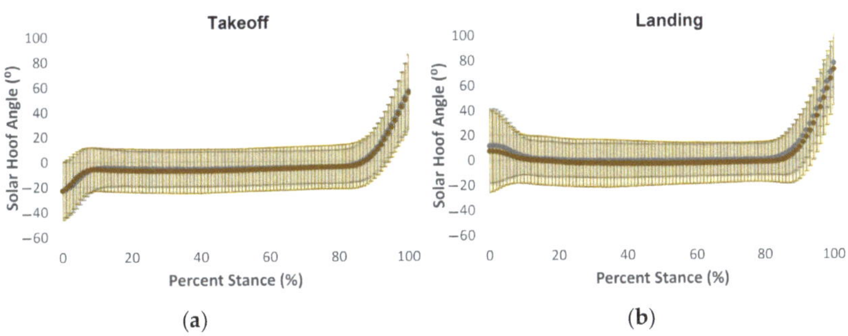

Figure 6. Average SHA normalized to percent stance for dirt (brown) and synthetic (gray) surfaces at (**a**) takeoff; (**b**) landing. Bars indicate a 95% confidence interval for joint angle at each percent stance.

Hoof angle was maximal ("toe down" orientation) at the end of the stance phase for all trials (100 ± 0%). Hoof angle was minimal ("toe up" orientation) near the beginning of the stance phase for takeoff (location of minimum at 1.8 ± 8.4% stance) as the hoof started "toe up" during the stance phase of takeoff in all but 2 of the 139 takeoff jump trials (98.6% of trials "toe up"). However, at landing, there was wide variation in the location of the minimum hoof angle amongst trials (38.0 ± 23.7% stance). At landing, the hoof started stance "toe down" in 103 of the 142 jump trials (72.5% of trials "toe down"), and the minimum SHA occurred during midstance rather than at hoof strike.

3.3. Hoof Movement during Slide

On average, the slide phase constituted the first 25.1 ± 9.2% of the stance phase. The slide phase constituted a greater percent of the stance phase on the trailing limb than on the leading limb (23.1 ± 1.1% of stance when leading, 27.0 ± 1.1% of stance when trailing, p = 0.004). However, surface type, jump phase, and jump lead did not have a significant effect on the duration of slide (Table 1).

Table 1. The effect of jump phase (takeoff, landing), jump lead (leading, trailing), and surface type (dirt, synthetic) on hoof movement during slide (LSMeans ± SE).

Variable	Takeoff (n = 139)	Landing (n = 142)	p-Value	Leading (n = 135)	Trailing (n = 146)	p-Value	Dirt (n = 111)	Synthetic (n = 170)	p-Value
Slide Time (s)	0.051 ± 0.003	0.052 ± 0.003	0.527	0.049 ± 0.003	0.055 ± 0.003	0.053	0.052 ± 0.003	0.052 ± 0.003	0.709
Average Hoof Angle (°)	−8.6 ± 3.0	2.2 ± 3.0	<0.001 *	−6.7 ± 3.0	0.3 ± 3.0	<0.001 *	−3.6 ± 3.0	−2.9 ± 3.0	0.289
Horizontal Hoof Motion									
Displacement of Toe (cm)	3.6 ± 0.5	2.1 ± 0.5	<0.001 *	4.1 ± 0.5	1.6 ± 0.5	<0.001 *	3.0 ± 0.5	2.7 ± 0.5	0.108
Displacement of Heel (cm)	2.6 ± 0.5	1.6 ± 0.5	<0.001 *	3.1 ± 0.5	1.0 ± 0.5	<0.001 *	2.3 ± 0.5	1.9 ± 0.5	0.105
Average Velocity of Toe (m/s)	0.71 ± 0.11	0.50 ± 0.11	<0.001 *	0.86 ± 0.11	0.35 ± 0.11	<0.001 *	0.65 ± 0.11	0.56 ± 0.11	0.081
Average Velocity of Heel (m/s)	0.52 ± 0.11	0.42 ± 0.11	0.038 *	0.67 ± 0.11	0.26 ± 0.11	<0.001 *	0.52 ± 0.11	0.42 ± 0.11	0.075
Average Deceleration of Toe (m/s^2)	33.4 ± 6.9	27.6 ± 6.9	0.087	46.2 ± 7.0	14.8 ± 7.0	<0.001 *	32.0 ± 7.0	28.9 ± 6.8	0.368
Average Deceleration of Heel (m/s^2)	21.1 ± 8.1	26.3 ± 8.1	0.143	36.0 ± 8.2	11.4 ± 8.2	<0.001 *	22.6 ± 8.2	24.9 ± 8.0	0.509
Vertical Hoof Motion									
Displacement of Toe (cm)	5.3 ± 2.5	1.6 ± 2.5	<0.001 *	4.0 ± 2.6	2.9 ± 2.6	<0.001 *	3.1 ± 2.6	3.8 ± 2.5	0.002 *
Displacement of Heel (cm)	2.0 ± 2.5	3.8 ± 2.5	<0.001 *	2.2 ± 2.5	3.5 ± 2.5	<0.001 *	2.6 ± 2.5	3.2 ± 2.4	0.058
Average Velocity of Toe (m/s)	1.06 ± 0.08	0.35 ± 0.08	<0.001 *	0.81 ± 0.08	0.59 ± 0.08	<0.001 *	0.63 ± 0.08	0.77 ± 0.08	0.002 *
Average Velocity of Heel (m/s)	0.38 ± 0.05	0.72 ± 0.05	<0.001 *	0.47 ± 0.05	0.63 ± 0.05	<0.001 *	0.49 ± 0.05	0.60 ± 0.05	0.044 *

* Result is statistically significant (p < 0.05).

During slide, hoof angle was significantly different at takeoff than landing, with a toe-up orientation at takeoff and a toe-down orientation at landing. Hoof angle during slide was also significantly different between the leading and trailing limb, with a toe-up orientation when the limb was leading and a very slight toe-down orientation when the limb was trailing.

Horizontal toe and heel displacement during slide were in the same direction as horse travel and were significantly greater at takeoff than landing and when the instrumented limb was leading. Average horizontal velocities of the toe and heel during slide were also significantly greater at takeoff and on the leading limb. Surface type (dirt, synthetic) did not have a significant effect on horizontal hoof displacement and velocity during slide.

The horizontal deceleration of both the toe and heel was significantly greater when the instrumented limb was leading. The horizontal deceleration was not significantly different between takeoff and landing or between dirt and synthetic surface types; however, there was a significant combined effect of jump phase and surface type on the horizontal deceleration at the heel, where deceleration was higher at landing than takeoff on dirt surfaces but lower at landing than takeoff on synthetic surfaces (p = 0.034).

The toe and heel moved deeper into the surface during slide (reported as positive numbers). The vertical displacement and average vertical velocity of the toe during slide were greater for the leading limb, at takeoff, and on synthetic surfaces, while vertical displacement and average vertical velocity of the heel during slide were greater for the trailing limb at landing. The average vertical velocity of the heel during slide was also greater on synthetic than dirt surfaces.

3.4. Hoof Movement during Support

On average, the support phase constituted the middle 55.0 ± 13.4% of the stance phase. The support phase was significantly longer and a greater percent of stance at takeoff than landing (56.5 ± 1.4% of stance at takeoff, 53.7 ± 0.9% of stance at landing, $p = 0.025$) and when the instrumented limb was the leading limb than the trailing limb (57.6 ± 0.9% of stance when leading, 52.6 ± 0.9% of stance when trailing, $p < 0.001$). The hoof angle during support was significantly lower (more "toe up") for the leading limb, at takeoff, and on dirt surfaces.

The horizontal toe and heel displacement during support was opposite to the direction of forward movement of the horse's center of mass (reported as negative numbers). The horizontal toe and heel displacement was significantly greater at landing than at takeoff (Table 2), and horizontal heel displacement was also significantly greater on the leading limb. The average horizontal velocity of the toe and heel during support was also significantly greater at landing than takeoff. Surface type (dirt, synthetic) did not have a significant effect on horizontal hoof displacement and velocity during support.

Table 2. The effect of jump phase (takeoff, landing), jump lead (leading, trailing), and surface type (dirt, synthetic) on hoof movement during support (LSMeans ± SE; [min, max], median).

Variable	Takeoff (n = 139)	Landing (n = 142)	p-Value	Leading (n = 135)	Trailing (n = 146)	p-Value	Dirt (n = 111)	Synthetic (n = 170)	p-Value
Support Time (s)	0.120 ± 0.003	0.108 ± 0.003	<0.001 *	0.122 ± 0.003	0.107 ± 0.003	<0.001 *	0.115 ± 0.003	0.114 ± 0.003	0.436
Average Hoof Angle (°)	−5.9 ± 2.9	−1.9 ± 2.9	<0.001 *	−5.5 ± 2.9	−2.2 ± 2.9	<0.001 *	−4.7 ± 2.9	−3.1 ± 2.9	0.008 *
Horizontal Hoof Motion									
Displacement of Toe (cm)	Range: [−0.6, 0.9] Median: −0.03	Range: [−2.3, 0.6] Median: −0.11	<0.001 *	Range: [−0.6, 0.6] Median: −0.11	Range: [−2.3, 0.9] Median: −0.03	0.122	Range: [−2.3, 0.9] Median: −0.08	Range: [−0.9, 0.3] Median: −0.05	0.958
Displacement of Heel (cm)	Range: [−0.8, 0.9] Median: −0.06	Range: [−2.3, 0.5] Median: −0.12	0.004 *	Range: [−0.8, 0.3] Median: −0.16	Range: [−2.3, 0.9] Median: −0.03	0.015 *	Range: [−2.3, 0.9] Median: −0.13	Range: [−0.9, 0.2] Median: −0.08	0.184
Average Velocity of Toe (m/s)	Range: [−0.05, 0.08] Median: −0.003	Range: [−0.41, 0.06] Median: −0.011	<0.001 *	Range: [−0.05, 0.06] Median: −0.010	Range: [−0.41, 0.08] Median: −0.003	0.577	Range: [−0.41, 0.08] Median: −0.007	Range: [−0.09, 0.04] Median: −0.006	0.779
Average Velocity of Heel (m/s)	Range: [−0.07, 0.08] Median: −0.006	Range: [−0.41, 0.05] Median: −0.011	<0.001 *	Range: [−0.07, 0.03] Median: −0.013	Range: [−0.41, 0.08] Median: −0.004	0.168	Range: [−0.41, 0.08] Median: −0.011	Range: [−0.09, 0.02] Median: −0.008	0.148
Vertical Hoof Motion									
Displacement of Toe (cm)	Range: [−0.2, 2.9] Median: 0.32	Range: [−0.3, 1.9] Median: 0.20	<0.001 *	Range: [−0.1, 2.9] Median: 0.36	Range: [−0.3, 2.1] Median: 0.18	<0.001 *	Range: [−0.3, 2.9] Median: 0.27	Range: [−0.9, 2.2] Median: 0.08	0.515
Displacement of Heel (cm)	0.13 ± 0.04	0.22 ± 0.04	<0.001 *	0.07 ± 0.04	0.22 ± 0.04	<0.001 *	0.17 ± 0.04	0.18 ± 0.04	0.923
Average Velocity of Toe (m/s)	Range: [−0.02, 0.29] Median: 0.026	Range: [−0.02, 0.16] Median: 0.018	<0.001 *	Range: [−0.02, 0.29] Median: 0.028	Range: [−0.02, 0.20] Median: 0.015	0.002 *	Range: [−0.02, 0.29] Median: 0.023	Range: [−0.02, 0.07] Median: 0.023	0.871
Average Velocity of Heel (m/s)	0.009 ± 0.003	0.021 ± 0.003	<0.001 *	0.004 ± 0.004	0.025 ± 0.004	<0.001 *	0.015 ± 0.004	0.014 ± 0.003	0.473

* Result is statistically significant ($p < 0.05$).

The toe and heel also moved deeper into the surface during support (reported as positive numbers). The vertical displacement and vertical velocity of the toe during support were greater for the leading limb at takeoff, while the vertical displacement and vertical velocity of the heel during support were greater for the trailing limb at landing. Surface type (dirt, synthetic) did not have a significant effect on the vertical hoof displacement and velocity during support.

3.5. Hoof Movement during Grab

On average, the grab phase constituted the last 20.0 ± 3.3% of the stance phase. The grab phase was significantly longer and a greater percent of stance on synthetic surfaces than dirt surfaces (20.3 ± 0.4% of stance on synthetic surfaces, 19.4 ± 0.5% of stance on dirt surfaces, $p = 0.023$). The grab phase was also a significantly greater percent of stance for the trailing limb (19.2 ± 0.5% of stance when leading, 20.5 ± 0.5% of stance when trailing, $p = 0.004$).

The horizontal toe displacement during grab was opposite to the direction of forward movement of the horse's center of mass, while the horizontal heel displacement during grab was in the same direction as the horse. This displacement trend is consistent with the positive ("toe-down") SHAs observed during grab. The horizontal toe displacement during grab was significantly greater (more negative) at landing (Table 3). The average horizontal velocity of the toe during grab was also significantly greater (more negative) at landing and on dirt surfaces. The horizontal heel displacement and velocity during grab were significantly greater (more positive) at landing with the trailing limb. The horizontal heel displacement was also greater (more positive) on synthetic than dirt surfaces.

Table 3. The effect of jump phase (takeoff, landing), jump lead (leading, trailing), and surface type (dirt, synthetic) on hoof movement during grab (LSMeans ± SE).

Variable	Takeoff (n = 139)	Landing (n = 142)	p-Value	Leading (n = 135)	Trailing (n = 146)	p-Value	Dirt (n = 111)	Synthetic (n = 170)	p-Value
Grab Time (s)	0.042 ± 0.002	0.040 ± 0.002	0.092	0.041 ± 0.002	0.041 ± 0.002	0.940	0.040 ± 0.002	0.042 ± 0.002	0.017*
Average SHA (°)	14.7 ± 2.9	21.6 ± 3.0	<0.001 *	15.8 ± 3.0	20.5 ± 3.0	<0.001 *	17.8 ± 3.0	18.6 ± 2.9	0.304
Horizontal Hoof Motion									
Displacement of Toe (cm)	−2.0 ± 0.3	−4.1 ± 0.3	<0.001 *	−2.9 ± 0.4	−3.3 ± 0.3	0.210	−3.2 ± 0.3	−2.9 ± 0.3	0.054
Displacement of Heel (cm)	3.5 ± 0.7	4.9 ± 0.7	<0.001 *	3.6 ± 0.7	4.8 ± 0.7	<0.001 *	3.8 ± 0.7	4.7 ± 0.7	0.019 *
Average Velocity of Toe (m/s)	−0.48 ± 0.07	−0.98 ± 0.07	<0.001 *	−0.70 ± 0.07	−0.76 ± 0.07	0.419	−0.79 ± 0.07	−0.67 ± 0.07	0.026 *
Average Velocity of Heel (m/s)	1.00 ± 0.20	1.54 ± 0.20	<0.001 *	1.10 ± 0.20	1.44 ± 0.20	<0.001 *	1.19 ± 0.20	1.35 ± 0.20	0.145
Vertical Hoof Motion									
Displacement of Toe (cm)	0.1± 0.4	0.1 ± 0.4	0.830	0.3 ± 0.4	−0.1 ± 0.4	0.046 *	0.5 ± 0.4	−0.3 ± 0.4	<0.001 *
Displacement of Heel (cm)	−10.9 ± 0.4	−11.9 ± 0.4	<0.001 *	−11.0 ± 0.4	−11.9 ± 0.4	0.001 *	−11.2 ± 0.4	−11.7 ± 0.4	0.250
Average Velocity of Toe (m/s)	−0.12 ± 0.11	−0.20 ± 0.11	0.117	−0.11 ± 0.11	−0.21 ± 0.11	0.015 *	−0.07 ± 0.11	−0.25 ± 0.11	0.002 *
Average Velocity of Heel (m/s)	−2.82 ± 0.17	−3.19 ± 0.17	<0.001 *	−2.88 ± 0.17	−3.14 ± 0.17	<0.001 *	−3.03 ± 0.17	−2.98 ± 0.16	0.344

* Result is statistically significant ($p < 0.05$).

The heel displaced out of the surface during grab, while the toe sometimes penetrated deeper into the surface (positive) and sometimes further out of the surface (negative) by the end of the grab phase. The toe displacement during grab was significantly related to the surface type, where the toe displaced further out of synthetic surfaces and further into dirt surfaces during grab. Additionally, the toe of the leading limb displaced into the surface and the toe on the trailing limb displaced out of the surface during grab. The heel displacement out of the surface was significantly greater for the trailing limb at landing. The average vertical velocity of the toe was significantly greater for the trailing limb and on synthetic surfaces with a direction out of the surface. The average vertical velocity of the heel was significantly greater for the trailing limb and at landing with a direction out of the surface.

When considering the combined effects of surface type and leading limb, the toe moved further backward and had a larger horizontal velocity with the leading limb than the trailing limb on synthetic surfaces, while the toe moved further backward and had a larger horizontal velocity with the trailing limb than the leading limb on dirt surfaces ($p = 0.006$ displacement; $p = 0.004$ velocity).

3.6. Multivariate Stepwise Regression of Surface Properties with Hoof Movement Parameters

Descriptive statistics for all surface composition variables (fiber content, sand content, silt content, clay content, average particle size, particle size deviation, average fiber length, and fiber length deviation), manageable properties (temperature, cushion depth, and moisture content), shear properties (adhesion, coefficient of friction, and normalized maximum shear force), and vertical impact properties (maximum vertical impact force, impulse, loading rate, maximum vertical displacement, soil rebound, energy dissipated during impact, stiffness, and maximum deceleration) as reported by Rohlf et al. [19,20] are depicted in Table 4.

Table 4. Descriptive statistics of compositional, manageable, shear, and vertical impact properties of dirt and synthetic surfaces (LSMeans ± SE).

Variable	Observations	Dirt	Synthetic	*p*-Value
Compositional Properties				
Fiber Content (%) [1]	12	0.12 ± 0.98 Median 0 Range [0, 0.6]	4.03 ± 0.83 Median 3.4 Range [1.5, 10]	<0.001 [2]
Sand Content (%)	12	84.6 ± 3.67	78.14 ± 3.11	0.210
Silt Content (%)	12	10.46 ± 2.54	12.31 ± 2.15	0.590
Clay Content (%)	12	4.83 ± 1.08	5.51± 0.91	0.639
Average Particle Size (mm)	12	0.74 ± 0.12	0.40 ± 0.10	0.051
Standard Deviation of Particle Size (mm)	12	1.00 ± 0.13	0.60 ± 0.11	0.042 [2]
Average Fiber Length (mm) [1]	7	N/A	27.7 ± 2.0 Median 24.8 Range [23.6, 38.3]	N/A
Standard Deviation of Fiber Length (mm) [1]	7	N/A	11.8 ± 1.8 Median 10.7 Range [6.0, 20.9]	N/A
Manageable Properties				
Surface Temperature (°C)	59	26.0 ± 2.3	13.9 ± 1.9	0.002 [2]
Cushion Depth (mm)	59	34.9 ± 7.5	53.2 ± 6.3	0.090
Moisture Content (%)	59	3.30 ± 2.37	9.84 ± 2.00	0.062
Shear Properties				
Adhesion (N)	46	30.0 ± 10.0	3.5 ± 8.4	0.078
Coefficient of Friction	46	0.37 ± 0.03	0.44 ± 0.02	0.065
Normalized Maximum Shear Force (F_{max}/F_N)	46	0.43 ± 0.02	0.46 ± 0.02	0.322
Vertical Impact Properties				
Maximum Vertical Impact Force (kN)	58	15.2 ± 1.3	13.7 ± 1.1	0.379
Impulse (N × s)	58	69.0 ± 1.0	72.1 ± 0.8	0.039 [2]
Loading Rate (kN/s)	58	4679 ± 568	3155 ± 473	0.066
Maximum Vertical Displacement (cm)	58	1.76 ± 0.18	2.07 ± 0.15	0.157
Soil Rebound (cm)	58	0.11 ± 0.03	0.23 ± 0.02	0.010 [2]
Dissipated Energy (J)	58	80.9 ± 1.5	79.8 ± 1.3	0.591
Stiffness (kN/m)	58	2477 ± 332	1602 ± 273	0.069
Maximum Deceleration (g)	58	63.6 ± 5.1	56.7 ± 4.3	0.322

[1] Indicates that the ANOVA was performed on the ranked data because the residuals of the ANOVA were not normally distributed. [2] Result is statistically significant ($p < 0.05$).

The relationships between surface properties and hoof translation parameters were analyzed with a multivariate stepwise regression (see Supplementary Material Table S4). Clay content was significantly related to many hoof movement variables at both takeoff and landing. At takeoff, surfaces with greater clay content had less displacement (r = −0.33; $p = 0.022$) and velocity (r = −0.49; $p = 0.004$) of the heel into the surface during slide. At landing, surfaces with higher clay content were significantly related to less vertical displacement (r = −0.33; $p = 0.031$) and velocity (r = −0.45; $p = 0.003$) of the toe into the surface during slide. During the grab phase of landing, surfaces with higher clay content exhibited a reduced SHA (less "toe down" orientation) (r = −0.42; $p = 0.004$), reduced horizontal heel displacement (r = −0.39; $p = 0.009$) and velocity (r = −0.5; $p < 0.001$), less vertical heel displacement (r = −0.46; $p = 0.002$; out of the surface), and less vertical toe velocity (r = −0.42; $p = 0.005$; out of the surface). Soils with more variable particle size distributions were also related to reduced horizontal heel displacement (r = −0.32; $p = 0.038$) and lower vertical toe velocity (r = −0.33; $p = 0.030$; out of the surface) during the grab phase at takeoff, and less vertical displacement of the toe out of the surface (r = −0.37; $p = 0.013$) during the grab phase at landing.

The horizontal deceleration of the hoof during slide was also related to surface characteristics. At takeoff, surfaces with greater variation in soil particle size exhibited less horizontal heel deceleration (r = −0.41; $p = 0.005$), while surfaces with higher temperatures exhibited less horizontal toe deceleration (r = −0.41; $p = 0.005$). At landing, surfaces with higher adhesion increased the deceleration of both the toe and heel (r = 0.33; $p = 0.027$).

Several surface properties were only related to hoof movement variables at takeoff. Surfaces with greater soil rebound exhibited more vertical heel displacement (r = 0.39; $p = 0.010$) and velocity (r = 0.33; $p = 0.012$) during slide. Additionally, higher surface temperatures were related to greater vertical displacement (r = 0.35; $p = 0.023$) and velocity (r = 0.41; $p = 0.007$) of the toe during support, but reduced vertical velocity (r = −0.42; $p = 0.005$) of the toe during slide. Surfaces with deeper cushion layers were also related to greater vertical displacement (r = 0.44; $p = 0.002$) and velocity (r = 0.40; $p = 0.004$) of the toe during support and a lower average SHA (r = −0.35; $p = 0.018$; more "toe up"). Surfaces with higher vertical deceleration rates were related to less vertical displacement of the heel (r = −0.33; $p = 0.027$; out of the surface) and less horizontal displacement of the toe (r = −0.32; $p = 0.041$) during grab. Surfaces with greater impulse during vertical impact (factor of impact force and duration of impact) exhibited less vertical toe displacement (r = −0.40; $p = 0.008$; into the surface) during grab. Finally, synthetic surfaces with longer fibers exhibited more vertical heel displacement into the surface during the slide phase (r = 0.62; $p < 0.001$) and more vertical heel displacement out of the surface during the grab phase (r = 0.40; $p = 0.041$).

Additionally, some surface properties were only related to hoof movement variables at landing. Surfaces with higher adhesion exhibited greater horizontal toe and heel displacement (toe: r = 0.33; $p = 0.031$, heel: r = 0.32; $p = 0.041$) and velocity (toe: r = 0.36; $p = 0.015$, heel: r = 0.36; $p = 0.020$) during slide, as well as greater horizontal heel displacement opposite the forward momentum of the horse (r = 0.32; $p = 0.030$) during support and greater vertical velocity of the heel out of the surface during grab (r = 0.41; $p = 0.005$). Surfaces with greater dissipated energy at impact (factor of impact force and vertical displacement into the surface) exhibited less horizontal toe displacement and velocity (opposite the forward momentum of the horse) during support (displacement: r = −0.32; $p = 0.042$, velocity: r = −0.32; $p = 0.041$) and grab (displacement: r = −0.46; $p = 0.002$, velocity: r = −0.37; $p = 0.014$). Stiffer surfaces (r = −0.33; $p = 0.011$), surfaces with higher loading rates during vertical impact (r = −0.28; $p = 0.042$), and surfaces with less sand content (r = 0.28; $p = 0.019$) were related to less heel displacement out of the surface during grab. Finally, surfaces with larger soil particles exhibited less vertical velocity of the toe out of the surface during grab (r = −0.28; $p = 0.044$).

Fiber content, silt content, fiber length variation, moisture content, coefficient of friction, maximum normalized shear force, maximum vertical impact force, and maximum vertical displacement of the impact tester were not related to any hoof movement properties.

4. Discussion

Our results appear to agree well with the previous research. Although surface type, jump phase, and leading limb were all identified as factors that may affect the horizontal deceleration of the hoof during slide and injury risk [5,6], only the leading limb had a statistically significant effect on the horizontal hoof deceleration. Furthermore, while surface properties were significantly related to some hoof movement variables, expected negative relationships between shear properties and horizontal hoof movement and expected positive relationships between vertical movement of the hoof and surface tester were not observed.

The methods used to determine slide, support, and grab in this study appear to be reasonable, since the timing of these phases matches the timings presented in previous research. In this study, the slide phase constituted the first 25% of the stance phase on average, which is in line with previous reports of secondary impact occurring in the first 30% of stance [2]. Furthermore, the timing of grab, also called breakover, in this study agreed with the timing observed in previous studies (80–100% stance in present study; 85–100% stance in Thomason et al. [2]).

The leading limb had a significant effect on many hoof movement parameters during slide. As expected, average horizontal deceleration in the leading limb was significantly greater than horizontal deceleration in the trailing limb during slide, which is also aligned with previous research findings [18]. Rapid deceleration has been linked to a greater risk of subchondral bone and cartilage damage by increasing the bending moment, longitudinal deceleration, and high-frequency oscillations of the third metacarpal bone [5,6]. Therefore, our findings suggest that the leading limb may be at greater risk of musculoskeletal injury. The finding that SHA was significantly greater for the trailing limb during all three jump phases also aligns with the results of Hernlund et al. [18]. Results from the present study also show that the horizontal velocity of the hoof is significantly greater in the leading limb during slide. Greater horizontal velocity in the leading limb at jump landing has also been reported in the literature [18]; however, in the previous study, velocity was reported for the entire stance phase and was not subdivided into slide, support, and grab.

In contrast, surface type had few significant effects on hoof motion during slide, support, and grab. Although a previous study of galloping horses found a longer support duration on a synthetic surface compared to a dirt surface [17], this was not observed in the present study. Support duration was longer and comprised a greater percent of stance on the leading limb at takeoff (the last forelimb to leave the ground), possibly to provide additional stability and time at takeoff for the horse to plant the hindlimbs. Grab time was significantly greater and comprised a larger percent of stance on synthetic surfaces; however, this finding could be explained by the fact that vertical hoof displacement was also significantly greater on synthetic surfaces and the time required for the horse to remove their hoof from deeper within the surface while pushing off was greater. A previous study also found significantly greater horizontal hoof displacement on a synthetic surface during slide [17]; however, no surface type effects on horizontal hoof motion during slide were observed in the current study. However, this previous study only evaluated one surface of each type and may have underestimated the variation in mechanical behavior within a surface type category (dirt, synthetic). The evaluation of five dirt and seven synthetic surfaces in the present study likely captured more variation and demonstrated that surface type, as a categorical variable, does not sufficiently describe the hoof–surface interaction. Additionally, since horizontal hoof motion is expected to be related to shear properties of arena surfaces [1], the lack of surface type effects on horizontal deceleration during slide agrees with our hypothesis because shear properties of these dirt and synthetic surfaces were not significantly different [19].

Our analysis of SHA also suggests a secondary mechanism of injury in show jumping in addition to rapid horizontal deceleration. During initial impact and slide, the SHA was heel-down at takeoff and toe-down at landing. Researchers have suggested that injury risk may be reduced when the hoof impacts the surface in a heel-first configuration because the structure of the hoof provides more elasticity in the heel area to dampen impact loads [23]. Furthermore, in a heel-first impact, tension in the flexor tendons decreases as the hoof rotates to a flat orientation during stance, which partially counteracts the increase in flexor tendon force due to fetlock extension [24]. In contrast, toe-first impacts have been suggested as a contributing factor for navicular disease because rotation of the hoof and fetlock extension both increase the forces applied to the deep digital flexor tendon and navicular bone [24]. Since the toe impacted first at jump landing, when impact forces are maximized, this supports a possible mechanism for the high prevalence of navicular injuries observed in non-elite show-jumping horses in the United Kingdom [25].

Finally, several significant relationships between hoof movement during jumping and arena surface properties were also identified. Surface clay content had the most significant relationships with hoof movement on arena surfaces. In general, surfaces with more clay content reduced or slowed hoof movement. The effect of clay on hoof movement is similar to the effect of clay courts on tennis balls, as the high coefficient of sliding friction of clay reduces the ball speed [26]. Additionally, surfaces with greater surface temperatures, more variably sized particles, and less adhesion were associated with less deceleration of the hoof during the sliding phase. These findings suggest that surfaces with these characteristics may also reduce the risk of injury to the horse by reducing the bending moment on the third metacarpal bone [5]. However, compositional and manageable properties were not systematically adjusted within a single arena surface. Therefore, future research is needed to understand the individualized effects of changing a single surface management or compositional parameter on hoof deceleration.

Although shear properties (adhesion, coefficient of friction, and maximum shear force) were expected to be strongly and negatively correlated with horizontal displacement of the hoof, especially during the slide phase, adhesion was the only shear property correlated with hoof movement. This hypothesis was based on previous research which showed that high shear forces (traction) restricted the amount of hoof movement [27,28]. Both adhesion and coefficient of friction have been defined as important metrics to assess friction between the playing surface and footwear of human athletes [29], where higher adhesion and/or a greater coefficient of friction are expected to reduce slip. Although adhesion was related to several horizontal hoof movement variables at landing, in all cases, adhesion was positively correlated with horizontal hoof motion (e.g., surfaces with higher adhesion exhibited more horizontal hoof motion). This result was very counterintuitive considering the mechanical nature of adhesion to prevent hoof movement.

Vertical hoof displacement was also expected to be strongly and positively correlated with vertical displacement of the vertical impact tester because the vertical impact testing device was designed to simulate the interaction of the hoof and the ground [22]. However, no relationships between vertical displacement of the hoof and vertical displacement of the tester were found. In all but 4 jumping trials (96%), hoof vertical displacement exceeded the maximum displacement of the vertical tester into the surface. Furthermore, the hoof penetrated the base surface layer (a compacted mixture of sand and gravel with a much higher stiffness than the sandy, aerated cushion layer on the top of the surface) in 63.4% of trials, while the vertical impact device only penetrated the base layer during 6 of the impact trials (6.7%). Previous studies of human playing surfaces have also found few correlations between the results of material testing devices and results from experimental subjects [30].

The counterintuitive and unexpected correlation results between hoof movement and surface properties measured with the mechanical testing devices suggest that further experimentation and development of these devices are required to better represent surface–hoof interactions during a jump. While these devices are not expected to replicate the magnitude of forces during equine stance, it is important that these devices are further validated to ensure that surface properties as measured by these devices are representative of true hoof–surface interactions. The benefit of mechanical testing devices lies in their ability to create a more standardized testing environment than is possible from live animal studies, and to reduce the number of confounding variables when comparing the behavior between different surfaces. However, even with further development, mechanical testing devices will have limitations and may not be able to represent hoof movement accurately or precisely. Therefore, it may be preferable to focus on the enhancement and development of non-invasive and low-profile equipment that can measure movement and forces directly at the hoof (i.e., dynamometric horseshoes).

Another limitation of this study is related to possible vibration of the hoof extension bar at impact which is not consistent with the sagittal plane motion of the hoof. However, large vibrations would likely have been observed while reviewing video capture, and small vibrations were removed during the high-pass filtering of the motion capture data. Additionally, dirt and synthetic arena surfaces evaluated in this study were limited to the northern California region, which may not capture the variation in arena properties worldwide. However, our sample size (five dirt; seven synthetic) was larger than that of previous studies which compared only one to two surfaces of each type, and it likely captures more variation than these previous studies. Finally, compositional and manageable properties were not varied within a particular arena surface in this study. Thus, other compositional and manageable properties may be confounding factors when trying to determine the individualized effects of surface parameters on joint motion. The confounding effect of surface temperature is especially noteworthy as dirt surfaces had significantly higher temperatures than synthetic surfaces. Although multivariate stepwise regression was chosen to statistically account for possible relationships between surface properties when reporting correlations, future research studies should evaluate the individualized effects of changing a single surface management or compositional parameter on hoof motion.

5. Conclusions

Large surface property variation among synthetic and dirt surfaces precluded the ability for surface type, described categorically, to be a good predictor for hoof translation in the surface. However, hoof deceleration during slide was significantly dependent on the forelimb that was leading during the jump, where the leading leg had significantly greater deceleration than the trailing leg. This finding suggests that the leading leg may have a higher risk of musculoskeletal injury. To alleviate the increased risk of injury to the leading leg, it may be beneficial for trainers and riders to switch leads during training and competition to reduce the number of repetitions of high deceleration on a single forelimb.

Supplementary Materials: The following supporting information can be downloaded at: https://www.mdpi.com/article/10.3390/ani13132122/s1, Figure S1: subphases of stance at landing; Table S1: correlations between compositional surface properties and hoof movement; Table S2: correlations between manageable surface properties and hoof movement; Table S3: correlations between vertical impact properties and hoof movement; Table S4: multivariate stepwise regression results.

Author Contributions: Conceptualization, C.M.R., T.C.G. and S.M.S.; methodology, C.M.R., T.C.G., L.J.M. and S.M.S.; software, C.M.R. and T.C.G.; validation, C.M.R., T.C.G. and L.J.M.; formal analysis, C.M.R.; investigation, C.M.R., T.C.G., L.J.M., E.V.A., S.S.l.J. and S.M.S.; resources, T.C.G., S.S.l.J. and S.M.S.; data curation, C.M.R. and L.J.M.; writing—original draft preparation, C.M.R.; writing—review and editing, C.M.R., T.C.G., L.J.M., E.V.A., S.S.l.J. and S.M.S.; visualization, C.M.R.; supervision, S.M.S.; project administration, S.M.S.; funding acquisition, C.M.R. and S.M.S. All authors have read and agreed to the published version of the manuscript.

Funding: This research was funded by the Center for Equine Health at University of California, Davis, grant number 17-01, with funds provided by the State of California satellite wagering fund and contributions by private donors.

Institutional Review Board Statement: The animal study protocol was approved by the Institutional Review Board of the University of California Davis (protocol 19843-Effect of Jumping Arena Surfaces on Equine Forelimb Biomechanics approved 3 April 2017).

Informed Consent Statement: Written informed consent was obtained from the owner of all horses involved in the study.

Data Availability Statement: The data presented in this study are available on request from the corresponding author.

Acknowledgments: Special thanks to Kaleb Dempsey from the Racing Surfaces Testing Laboratory for determining soil compositional properties.

Conflicts of Interest: The authors declare no conflict of interest.

References

1. Hobbs, S.J.; Northropp, A.J.; Mahaffey, C.; Martin, J.H.; Murray, R.; Roepstorff, L.; Peterson, M. *Equine Surfaces white Paper*; Federation Equestre Internationale: Lausanne, Switzerland, 2014.
2. Thomason, J.J.; Peterson, M.L. Biomechanical and mechanical investigations of the hoof-track interface in racing horses. *Vet. Clin. N. Am. Equine Pract.* **2008**, *24*, 53–77. [CrossRef]
3. Johnston, C.; Roepstorff, L.; Drevemo, S.; Kallings, P. Kinematics of the distal hindlimb during stance phase in the fast trotting standardbred. *Equine Vet. J.* **1996**, *28*, 263–268. [CrossRef]
4. Gustås, P.; Johnston, C.; Hedenström, U.; Roepstorff, L.; Drevemo, S. A field study on hoof deceleration at impact in standardbred trotters at various speeds. *Equine Comp. Exerc. Physiol.* **2006**, *3*, 161–168. [CrossRef]
5. Pratt, G.W. Model for injury to the foreleg of the thoroughbred racehorse. *Equine Vet. J. Suppl.* **1997**, *29*, 30–32. [CrossRef] [PubMed]
6. Gustås, P.; Johnston, C.; Roepstorff, L.; Drevemo, S. In vivo transmission of impact shock waves in the distal forelimb of the horse. *Equine Vet. J. Suppl.* **2001**, *33*, 11–15. [CrossRef]
7. Gustås, P.; Johnston, C.; Drevemo, S. Ground reaction force and hoof deceleration patterns on two different surfaces at the trot. *Equine Comp. Exerc. Physiol.* **2006**, *3*, 209–216. [CrossRef]
8. Crevier-Denoix, N.; Robin, D.; Pourcelot, P.; Falala, S.; Holden, L.; Estoup, P.; Desquilbet, L.; Denoix, J.M.; Chateau, H. Ground reaction force and kinematic analysis of limb loading on two different beach sand tracks in harness trotters. *Equine Vet. J.* **2010**, *42*, 544–551. [CrossRef]
9. Riemersma, D.J.; Van Den Bogert, A.J.; Jansen, M.O.; Schamhardt, H.C. Influence of shoeing on ground reaction forces and tendon strains in the forelimbs of ponies. *Equine Vet. J.* **1996**, *28*, 126–132. [CrossRef]
10. Egenvall, A.; Roepstorff, L.; Peterson, M.; Lundholm, M.; Hernlund, E. The descriptions and attitudes of riders and arena owners to 656 equestrian sport surfaces in Sweden. *Front. Vet. Sci.* **2021**, *8*, 798910. [CrossRef] [PubMed]
11. Schamhardt, H.C.; Merkens, H.W.; Vogel, V.; Willekens, C. External loads on the limbs of jumping horses at take-off and landing. *Am. J. Vet. Res.* **1993**, *54*, 675–680.
12. Deuel, N.R.; Park, J. Kinematic analysis of jumping sequences of olympic show jumping horses. *Equine Exerc. Physiol.* **1991**, *3*, 158–166.
13. Deuel, N.R.; Park, J.-J. The gait patterns of olympic dressage horses. *J. Appl. Biomech.* **1990**, *6*, 198–226. [CrossRef]
14. Barrey, E.; Landjerit, B.; Wolter, R. Shock and vibration during the hoof impact on different track surfaces. In Proceedings of the Third International Conference on Equine Physiology, Uppsala, Sweden, 15–19 July 1990; pp. 97–106.
15. Chateau, H.; Robin, D.; Falala, S.; Pourcelot, P.; Valette, J.P.; Ravary, B.; Denoix, J.M.; Crevier-Denoix, N. Effects of a synthetic all-weather waxed track versus a crushed sand track on 3D acceleration of the front hoof in three horses trotting at high speed. *Equine Vet. J.* **2009**, *41*, 247–251. [CrossRef]
16. Crevier-Denoix, N.; Pourcelot, P.; Holden-Douilly, L.; Camus, M.; Falala, S.; Ravary-Plumioën, B.; Vergari, C.; Desquilbet, L.; Chateau, H. Discrimination of two equine racing surfaces based on forelimb dynamic and hoof kinematic variables at the canter. *Vet. J.* **2013**, *198*, e124–e129. [CrossRef]
17. Symons, J.E.; Garcia, T.C.; Stover, S.M. Distal hindlimb kinematics of galloping thoroughbred racehorses on dirt and synthetic racetrack surfaces. *Equine Vet. J.* **2014**, *46*, 227–232. [CrossRef]
18. Hernlund, E.; Egenvall, A.; Roepstorff, L. Kinematic characteristics of hoof landing in jumping horses at elite level. *Equine Vet. J. Suppl.* **2010**, *42*, 462–467. [CrossRef]
19. Rohlf, C.M.; Garcia, T.C.; Fyhrie, D.P.; le Jeune, S.S.; Peterson, M.L.; Stover, S.M. Shear ground reaction force variation among equine arena surfaces. *Vet. J.* **2023**, *291*, 105930. [CrossRef] [PubMed]
20. Rohlf, C.M.; Garcia, T.C.; Fyhrie, D.P.; le Jeune, S.S.; Peterson, M.L.; Stover, S.M. Arena surface vertical impact forces vary with surface compaction. *Vet. J.* **2023**, *293*, 105955. [CrossRef] [PubMed]
21. Hernlund, E.; Egenvall, A.; Hobbs, S.J.; Peterson, M.L.; Northrop, A.J.; Bergh, A.; Martin, J.H.; Roepstorff, L. Comparing subjective and objective evaluation of show jumping competition and warm-up arena surfaces. *Vet. J.* **2017**, *227*, 49–57. [CrossRef]
22. Setterbo, J.J.; Chau, A.; Fyhrie, P.B.; Hubbard, M.; Upadhyaya, S.K.; Symons, J.E.; Stover, S.M. Validation of a laboratory method for evaluating dynamic properties of reconstructed equine racetrack surfaces. *PLoS ONE* **2012**, *7*, e50534. [CrossRef]
23. Back, W.; Pille, F. The role of the hoof and shoeing. In *Equine Locomotion*; Back, W., Clayton, H.M., Eds.; Saunders Elsevier: Philadelphia, PA, USA, 2013; pp. 147–174.
24. Rooney, J.R. Functional anatomy of the hoof. In *Equine Podiatry*; Floyd, A., Mansmann, R., Eds.; Saunders Elsevier: St. Louis, MO, USA, 2007; pp. 57–73.

25. Murray, R.C.; Dyson, S.J.; Tranquille, C.; Adams, V. Association of type of sport and performance level with anatomical site of orthopaedic injury diagnosis. *Equine Vet. J.* **2006**, *38*, 411–416. [CrossRef] [PubMed]
26. Cross, R. Measurements of the horizontal and vertical Speeds of tennis courts. *Sports Eng.* **2003**, *6*, 95–111. [CrossRef]
27. Chateau, H.; Holden, L.; Robin, D.; Falala, S.; Pourcelot, P.; Estoup, P.; Denoix, J.-M.; Crevier-Denoix, N. Biomechanical analysis of hoof landing and stride parameters in harness trotter horses running on different tracks of a sand beach (from wet to dry) and on an asphalt road. *Equine Vet. J.* **2010**, *42*, 488–495. [CrossRef]
28. Orlande, O.; Hobbs, S.J.; Martin, J.H.; Owen, A.G.; Northrop, A.J. Measuring hoof slip of the leading limb on jump landing over two different equine arena surfaces. *Comp. Exerc. Physiol.* **2012**, *8*, 33–39. [CrossRef]
29. Medoff, H. Problems in defining and measuring friction on natural and artificial playing surfaces. In Proceedings of the 1995 Fourteenth Southern Biomedical Engineering Conference, Shreveport, LA, USA, 7–9 April 1995; pp. 171–174. [CrossRef]
30. Nigg, B.M.; Yeadon, M.R. Biomechanical aspects of playing surfaces. *J. Sports Sci.* **1987**, *5*, 117–145. [CrossRef]

animals

MDPI

Article

Investigation of Thresholds for Asymmetry Indices to Represent the Visual Assessment of Single Limb Lameness by Expert Veterinarians on Horses Trotting in a Straight Line

Claire Macaire [1,2,3,*], Sandrine Hanne-Poujade [1], Emeline De Azevedo [2], Jean-Marie Denoix [2], Virginie Coudry [2], Sandrine Jacquet [2], Lélia Bertoni [2], Amélie Tallaj [2], Fabrice Audigié [2], Chloé Hatrisse [2], Camille Hébert [1], Pauline Martin [1], Frédéric Marin [3] and Henry Chateau [2]

1 LIM France, Labcom LIM-ENVA, 24300 Nontron, France
2 Ecole Nationale Vétérinaire d'Alfort, USC INRAE-ENVA 957 BPLC, CIRALE, 94700 Maisons-Alfort, France
3 Laboratoire de BioMécanique et BioIngénierie (UMR CNRS 7338), Centre of Excellence for Human and Animal Movement Biomechanics (CoEMoB), Université de Technologie de Compiègne (UTC), Alliance Sorbonne Université, 60200 Compiègne, France
* Correspondence: claire.macaire@vet-alfort.fr

Simple Summary: Visual gait evaluation made by the equine veterinarian is an essential part of the diagnosis of locomotor disorders. Measurement of movement asymmetry can provide objective support for diagnosis. However, their interpretation remains complex as horses considered to be healthy may show some degree of asymmetry. This study aims to establish and analyze the threshold values for different indices that can be used to discriminate a healthy horse from a horse considered lame by expert clinicians in their daily practice. At least 88% of healthy horses had an upward range of movement of the withers between −10% and 7% of asymmetry. The withers asymmetry of at least 84% of the forelimb lame horses was out of these thresholds. As well, at least 86% of healthy horses had an upward range of movement of the pelvis between −7% and 18% of asymmetry. At least 83% of the hindlimb lame horses were out of these pelvis asymmetry thresholds. Despite the quite low number of horses included in this study (224), these thresholds provide a first help to avoid overinterpretation of asymmetry when using objective gait analysis systems.

Abstract: Defining whether a gait asymmetry should be considered as lameness is challenging. Gait analysis systems now provide relatively accurate objective data, but their interpretation remains complex. Thresholds for discriminating between horses that are visually assessed as being lame or sound, as well as thresholds for locating the lame limb with precise sensitivity and specificity are essential for accurate interpretation of asymmetry measures. The goal of this study was to establish the thresholds of asymmetry indices having the best sensitivity and specificity to represent the visual single-limb lameness assessment made by expert veterinarians as part of their routine practice. Horses included in this study were evaluated for locomotor disorders at a clinic and equipped with the EQUISYM® system using inertial measurement unit (IMU) sensors. Visual evaluation by expert clinicians allocated horses into five groups: 49 sound, 62 left forelimb lame, 67 right forelimb lame, 23 left hindlimb lame, and 23 right hindlimb lame horses. 1/10 grade lame horses were excluded. Sensors placed on the head (_H), the withers (_W), and the pelvis (_P) provided vertical displacement. Relative difference of minimal (AI-min) and maximal (AI-max) altitudes, and of upward (AI-up) and downward (AI-down) amplitudes between right and left stance phases were calculated. Receiver operating characteristic (ROC) curves discriminating the sound horses from each lame limb group revealed the threshold of asymmetry indice associated with the best sensitivity and specificity. AI-up_W had the best ability to discriminate forelimb lame horses from sound horses with thresholds (left: −7%; right: +10%) whose sensitivity was greater than 84% and specificity greater than 88%. AI-up_P and AI-max_P discriminated hindlimb lame horses from sound horses with thresholds (left: −7%; right: +18% and left: −10%; right: +6%) whose sensitivity was greater than 78%, and specificity greater than 82%. Identified thresholds will enable the interpretation of quantitative data from lameness quantification systems. This study is mainly limited by the number of included horses and deserves further investigation with additional data, and similar studies on circles are warranted.

Keywords: horse; lameness; symmetry; ROC curves; IMU

1. Introduction

Movement asymmetry is commonly used as an indicator of locomotor disorders by horses. Indeed, the aim of locomotor examination is to identify any impairment and to locate its source. Currently, lameness is visually evaluated by veterinarians. However agreement between veterinarians about lameness grade assessment is low, particularly for subtle lameness detection [1,2]. Modern gait analysis tools provide quantitative measures of asymmetry. The most versatile tool, the inertial measurement units (IMUs), can be used in a clinical setting [3,4]. The issue about the relationship between visual lameness assessment and gait asymmetries measurement systems has been raised. Asymmetry of vertical displacement of the head and pelvis has shown relevant increase with induced lameness [5–7]. But even horses perceived by the veterinarian to be sound have demonstrated physiological asymmetrical gait [8–10]. Despite the known capacity of withers asymmetry for detecting compensatory movements, it has been studied relatively less than the head [11,12].

In this context, thresholds of asymmetry parameters which correspond to visual evaluation of lameness by veterinarians have been studied. Asymmetry thresholds of the head (>6 mm) and the pelvic (>3 mm) vertical displacement were used for the first time by McCracken et al. [13]. They were probably based on a confidence interval calculated with two repeated measures on 236 horses [14]. These thresholds have been adjusted to the method of data construction used in other IMU systems [15]. A growing number of studies have used these thresholds as an objective lameness detection [11,12,16]. However numerous asymmetry values of sound horses have been over these thresholds [8,17,18]. This might be explained by undetected subclinical, pain-mediated disease or by biological variation, but no consensus has yet been reached [19,20]. Recently, a discrimination method of statistical analysis was applied on 25 Thoroughbred racehorses to redefine higher thresholds, (14.5 mm for the head and 7.5 mm for the pelvis) [21]. In this study, the focus was on specificity because the objective was to screen horses before racing. These results have given guidelines but require further investigations with heterogeneous horses and lameness types using a clinical environment faced by practitioners.

The goals of this clinical observational study were (i) to establish which asymmetry indices have the best sensitivity and specificity to reflect the visual assessment of single-limb lameness made by expert clinicians as part of their routine practice. (ii) Then, for the relevant indices, the aim was to determine the threshold of lameness detection and lame limb identification. This first study was limited to the following conditions: at trot, in hand, on a straight line and on a hard surface.

2. Materials and Methods

This clinical observational retrospective study was approved by the clinical research ethics committee (ComERC n○2022-01-19).

2.1. Horses

This study was conducted on horses (n = 224), presented at a clinic for locomotor evaluation from August 2019 until October 2021. The sample was composed of 46% females, 47% geldings and 7% stallions; 48% Selle Français, 7% KWPN, 5% trotters and 40% other breeds; 62% showjumpers, 11% dressage, 10% eventing, and 17% other disciplines; aged from 2 to 20 years (mean ± SD, 9 ± 3 years).

2.2. Locomotor Examination

After collecting the anamnesis and performing the examination of the locomotor system, the veterinarian evaluated the horse locomotion without warm-up. As part of the dynamic locomotor examination, horses were trotted by their owner/groom on a straight line of 25 meters long. The handler was asked to run at adequate speed and to keep a steady pace. The ground surface was made of asphalt. Visual evaluation was performed by one of the five expert veterinarians graduated as DESV (French certification as a specialist in equine locomotor pathology) and certified ISELP (International Society of Equine Locomotor Pathology). Based on this evaluation on the straight line, horses were classified into five groups: right forelimb (RF) lame, left forelimb (LF) lame, right hindlimb (RH) lame, left hindlimb (LH) lame, and sound horses.

In total, 381 horses were screened and were evaluated lame on a straight line. Among them, 209 horses showed lameness grade ranging between 2/10 (inclusive) and 6/10 (inclusive) on a 11-grades scale equivalent to the UK scale (where 0 is: Sound and 10 is: Non-weight bearing lameness) [22–24]. Horses showing lameness on multiple limbs on the straight line were excluded (n = 33). With these criteria, 67 horses showed RF lameness, 62 horses showed LF lameness, 23 horses showed RH lameness, and 23 horses showed LH lameness. Flowchart is provided as Figure S1. Lameness grades included in each group are summarized in Table 1.

Table 1. Number of horses showing a lameness depending on the location and the grade according to the 11-grades UK lameness scale. Mean ± SD[1] of lameness grade in each lame horses group.

Clinical Lameness Grade	2/10	3/10	4/10	5/10	6/10	Total	Mean ± SD
Right Forelimb lameness	35	9	17	4	2	67	1.5 ± 0.7
Left Forelimb lameness	40	9	7	4	2	62	1.4 ± 0.8
Right Hindlimb lameness	7	4	11	0	1	23	1.7 ± 0.5
Left Hindlimb lameness	7	6	5	1	4	23	1.8 ± 0.6

SD[1]—standard deviation.

Forty-nine horses were included in the group of "sound" horses. These sound horses have been presented at the clinic for pre-purchase examination or for gait evaluation prior to further training. In this group were included individuals who met all of the following criteria (1) and (2). (1) The sound horses were in training and judged by their owners to be capable of performing all the exercises required for their sport level. (2) A full locomotor examination of these horses by an expert clinician revealed no abnormalities deemed significant under any of the examination conditions. This examination included: walk, trot on a hard circle at both reins, on a hard straight line, four flexion tests (one for each limb), trot on a soft circle at both reins.

2.3. Data Collection

During the locomotor examination, as part of the clinical routine, horses were systematically equipped with the EQUISYM® (Arioneo, LIM France, Nouvelle-Aquitaine, France) system consisting of seven wireless IMUs placed on the head, the withers, the pelvis, and the four cannon bones (Figure 1). They recorded tri-axial angular velocity within a range of 2000°/s and tri-axial acceleration within a range of 16 g, at a frequency of 200 Hz during approximately two trot-ups, corresponding to a mean of 14.7 ± 7.8 trot strides on a straight line. Data were recorded on the sensors and downloaded wirelessly.

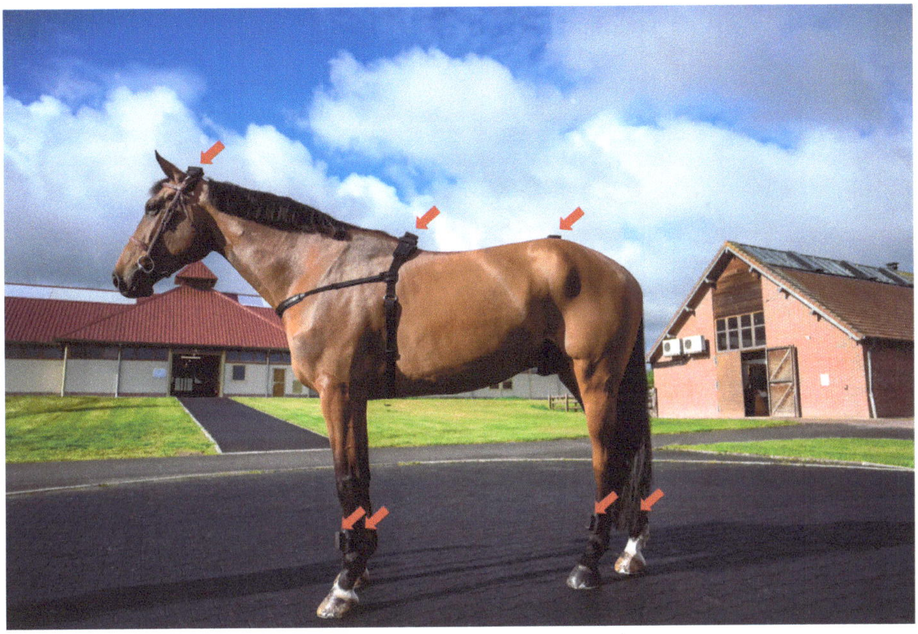

Figure 1. Horse equipped with EQUISYM® system, composed by sensors placed on the head, the withers, the pelvis and the four cannon bones (shown by the red arrows).

2.4. Data Processing

First, stance phase periods, e.g., foot-on and foot-off times, were determined based on the analysis of the gyroscopic signals recorded on the four cannon bones owing to the method developed by Hatrisse et al. [25]. One stride was defined as the time between two consecutive foot-on of the left forelimb.

Then vertical displacements of the head, withers and pelvis were segmented into strides. The acceleration signal measured along the dorso-ventral axis of the horse was integrated twice and high-pass filtered using a fourth-order Butterworth filter with a cut-off frequency set to 1 Hz to obtain displacement curves [4,26].

Based on the vertical displacement of the head (_H), withers (_W) and pelvis (_P) occurring along a stride, four variables were calculated for each sensor location. The following asymmetry indices (AI), expressed as a percentage of the maximal range of motion within a stride, were used to compare left vs. right part of the stride (Figure 2): AI-Min was the left-right difference of the lowest point of the vertical excursion; AI-Max was the left-right difference of the highest point of the vertical excursion; AI-up was the left-right difference of the upward range of motion during the propulsion phase; and AI-down was the left-right difference of the downward range of motion during the damping phase. Positive AI value indicated a smaller movement amplitude during the right stance than during left stance, and negative AI value indicated the opposite.

All calculations were performed with custom-made Matlab2020a (The MathWorks, Natick, MA, USA) scripts.

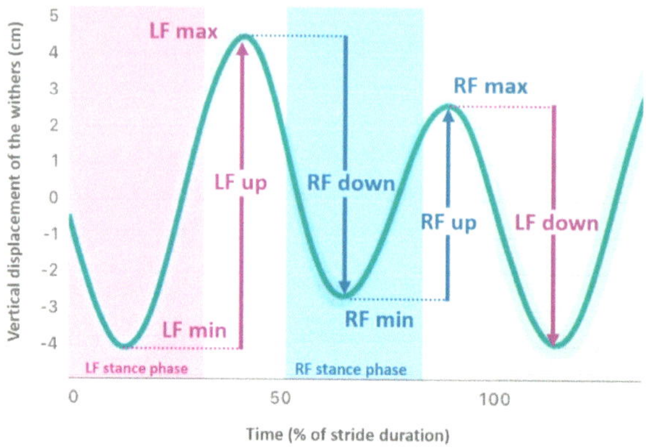

Figure 2. Mean vertical displacement (cm) of the withers plotted against time (expressed as % of stride duration) of a horse showing right forelimb (RF) lameness. Asymmetry Indices (AI) are: AI-min = RFmin-LFmin/LFup; AI-max = LFmax-RFmax/LFup; AI-up = LFup-RFup/LFup; AI-down = LFdown-RFdown/LFdown. (LF—Left Forelimb).

2.5. Data Analysis

Mean and standard deviation (SD) were calculated from data collected in each group. Normality was assessed using graphical methods [27]. Open software RStudio (RStudio Inc., Boston, MA, USA, version 4.1.3) was used, including the packages ROCR, pROC and boot. The four AIs calculated from head, withers, and pelvis were analyzed. Receiver operating characteristic (ROC) curves were plotted to discriminate each lame limb group (RF, LF, RH, LH) from the control group (sound horses). Area under curve (AUC) of the ROC curves was calculated. Then, thresholds with highest specificity and sensitivity using the top-left method were calculated. The top-left method involves choosing the threshold related to the curve point closest to the upper-left corner of the graph. 95% confidence interval (95% CI, which values are expressed into [;] in the text) was obtained from the repartition of the best specificities and sensitivities calculated for 400 samples, using the bootstrap method based on resampling to estimate the confidence interval [28]. In this study, indices were considered having good discrimination capacity if the sum of sensitivity and specificity was strictly higher than 150% [29].

3. Results

3.1. Descriptive Results

Mean ± SD for each AI and for each horse group are summarized in Table 2 and boxplots are plotted in Figure 3.

Means of the AIs in sound horses were close to 0% of asymmetry, particularly for the withers (AI-min = −3% ± 8%; AI-max = 2% ± 8%; AI-up = −1% ± 9% and AI-down = −3% ± 11%). The head (AI-min = −7% ± 29% and AI-up = −11% ± 29%) and pelvis (AI-min = 6% ± 8%, AI-up = 5% ± 13 % and AI-down = 5% ± 11%) showed higher absolute mean values than the withers. The negative sign of AIs for the withers and the positive sign of AIs for the pelvis expressed reduced range of movement during the LF and RH stance phase.

RF lame horses showed higher mean values (sign of a reduced movement on the right) than sound horses for all AIs of the head and withers, and discrete lower mean values (sign of a reduced movement on the left) for all AIs of the pelvis, except AI-down_P. Like a mirror, LF lame horses showed lower mean values than sound horses for all AIs of the head and withers, and higher mean values for all AIs of the pelvis, except AI-max_H and AI-down_P.

Horses with RH lameness showed higher mean values (sign of a reduced movement on the right) than sound horses for all AIs of the head and pelvis, except AI-down_P, and showed discrete lower mean values (sign of a reduced movement on the left) for all AIs of the withers. Like a mirror, LH lame horses showed lower mean values than sound horses for all AIs of the head and pelvis, except AI-max_H and AI-down_P, and they showed higher mean values for all AIs of the withers.

Table 2. Mean ± SD of AIs of the head, the withers and the pelvis in sound, RF lame, LF lame, RH lame, and LH lame horses trotting on a hard straight line.

Location	AI[1]	Sound	RF[2]	LF[3]	RH[4]	LH[5]
Head (_H)	AI-min_H (%)	−7 ± 29	34 ± 30	−41 ± 38	22 ± 18	−27 ± 33
	AI-max_H (%)	−4 ± 12	10 ± 17	−1 ± 27	−2 ± 16	−1 ± 27
	AI-up_H (%)	−11 ± 29	44 ± 36	−42 ± 36	21 ± 21	−28 ± 36
	AI-down_H (%)	−2 ± 29	31 ± 35	−29 ± 37	25 ± 21	−19 ± 32
Withers (_W)	AI-min_W (%)	−3 ± 8	16 ± 15	−17 ± 18	−6 ± 8	9 ± 13
	AI-max_W (%)	2 ± 8	8 ± 9	−5 ± 14	−2 ± 7	6 ± 12
	AI-up_W (%)	−1 ± 9	24 ± 20	−22 ± 14	−7 ± 13	15 ± 18
	AI-down_W (%)	−3 ± 11	9 ± 14	−10 ± 24	−4 ± 7	2 ± 15
Pelvis (_P)	AI-min_P (%)	6 ± 8	1 ± 8	7 ± 10	16 ± 12	−13 ± 19
	AI-max_P (%)	−1 ± 9	−8 ± 11	6 ± 12	14 ± 10	−25 ± 16
	AI-up_P (%)	5 ± 13	−7 ± 15	13 ± 16	30 ± 17	−38 ± 27
	AI-down_P (%)	5 ± 11	7 ± 11	0 ± 14	1 ± 15	10 ± 18

AI[1]—asymmetry indice, RF[2]—right forelimb, LF[3]—left forelimb, RH[4]—right hindlimb, LH[5]—left hindlimb.

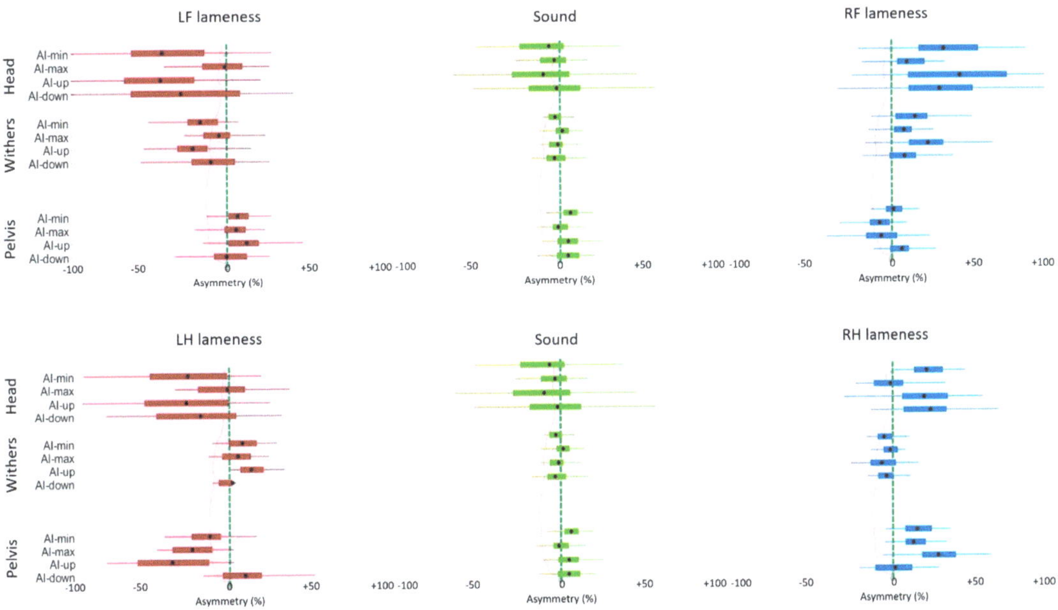

Figure 3. Boxplots of asymmetry indice (AI) in % for sound, left forelimb (LF), right forelimb (RF), left hindlimb (LH), and right hindlimb (RH) lame horses. The black dot represents the mean, the 2 extremities of the box are 25th and 75th percentiles, and extremities of the whiskers represent extreme data points not considered outliers. Negative value represents smaller movement on the left limb.

3.2. Forelimb Lameness Discrimination

ROC curves are presented in Figure 4 for forelimbs lameness discrimination. Calculated from these ROC curves, AUC, best sensitivity and specificity, and threshold associated are summarized in Table 3. ROC curves for RF lameness discrimination showed highest AUC values of 91% [95% CI, 85;96] (AI-up_W), 90% [84;95] (AI-up_H), 90% [83;95] (AI-min_W), and 86% [78;93] (AI-min_H). The lowest AUC values were of 55% (AI-down_P), 70% (AI-min_P), 72% (AI-max_P), and 72% (AI-down_W).

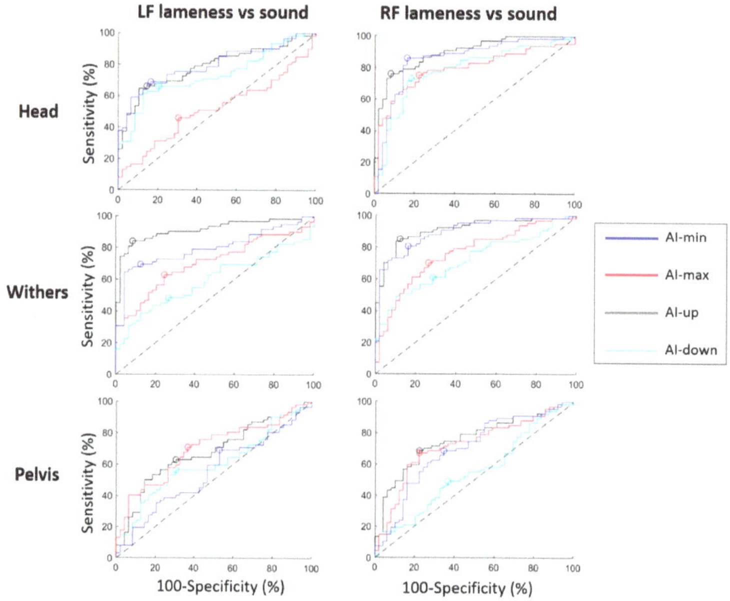

Figure 4. ROC curves discriminating horses with left forelimb (LF) lameness from sound horses; and discriminating horses with right forelimb (RF) lameness from sound horses, plotted for each sensor location (head, withers, pelvis); and plotted for asymmetry indice: AI-min (blue), AI-max (red), AI-up (black) and AI-down (cyan). The best specificity and sensitivity point of each curve is represented by a circle. The dashed black line is the hypothesized ROC curve with discrimination capacity only due to perfect chance.

Table 3. Area under the curve (AUC) of the receiver operating characteristic (ROC) curve discriminating sound and forelimb lame horses, for each asymmetry indice (AI). Best sensitivity, specificity, and associated threshold were calculated using top-left method of ROC analysis. [95% confidence interval] were calculated plotting ROC analysis on 400 population resamplings (bootstraps). Results for which the sum of sensitivity and specificity is over 150% for both sides are in bold.

AI	AUC RF[1] (%)	Sensitivity RF (%)	Specificity RF (%)	Threshold RF (%)	AUC LF[2] (%)	Sensitivity LF (%)	Specificity LF (%)	Threshold LF (%)
AI-min_H	**86 [78;93]**	**86 [78;95]**	**84 [73;92]**	**6 [−6;13]**	**79 [71;87]**	**69 [54;78]**	**84 [73;96]**	**−30 [−38;−24]**
AI-max_H	79 [70;87]	75 [64;86]	78 [63;87]	5 [−1;10]	48 [38;59]	46 [29;53]	69 [53;87]	−10 [−24;−4]
AI-up_H	**90 [84;95]**	**76 [62;81]**	**92 [85;100]**	**24 [14;45]**	**79 [70;87]**	**66 [51;76]**	**86 [74;100]**	**−36 [−49;−26]**
AI-down_H	79 [70;87]	73 [61;81]	82 [70;94]	17 [10;25]	73 [65;83]	66 [56;79]	80 [66;85]	−25 [−29;−18]
AI-min_W	**90 [83;95]**	**81 [68;90]**	**84 [71;93]**	**3 [−2;6]**	**79 [71;87]**	**69 [57;79]**	**88 [77;98]**	**−10 [−14;−8]**
AI-max_W	77 [68;86]	70 [56;81]	73 [59;85]	6 [3;9]	71 [61;79]	63 [48;72]	76 [65;89]	−2 [−6;0]
AI-up_W	**91 [85;96]**	**85 [77;93]**	**88 [78;95]**	**7 [1;10]**	**91 [85;95]**	**84 [74;91]**	**92 [84;100]**	**−10 [−13;−8]**
AI-down_W	72 [61;80]	61 [41;75]	71 [49;89]	1 [−7;7]	58 [48;69]	48 [22;58]	73 [56;100]	−8 [−16;−4]
AI-min_P	70 [59;78]	69 [56;85]	65 [45;74]	4 [1;7]	55 [43;64]	69 [59;95]	47 [18;54]	5 [−2;7]
AI-max_P	72 [63;81]	67 [55;77]	78 [66;89]	−5 [−7;−4]	70 [60;79]	71 [58;86]	63 [44;73]	1 [−2;4]
AI-up_P	76 [67;84]	69 [55;78]	78 [66;90]	−3 [−7;0]	67 [57;77]	63 [52;77]	69 [48;76]	10 [6;13]
AI-down_P	55 [44;67]	49 [32;59]	63 [48;78]	7 [4;12]	61 [50;71]	56 [47;68]	69 [53;81]	1 [−3;6]

RF[1]—right forelimb, LF[2]—left forelimb. Results for which the sum of sensitivity and specificity is over 150% for both sides are in bold.

As well, ROC curves for LF lameness discrimination showed highest AUC values of 91% [85;95] (AI-up_W), 79% [71;87] (AI-min_W), 79% [71;87] (AI-min_H), and 79% [70;87] (AI-up_H). The lowest AUC values were of 48% (AI-max_H), 55% (AI-min_P), 58% (AI-down_W), and 61% (AI-down_P).

For RF and LF lameness respectively, thresholds of +7% [+1;+10] and −10% [−13;−8] of asymmetry for AI-up_W resulted in 85% [77;93] and 84% [74;91] sensitivity and 88% [78;95] and 92% [84;100] specificity respectively.

3.3. Hindlimb Lameness Discrimination

ROC curves are presented in Figure 5 for hindlimbs lameness discrimination. Calculated from these ROC curves, AUC, best sensitivity and specificity, and threshold associated are summarized in Table 4. ROC curves for RH lameness discrimination showed highest AUC values of 88% [77;95] (AI-max_P), 86% [74;95] (AI-up_P), 84% [75;93] (AI-min_H), 81% [71;91] (AI-up_H), and 80% [69;89] (AI-down_H). The lowest AUC values were of 51% (AI-max_H), 54% (AI-down_W), 59% (AI-max_W), 62% (AI-up_W and AI-min_W).

As well, ROC curves for LH lameness discrimination showed highest AUC values of 96% [90;99] (AI-up_P), 89% [80;96] (AI-max_P), 89% [77;98] (AI-min_P). The lowest AUC values were of 48% (AI-max_H), 55% (AI-down_W), 57% (AI-down_P), and 58% (AI-down_H).

For RH and LH lameness respectively, a threshold of +18% [+16;+27] and −7% [−12;+2] of asymmetry for AI-up_P resulted in 83% [65;91] and 91% [82;100] sensitivity, and 90% [82;100] and 86% [69;91] specificity. Thresholds of +6% [+2;+8] and −10% [−19;−6] of asymmetry for AI-max_P resulted in 87% [75;100] and 78% [59;86] sensitivity, and 82% [64;88] and 88% [78;100] specificity respectively.

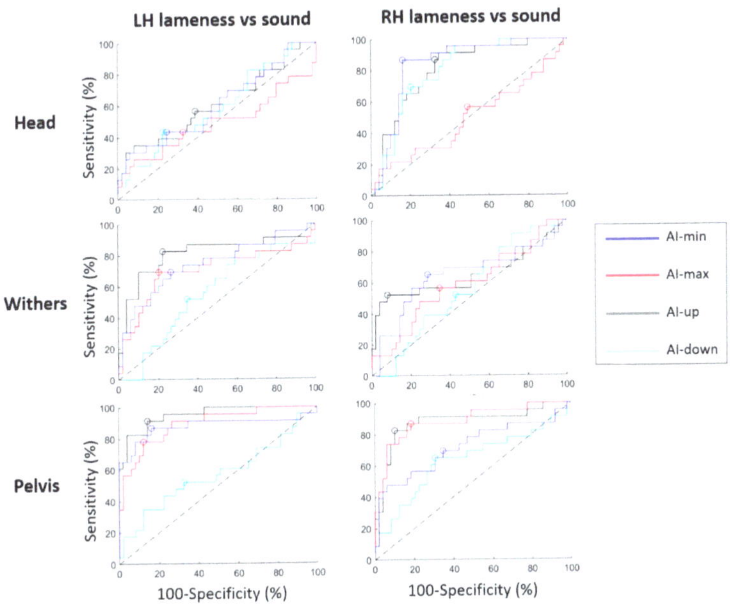

Figure 5. ROC curves discriminating horses with left hindlimb (LH) lameness from sound horses; and discriminating horses with right hindlimb (RH) lameness from sound horses, plotted for each sensor location (head, withers, pelvis); and plotted for asymmetry indice: AI-min (blue), AI-max (red), AI-up (black), and AI-down (cyan). The best specificity and sensitivity point of each curve is represented by a circle. The dashed black line is the hypothesized ROC curve with discrimination capacity only due to perfect chance.

Table 4. Area under the curve (AUC) of the receiver operating characteristic (ROC) curve discriminating sound and hindlimb lame horses, for each asymmetry indice (AI). Best sensitivity, specificity and associated threshold were calculated using top-left method of ROC analysis. [95% Confidence Interval] were calculated plotting ROC analysis on 400 population resamplings (bootstraps). Results for which the sum of sensitivity and specificity is over 150% for both sides are in bold.

AI	AUC RH[1] (%)	Sensitivity RH (%)	Specificity RH (%)	Threshold RH (%)	AUC LH[2] (%)	Sensitivity LH (%)	Specificity LH (%)	Threshold LH (%)
AI-min_H	84 [75;93]	87 [73;100]	84 [73;95]	8 [4;11]	60 [45;76]	43 [6;47]	76 [64;100]	−25 [−53;−16]
AI-max_H	51 [36;66]	57 [34;70]	51 [23;63]	−5 [−14;3]	48 [32;66]	43 [17;45]	67 [47;84]	3 [−2;24]
AI-up_H	81 [71;91]	87 [74;100]	67 [47;75]	−1 [−18;7]	60 [46;75]	57 [37;73]	61 [33;78]	−19 [−42;6]
AI-down_H	80 [69;89]	70 [41;77]	80 [67;100]	16 [8;35]	58 [43;73]	43 [8;49]	78 [66;100]	−22 [−53;−14]
AI-min_W	62 [47;76]	65 [46;82]	71 [55;83]	−6 [−10;−3]	75 [61;86]	70 [50;85]	73 [57;86]	0 [−4;3]
AI-max_W	59 [43;72]	57 [37;70]	65 [46;79]	0 [−4;3]	70 [55;84]	70 [51;88]	80 [66;92]	7 [4;9]
AI-up_W	62 [46;76]	52 [29;64]	92 [74;100]	−11 [−21;−5]	81 [67;92]	83 [70;100]	78 [59;87]	3 [−6;7]
AI-down_W	54 [41;68]	52 [20;64]	57 [37;75]	−5 [−12;−1]	55 [41;69]	52 [19;59]	65 [53;90]	−7 [−13;−4]
AI-min_P	72 [58;84]	70 [53;91]	65 [33;78]	10 [1;15]	89 [77;98]	87 [76;100]	84 [68;90]	−1 [−4;5]
AI-max_P	**88 [77;95]**	**87 [75;100]**	**82 [64;88]**	**6 [2;8]**	**89 [80;96]**	**78 [59;86]**	**88 [78;100]**	**−10 [−19;−6]**
AI-up_P	**86 [74;95]**	**83 [65;91]**	**90 [82;100]**	**18 [16;27]**	**96 [90;99]**	**91 [82;100]**	**86 [69;91]**	**−7 [−12;2]**
AI-down_P	64 [49;77]	65 [47;84]	69 [54;81]	0 [−3;4]	57 [42;71]	52 [33;63]	67 [47;82]	9 [2;17]

RH[1]—right hindlimb, LH[2]—left hindlimb. Results for which the sum of sensitivity and specificity is over 150% for both sides are in bold.

3.4. Asymmetry Thresholds of Reliable Indices

With a sum of sensitivity and specificity over 150%, head (AI-min_H and AI-up_H) and withers (AI-min_W and AI-up_W) indices discriminated the LF lame horses from sound horses. As well, head (AI-min_H, AI-max_H, AI-up_H, and AI-down_H) and withers (AI-min_W and AI-up_W) indices discriminated the RF lame horses from sound horses.

With a sum of sensitivity and specificity over 150%, withers (AI-up_W) and pelvis (AI-min_P, AI-max_P, and AI-up_P) indices discriminated the LH lame horses from sound horses. As well, head (AI-min_H and AI-up_H) and pelvis (AI-max_P and AI-up_P) indices discriminated the RH lame horses from sound horses.

Thresholds and their 95% CI associated with a sum of sensitivity and specificity over 150% for both right and left lameness discrimination were plotted in Figure 6.

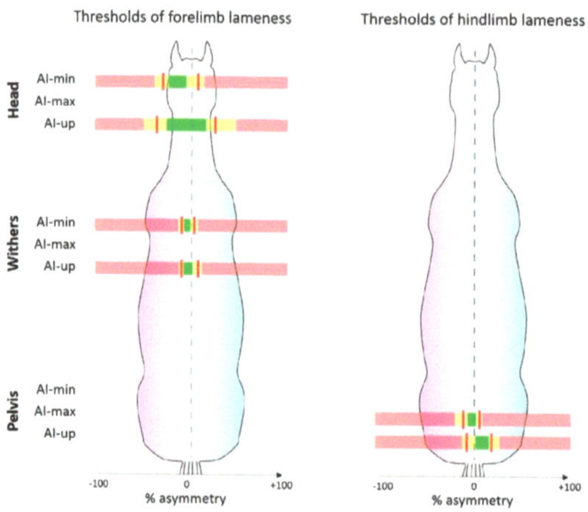

Figure 6. Thresholds (red line) of asymmetry indices (AI) (in % of asymmetry) for forelimb and hindlimb lameness discrimination. Only the AIs with the sum of sensitivity and specificity over 150% for both right and left lameness are plotted. Three range of values are represented: yellow for 95% confidence interval (95% CI) around the threshold, green for values below the 95% CI ("sound" horses) and red for values beyond the 95% CI ("lame" horses).

4. Discussion

Description of AIs provided by the head, withers, and pelvis from sound horses showed that almost no asymmetry was detected on the withers, whereas head and pelvis showed slightly lower range of movement during the RF-LH stance phase. In lame horses, the withers and pelvis showed reduced range of movement during the stance phase of respectively the front and hind lame limb. The head also showed reduced movement during the stance phase of a lame forelimb. Conversely, the head showed increased movement during the stance phase of a lame hindlimb.

Our study confirms the hypothesis that head and withers vertical displacements are indicators of forelimb lameness. Indeed, head indices (AI-min_H, AI-up_H) and withers indices (AI-min_W and AI-up_W) are the indices with the highest sensitivity and specificity (sum of sensitivity and specificity greater than 150%) for discriminating horses with forelimb lameness from sound horses. Among them, AI-up_W discriminated forelimb lameness with the highest sensitivity (>84%) and specificity (>88%).

For hindlimb lameness, pelvic vertical displacement was the most consistent indicator. Withers and head vertical displacement were also modified, with compensatory movements but only indices from the pelvis (AI-max_P and AI-up_P) discriminated both sides hindlimb lameness with sensitivity over 78% and specificity over 82%.

Among the four indices (AI-up, AI-max, AI-min, AI-down) used in this study, it was shown that AI-down indice has systematically a low sensitivity and specificity for discriminating both hindlimb and forelimb lame horses from sound horses. This result suggests that the AI-down indice should not be considered as the most useful indice in future work.

Main results give the following guidelines: associated with the highest sensitivity and specificity, AI-up_W discriminates LF lame horses under −10% of asymmetry and RF lame horses over +7% of asymmetry from sound horses. Associated with the highest sensitivity and specificity, AI-up_P discriminates LH lame horses under −7% of asymmetry and RH lame horses over +18% of asymmetry from sound horses. These observations confirm that the upward movement of the pelvis has the highest power to discriminate hindlimb lameness [30].

Higher relevance of the withers data than the head data contradicts previous studies [5,21]. Head shows greater movement asymmetry than withers, helping the visual assessment for forelimb lameness. However, the head is subjected to random movements existing in restless horses [7,8,10,31]. This study demonstrates that the withers movement provides useful and relevant information to detect forelimb lameness. Although having a lower reliability, head movement indices provide additional information useful to differentiate forelimb and hindlimb lameness [11,32].

Moreover, absolute threshold values of the head asymmetry were different in our study between the right and the left side of lameness discrimination (AI-up_H: +24% for RF vs. −36% for LF; AI-min_H: +6% for RF vs. −33% for LF). This difference may reflect different types of lameness between the RF and the LF lame horses in our reference population. This difference could also reflect an artefactual reduced movement of the head during the LF stance phase, compared to the RF stance phase for sound horse. Explanation could be found because horses were trotted in-hand on their left side by their owner or groom. This artefactual asymmetry may be induced by the handler despite instructions not to hold the head too firmly and to release the lunge. The head was either pulled forward, either hold backward depending on the spontaneous speed of the horse. This difference was not highlighted in other studies, which were maybe performed under more standardized conditions [33]. To a lesser extent, a similar phenomenon to the other side appeared on the pelvis in sound horses (AI-min_P mean of +6%; AI-up_P +5%; AI-down_P +5%).

Here AIs were divided by the range of movement, generating relative indices expressed in %. Values in millimeters are also provided in Table S1. Normalizing values seems natural in order to compare movement measured in a heterogeneous population, possibly including ponies. In addition, normalizing may lead to an easier comparison of asymmetry indices processed by different gait analysis systems [15,34]. Previous studies [13,21] have however expressed thresholds in millimeters. Pfau et al. [21] found that the threshold of HDmin was 14.5 mm for forelimb lameness discrimination. As well, PDmax discriminated hindlimb lameness from 10 mm with a low sensitivity. Contrary to our results, PDmin was more reliable than PDmax, and the head was more reliable than the withers. Pfau et al. focused on specificity in a selection context (racing Thoroughbreds for the purpose of "lameness screening") where false positives should be avoided. Conversely, in a clinical context, a fair balance between sensitivity and specificity must be found to limit both false positives (inducing unnecessary costly investigations and anxiety of the owner) and false negatives [21]. This choice may explain differences with the results of Pfau et al. [21]. Other differences were: the lack of differentiation between right and left lameness, the study of a homogeneous population, and the subjective evaluation made by five assessors using video.

In the present study, we noticed that forelimb lameness also decreased the pelvic vertical range of motion during the lame limb stance phase. This observation has been previously noticed in other studies [35,36]. LH lameness showed a small impact on the head but decreased the withers movement during RF stance phase. Contrary to LH lameness, RH lameness increased the head movement during LF stance phase. This supports the hypothesis that the head, the withers, and the pelvis provide complementary information about the lameness location [11,37].

The low number of hindlimb lame horses (23 RH and 23 LH) may induce a bias. Furthermore, all lameness were included regardless of the type of injury diagnosed. It is obvious that some indices may be more or less modified according to the type of injury. To go further, more horses and specific groups for each type of diagnosed injury or clinical manifestation will be needed. This must be in the future roadmap.

Another limitation of this study is the clinical reference used to detect lame horses from non-lame horses and single limb lameness vs. multi-limbs lameness because this clinical assessment is recognized by definition as being subjective [2]. In the present study, visual examination of lameness by expert clinicians in the real context of the clinical examination, in the field, has been chosen as a reference to establish thresholds and calculate their sensitivity and specificity. This choice must, of course, be discussed as it is well known that visual assessment by experts is subject to many uncertainties (e.g., lack of repeatability and reproducibility) [1]. Visual assessment is not considered a "gold standard" in the present study, but only as a reference to what exists in the best possible conditions. In order for clinicians to appropriate the tools for quantifying locomotor asymmetries, it seems indeed necessary to give them an idea of the threshold values which, on these devices, correspond to what they are used to seeing and concluding subjectively with the classical (even imperfect) methods. This first step seems necessary because it is only once these benchmarks have been established that real progress can be made in interpreting the data from the quantification systems. The challenge here is to avoid the slightest asymmetry measured by a quantification system from being mistaken for lameness. It should indeed be remembered that the definition of lameness refers to a veterinarian's diagnosis and not to a machine. The machine can only be considered as a quantitative aid to a multi-factorial medical decision. In this study, the real condition of clinical routine was deliberately chosen in order to reflect the real-life examination of lame horses. Five highly experienced veterinarians were involved. Their experience and their identical and consistent method of assessment are likely to increase the agreement rate [35,38], although this result can be discussed [1]. The agreement could for example be slightly increased if the experts had not been informed of the owner's request. In this context, the lowest grade of lameness (1/10) was deliberately excluded because of weaker agreement for very subtle asymmetries [1].

5. Conclusions

Although quite small 95% CIs were found, an increased number of horses improved threshold accuracy. This study highlights the most relevant indices (AI-up_W for forelimb lameness and AI-up_P for hindlimb lameness) and indicates an order of magnitude of the thresholds and their 95% CIs. These thresholds can be used as a first support to discriminate between lame (from grade 2/10) and non-lame horses, bearing in mind the value of the 95% CIs which prohibits the use of these thresholds as an absolute cut-off value. In any case, these indicators can only be interpreted in the light of a global clinical expertise taking into account that there is not only one type of lameness but multiple clinical manifestations of locomotor disorders depending on the type of lesion. Subtle lameness (1/10 grade) have not been included here; further studies are warranted to refine the thresholds for horses with subtle lameness.

Moreover, forelimb and hindlimb lameness were analyzed separately and multi-limb lame horses were excluded. It should therefore be kept in mind that the interrelationship between the movements of the head, withers, and pelvis still requires further work. Future studies with multivariate analysis are needed to provide more information on the lame limb identification and relationship between the indices in various clinical circumstances.

In the longer term, the application of this study is aimed at a wider range of conditions in veterinary practice. A main limitation is that all measures were recorded under specific and standardized conditions. In the following years, further data are needed to refine lameness detection thresholds under conditions where physiological asymmetries are known to be higher (circles for instance) [38].

Supplementary Materials: The following supporting information can be downloaded at: https://www.mdpi.com/article/10.3390/ani12243498/s1. Figure S1: Flowchart of the exclusion/inclusion criteria of the screened horses, which were visually considered lame on a straight line by an expert veterinarian during his routine practice. Table S1: Table of the mean asymmetry indice (AI) in % and the mean of the non-normalized differences (Diff) in centimeters between minima and/or maxima of the vertical displacement of the head (_H), the withers (_W), and the pelvis (_P) for all horses included in the study at the trot on the straight line. These horses were visually assessed as sound, right forelimb (RF) lame, left forelimb (LF) lame, right hindlimb (RH) lame, or left hindlimb (LH) lame.

Author Contributions: Conceptualization, C.M., F.M., P.M. and H.C.; methodology, C.M., S.H.-P., F.M., P.M. and H.C.; software, C.M., S.H.-P., C.H. (Chloé Hatrisse) and C.H. (Camille Hébert); validation, C.M., S.H.-P., E.D.A. and C.H. (Camille Hébert); formal analysis, C.M. and S.H.-P.; investigation, E.D.A., J.-M.D., V.C., S.J., L.B. and A.T.; resources, E.D.A., J.-M.D., V.C., S.J., L.B., A.T., F.A., C.H. (Camille Hébert) and P.M.; data curation, C.M. and E.D.A.; writing—original draft preparation, C.M.; writing—review and editing, S.H.-P., F.A., F.M., P.M. and H.C.; visualization, C.M.; supervision, F.M., P.M. and H.C.; project administration, P.M. and H.C.; funding acquisition, P.M. All authors have read and agreed to the published version of the manuscript.

Funding: This research was funded by the Agence Nationale de la Recherche (LabCom "CWD-Vetlab", Contract ANR 16-LCV2-0002-01), the European Regional Development Fund (FEDER) and the Region Normandie (Project "EquiSym", Contract 20E01636).

Institutional Review Board Statement: The animal study protocol was approved by the Ethics Committee of COMITE D'ETHIQUE EN RECHERCHE CLINIQUE—ComERC (no2022-01-19).

Informed Consent Statement: Informed consent was obtained from the owner of all the subjects involved in the study.

Data Availability Statement: The data that support the findings of this study are available from the corresponding author upon reasonable request.

Acknowledgments: The authors thank the Centre d'Imagerie et de Recherche sur les Affections Locomotrices Equines (CIRALE). They also thank Alexandre Charles, Anne-Claire Idoux, Antoinette Terlinden and Alberto De la Rocha who actively contributed to the data collection.

Conflicts of Interest: The project was supported by the Agence Nationale de la Recherche (ANR) which sponsors a collaborative project between a company (LIM France) and the Ecole Nationale Vétérinaire d'Alfort (ENVA).

References

1. Keegan, K.G.; Dent, E.V.; Wilson, D.A.; Janicek, J.; Kramer, J.; Lacarrubba, A.; Walsh, D.M.; Cassells, M.W.; Esther, T.M.; Schiltz, P.; et al. Repeatability of subjective evaluation of lameness in horses: Repeatability of subjective evaluation of lameness in horses. *Equine Vet. J.* **2010**, *42*, 92–97. [CrossRef] [PubMed]
2. Starke, S.D.; Oosterlinck, M. Reliability of equine visual lameness classification as a function of expertise, lameness severity and rater confidence. *Vet. Rec.* **2019**, *184*, 63. [CrossRef] [PubMed]
3. Marin, F. Human and Animal Motion Tracking Using Inertial Sensors. *Sensors* **2020**, *20*, 6074. [CrossRef] [PubMed]
4. Warner, S.M.; Koch, T.O.; Pfau, T. Inertial sensors for assessment of back movement in horses during locomotion over ground: Inertial sensors for back movement. *Equine Vet. J.* **2010**, *42*, 417–424. [CrossRef]
5. Buchner, H.H.F.; Savelberg, H.H.C.M.; Schamhardt, H.C.; Barneveld, A. Head and trunk movement adaptations in horses with experimentally induced fore- or hindlimb lameness. *Equine Vet. J.* **1996**, *28*, 71–76. [CrossRef] [PubMed]
6. Kramer, J.; Keegan, K.G.; Kelmer, G.; Wilson, D.A. Objective determination of pelvic movement during hind limb lameness by use of a signal decomposition method and pelvic height differences. *Am. J. Vet. Res.* **2004**, *65*, 741–747. [CrossRef]
7. Keegan, K.G.; Pai, P.F.; Wilson, D.A.; Smith, B.K. Signal decomposition method of evaluating head movement to measure induced forelimb lameness in horses trotting on a treadmill. *Equine Vet. J.* **2010**, *33*, 446–451. [CrossRef]
8. Kallerud, A.S.; Fjordbakk, C.T.; Hendrickson, E.H.S.; Persson-Sjodin, E.; Hammarberg, M.; Rhodin, M.; Hernlund, E. Objectively measured movement asymmetry in yearling Standardbred trotters. *Equine Vet. J.* **2021**, *53*, 590–599. [CrossRef]
9. Greve, L.; Pfau, T.; Dyson, S. Thoracolumbar movement in sound horses trotting in straight lines in hand and on the lunge and the relationship with hind limb symmetry or asymmetry. *Vet. J.* **2017**, *220*, 95–104. [CrossRef]
10. Scheidegger, M.D.; Gerber, V.; Dolf, G.; Burger, D.; Flammer, A.; Ramseyer, A. Quantitative gait analysis before and after a cross-country test in a population of elite eventing horses. *J. Equine Vet. Sci.* **2022**, *117*, 104077. [CrossRef]
11. Rhodin, M.; Persson-Sjodin, E.; Egenvall, A.; Serra Bragança, F.M.; Pfau, T.; Roepstorff, L.; Weishaupt, M.A.; Thomsen, M.H.; van Weeren, P.R.; Hernlund, E. Vertical movement symmetry of the withers in horses with induced forelimb and hindlimb lameness at trot. *Equine Vet. J.* **2018**, *50*, 818–824. [CrossRef] [PubMed]
12. Reed, S.K.; Kramer, J.; Thombs, L.; Pitts, J.B.; Wilson, D.A.; Keegan, K.G. Comparison of results for body-mounted inertial sensor assessment with final lameness determination in 1224 equids. *J. Am. Vet. Med. Assoc.* **2020**, *256*, 590–599. [CrossRef] [PubMed]
13. McCracken, M.J.; Kramer, J.; Keegan, K.G.; Lopes, M.; Wilson, D.A.; Reed, S.K.; LaCarrubba, A.; Rasch, M. Comparison of an inertial sensor system of lameness quantification with subjective lameness evaluation: Comparison of inertial system with subjective lameness evaluation. *Equine Vet. J.* **2012**, *44*, 652–656. [CrossRef]
14. Keegan, K.G.; Kramer, J.; Yonezawa, Y.; Maki, H.; Pai, P.F.; Dent, E.V.; Kellerman, T.E.; Wilson, D.A.; Reed, S.K. Assessment of repeatability of a wireless, inertial sensor–based lameness evaluation system for horses. *Am. J. Vet. Res.* **2011**, *72*, 1156–1163. [CrossRef] [PubMed]
15. Pfau, T.; Boultbee, H.; Davis, H.; Walker, A.; Rhodin, M. Agreement between two inertial sensor gait analysis systems for lameness examinations in horses. *Equine Vet. Educ.* **2016**, *28*, 203–208. [CrossRef]
16. Kallerud, A.S.; Hernlund, E.; Byström, A.; Persson-Sjodin, E.; Rhodin, M.; Hendrickson, E.H.S.; Fjordbakk, C.T. Non-banked curved tracks influence movement symmetry in two-year-old Standardbred trotters. *Equine Vet. J.* **2021**, *53*, 1178–1187. [CrossRef]
17. Rhodin, M.; Egenvall, A.; Haubro Andersen, P.; Pfau, T. Head and pelvic movement asymmetries at trot in riding horses in training and perceived as free from lameness by the owner. *PLoS ONE* **2017**, *12*, e0176253. [CrossRef]
18. Movement asymmetries in 200 non-lame elite and non-elite horses during in-hand trot. *Equine Vet. J.* **2021**, *53*, 10. [CrossRef]
19. Weeren, P.R.; Pfau, T.; Rhodin, M.; Roepstorff, L.; Serra Bragança, F.; Weishaupt, M.A. Do we have to redefine lameness in the era of quantitative gait analysis? *Equine Vet. J.* **2017**, *49*, 567–569. [CrossRef]
20. Serra Bragança, F.M.; Rhodin, M.; van Weeren, P.R. On the brink of daily clinical application of objective gait analysis: What evidence do we have so far from studies using an induced lameness model? *Vet. J.* **2018**, *234*, 11–23. [CrossRef]
21. Pfau, T.; Sepulveda Caviedes, M.F.; McCarthy, R.; Cheetham, L.; Forbes, B.; Rhodin, M. Comparison of visual lameness scores to gait asymmetry in racing Thoroughbreds during trot in-hand. *Equine Vet. Educ.* **2020**, *32*, 191–198. [CrossRef]
22. May, S.A.; Wyn-Jones, G. Identification of hindleg lameness. *Equine Vet. J.* **1987**, *19*, 185–188. [CrossRef] [PubMed]
23. Dyson, S. Can lameness be graded reliably?: Can lameness be graded reliably? *Equine Vet. J.* **2011**, *43*, 379–382. [CrossRef] [PubMed]
24. Arkell, M.; Archer, R.M.; Guitian, F.J.; May, S.A. Evidence of bias affecting the interpretation of the results of local anaesthetic nerve blocks when assessing lameness in horses. *Vet. Rec.* **2006**, *159*, 346–348. [CrossRef] [PubMed]
25. Hatrisse, C.; Macaire, C.; Sapone, M.; Hebert, C.; Hanne-Poujade, S.; De Azevedo, E.; Marin, F.; Martin, P.; Chateau, H. Stance Phase Detection by Inertial Measurement Unit Placed on the Metacarpus of Horses Trotting on Hard and Soft Straight Lines and Circles. *Sensors* **2022**, *22*, 703. [CrossRef]
26. Pfau, T.; Witte, T.H.; Wilson, A.M. A method for deriving displacement data during cyclical movement using an inertial sensor. *J. Exp. Biol.* **2005**, *208*, 2503–2514. [CrossRef]
27. Oppong, F.B.; Agbedra, S.Y. Assessing Univariate and Multivariate Normality, A Guide For Non-Statisticians. *Math. Theory Model.* **2016**, *6*, 26–33.
28. Saporta, G. *Probabilités, Analyse des Données et Statistique*, 2nd ed.; révisée et augm.; Editions Technip: Paris, France, 2008; ISBN 978-2-7108-0814-5.

29. Power, M.; Fell, G.; Wright, M. Principles for high-quality, high-value testing. *Evid. Based Med.* **2013**, *18*, 5–10. [CrossRef]
30. Marunova, E.; Dod, L.; Witte, S.; Pfau, T. Smartphone-Based Pelvic Movement Asymmetry Measures for Clinical Decision Making in Equine Lameness Assessment. *Animals* **2021**, *11*, 1665. [CrossRef]
31. Hardeman, A.; Serra Braganca, F.M.; Koene, M.; Swagemakers, J.-H.; van Weeren, P.R.; Roepstorff, L. *Variation in Gait Symmetry Parameters in Sound Horses at Trot, on the Straight Line and on the Lunge*; Utrecht University: Utrecht, The Netherlands, 2018. [CrossRef]
32. Hardeman, A.M.; Egenvall, A.; Serra Bragança, F.M.; Koene, M.H.W.; Swagemakers, J.; Roepstorff, L.; Weeren, R.; Byström, A. Movement asymmetries in horses presented for prepurchase or lameness examination. *Equine Vet. J.* **2021**, evj.13453. [CrossRef]
33. Hopkins, S.; Pfau, T. Effect of Side of Handling on Movement Symmetry in Horses. *Equine Vet. J.* **2014**, *46*, 42. [CrossRef]
34. Serra Bragança, F.M.; Roepstorff, C.; Rhodin, M.; Pfau, T.; van Weeren, P.R.; Roepstorff, L. Quantitative lameness assessment in the horse based on upper body movement symmetry: The effect of different filtering techniques on the quantification of motion symmetry. *Biomed. Signal Process. Control* **2020**, *57*, 101674. [CrossRef]
35. Pfau, T.; Noordwijk, K.; Sepulveda Caviedes, M.F.; Persson-Sjodin, E.; Barstow, A.; Forbes, B.; Rhodin, M. Head, withers and pelvic movement asymmetry and their relative timing in trot in racing Thoroughbreds in training. *Equine Vet. J.* **2018**, *50*, 117–124. [CrossRef] [PubMed]
36. Audigié, F.; Pourcelot, P.; Degueurce, C.; Geiger, D.; Denoix, J.M. Fourier analysis of trunk displacements: A method to identify the lame limb in trotting horses. *J. Biomech.* **2002**, *35*, 1173–1182. [CrossRef] [PubMed]
37. Movement Symmetry of the Withers Can be Used to Discriminate Primary Forelimb Lameness From Compensatory Forelimb Asymmetry in Horses with Induced Lameness. *Equine Vet. J.* **2016**, *48*, 32–33. [CrossRef]
38. Pfau, T.; Jennings, C.; Mitchell, H.; Olsen, E.; Walker, A.; Egenvall, A.; Tröster, S.; Weller, R.; Rhodin, M. Lungeing on hard and soft surfaces: Movement symmetry of trotting horses considered sound by their owners: Movement symmetry on hard and soft surfaces on the lunge. *Equine Vet. J.* **2016**, *48*, 83–89. [CrossRef]

animals

MDPI

Article

Asymmetry Thresholds Reflecting the Visual Assessment of Forelimb Lameness on Circles on a Hard Surface

Claire Macaire [1,2,3], Sandrine Hanne-Poujade [1], Emeline De Azevedo [2], Jean-Marie Denoix [2], Virginie Coudry [2], Sandrine Jacquet [2], Lélia Bertoni [2], Amélie Tallaj [2], Fabrice Audigié [2], Chloé Hatrisse [2], Camille Hébert [1], Pauline Martin [1], Frédéric Marin [3] and Henry Chateau [2,*]

1 Labcom LIM-ENVA, LIM France, 24300 Nontron, France; claire.macaire@vet-alfort.fr (C.M.)
2 CIRALE, USC 957 BPLC, Ecole Nationale Vétérinaire d'Alfort, 94700 Maisons-Alfort, France
3 Laboratoire de BioMécanique et BioIngénierie (UMR CNRS 7338), Centre of Excellence for Human and Animal Movement Biomechanics (CoEMoB), Université de Technologie de Compiègne (UTC), Alliance Sorbonne Université, 60200 Compiègne, France
* Correspondence: henry.chateau@vet-alfort.fr

Simple Summary: Veterinary lameness examination commonly involves a visual evaluation of a horse trotting on a circle. Lameness detection can be aided by objective gait analysis, which is used to quantify the movement asymmetry of horses. However, the asymmetry thresholds defined for the trot on a straight line are not applicable to the circles because turning induces physiological asymmetric movement. Four Asymmetry Indices (AIs) were calculated to compare the vertical movement of the head and of the withers between the right limb movement and the left limb movement during a trot stride. This study aims to select the AIs with good discriminative power between a group of sound horses and a group of horses showing consistent unilateral lameness (grade > 1/10) across both circle directions (clockwise, counter clockwise) on a hard surface, and to define the optimal threshold value, based on sensitivity and specificity. Head vertical movement asymmetry showed the highest sensitivity and specificity to detect forelimb lameness when the lame limb was on the inside of the circle, while withers vertical movement asymmetry showed the highest sensitivity and specificity to detect forelimb lameness when the lame limb was on the outside of the circle.

Abstract: The assessment of lameness in horses can be aided by objective gait analysis tools. Despite their key role of evaluating a horse at trot on a circle, asymmetry thresholds have not been determined for differentiating between sound and lame gait during this exercise. These thresholds are essential to distinguish physiological asymmetry linked to the circle from pathological asymmetry linked to lameness. This study aims to determine the Asymmetry Indices (AIs) with the highest power to discriminate between a group of sound horses and a group of horses with consistent unilateral lameness across both circle directions, as categorized by visual lameness assessment conducted by specialist veterinarians. Then, thresholds were defined for the best performing AIs, based on the optimal sensitivity and specificity. AIs were calculated as the relative comparison between left and right minima, maxima, time between maxima and upward amplitudes of the vertical displacement of the head and the withers. Except the AI of maxima difference, the head AI showed the highest sensitivity (≥69%) and the highest specificity (≥81%) for inside forelimb lameness detection and the withers AI showed the highest sensitivity (≥72%) and the highest specificity (≥77%) for outside forelimb lameness detection on circles.

Keywords: horse; lameness; symmetry; receiver operating characteristic curves; inertial measurement unit; circle

1. Introduction

The evaluation of equine locomotion during a trot on a circle represents an essential component of the veterinary lameness assessment [1]. Indeed, the need to produce centripetal force on a circle and the resulting body lean angle induce specific forces on the limb and 3D joint movements compared to the straight line, like a higher loading force on the outside limb, and collateromotion and axial rotation in the digital joints [1,2]. These specific biomechanical constraints on the anatomical structures are considered to be responsible for a different symptomatology between the circle and the straight line [2]. Therefore, this condition provides key information to aid clinical decision making [1].

Nowadays, the assessment of lameness can be aided by objective gait analysis tools [3–6]. Essential for the clinical application of these tools, asymmetry thresholds have been defined to distinguish between non-lame and lame gait [7–12]. McCracken et al. [13] have determined a threshold of 6 mm for the difference in the vertical displacement of the head between the right stance phase and left stance phase for defining forelimb lameness on a straight line. Pfau et al. [14] have established another value for this threshold of 14.5 mm using another objective gait analysis system and in the specific context of screening Thoroughbreds in race training. Lastly, asymmetry thresholds for indices normalized with the Range Of Movement (ROM) have been determined for discriminating visually assessed forelimb lameness on the straight line [15]. In this study, it was shown that the asymmetry of the upward movement of the withers had the highest power to discriminate between sound and forelimb-lame horses. The associated thresholds were −7% asymmetry for left forelimb lameness and +10% asymmetry for right forelimb lameness. These thresholds were expressed in percentage contrary to the previous thresholds expressed in millimeters [13,14], as relative values can be seen as a better way of facilitating comparisons between horses of different sizes and between objective gait analysis systems with different signal processing [16]. Moreover, time-related indices of head movement have proven to be affected by forelimb lameness on a straight line [17–19].

Asymmetry thresholds for lameness detection determined on a straight line are not applicable on a circle [20]. Yet, their usefulness in this circumstance of locomotion is all the more crucial as a large proportion of the movements recorded on the circle must be considered as physiologically asymmetric [11,12,20–22]. It is therefore essential to highlight the boundary between the physiological asymmetric movement of the circle and an excessive asymmetric movement which should be considered pathological. Asymmetries measured in sound horses during lunging at trot have shown variation higher than previously defined threshold values [11,12,20–22]. This variation could be due to factors such as speed, radius and body lean angle, which have been identified as impacting the measurements [23,24].

Thresholds for lameness detection on circles would help the interpretation of asymmetry values provided by an objective gait analysis tool during the entire locomotor examination. The objectives of this study were (i) to select asymmetry indices with the highest sensitivity and specificity to reflect the visual assessment of a veterinary specialist and then (ii) to define the optimal asymmetry thresholds for the inside and outside forelimb lameness detection on circles on a hard surface.

2. Materials and Methods

This clinical observational retrospective study was approved by the Clinical Research Ethics Committee (ComERC n○2022-01-19).

2.1. Horses and Conditions

This study was conducted on horses that presented at the Equine Clinic (CIRALE) of the National Veterinary College of Alfort (Maisons-Alfort, France) for locomotor evaluation from April 2019 to February 2023. After collecting the anamnesis and performing the inspection and the palpation of the locomotor system, the veterinarian evaluated the horse locomotion without warm-up. As part of the dynamic locomotor examination, horses were trotted by their owner/groom on the lunge on a circle of 8–14 m diameter, on the left rein (counter clockwise direction) and then on the right rein (clockwise direction). The ground surface was made of hard rubber pavers. Visual evaluation was performed by one of the five veterinary specialists who graduated as DESV (French certification as a specialist in equine locomotor pathology) and were certified by the ISELP (International Society of Equine Locomotor Pathology).

In total, 574 horses were screened and were visually evaluated at lunge on the left rein and on the right rein on a hard surface. Among them, 95 horses showed left forelimb lameness (LF) and 122 horses showed right forelimb lameness (RF) on both reins. Horses showing a lameness grade of 1/10 or over 7/10 on a 0–10 grade scale equivalent to the UK scale (where 0 is sound and 10 is non-weight bearing lameness) on one rein were excluded [25–27]. After exclusion, 61 horses showed LF and 76 horses showed RF grade 2–7 lameness on both reins. Horses showing lameness on multiple limbs on one rein were excluded (n = 8). With these criteria, 57 horses showed LF lameness and 70 horses showed RF lameness on both reins. A flowchart is provided as a Supplementary Material (Figure S1). Lameness grades included in each group on both reins are summarized in Table 1.

Table 1. Number of horses showing lameness depending on the affected limb and the grade according to the 0–10 grade UK lameness scale. Mean ± SD [1] of lameness grade in each lame horse group.

Horses	Rein	2/10	3/10	4/10	5/10	6/10	7/10	Total	Mean ± SD [1]
Left forelimb lameness	Left rein (inside lameness)	18	8	23	3	4	1	57	3.5 ± 1.4
	Right rein (outside lameness)	30	10	10	1	5	1	57	3.0 ± 1.4
Right forelimb lameness	Left rein (outside lameness)	28	13	23	3	3	0	70	3.1 ± 1.2
	Right rein (inside lameness)	23	14	19	5	8	1	70	3.5 ± 1.4

SD [1]—Standard Deviation.

Thirty-one horses were included in the group of "sound" horses according to the following criteria: (1) the horses were in training and judged by their owners to be capable of performing all the exercises required for their sport level; (2) three of the five veterinary specialists independently watched blinded videos of the horse at walk and at trot, on a hard circle on both reins and on a hard straight line and did not notice any locomotion abnormalities in the entire video (<1/10 lameness grade).

2.2. Data Collection

During the locomotor examination, as part of the clinical routine, horses were systematically equipped with the EQUISYM® system (Arioneo, LIM France, Le Bouscat, France), described by Macaire et al. and Timmerman et al. [15,28]. Data were recorded during approximately 20 s of trot per direction (clockwise/counterclockwise). The trot is of particular interest because a stride is composed of two diagonal beats whether on a straight line or circling to left or right.

2.3. Data Processing

The data were processed following the methods described by Macaire et al. [15]. Briefly, based on the vertical displacement of the head (_H) and the withers (_W) occurring along a stride, the following asymmetry indices (AIs), expressed as a percentage of the maximal range of motion within a stride, were used to compare the left vs. right part of the stride (Figure 1): AI-Min, AI-Max and AI-up. Additionally, AI-Tmax was calculated as a time-related index, representing the left–right difference in the duration of the down–up cycle (the time between the two maxima) of the vertical displacement occurring before and after the stance phase. AI-Tmax was expressed as a percentage of the maximal time between two consecutive maxima. A positive AI value indicated a smaller movement amplitude or duration during the right stance than during the left stance, and a negative AI value indicated the opposite.

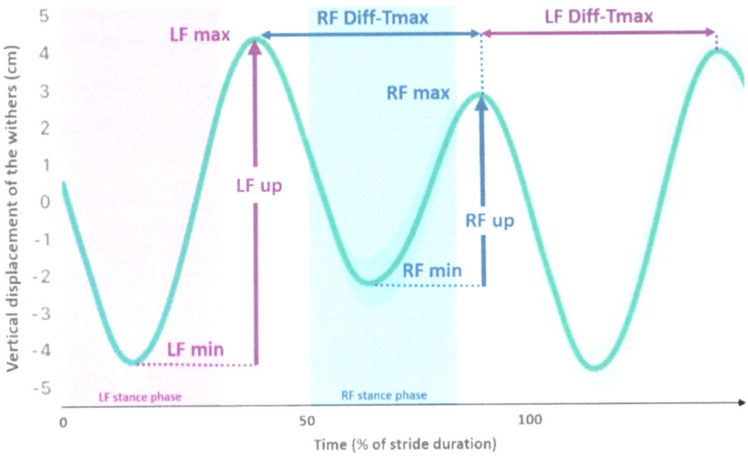

Figure 1. Mean vertical displacement (cm) of the withers plotted against time (expressed as percentage of stride duration) of a horse showing right forelimb (RF) lameness. Asymmetry Indices (AIs) are AI-min = RFmin−LFmin/LFup; AI-max = LFmax−RFmax/LFup; AI-up = LFup−RFup/LFup; and AI-Tmax = LFdiffTmax−RFdiffTmax/LFdiffTmax. (LF—Left Forelimb).

2.4. Data Analysis

Descriptive analyses, including mean and standard deviation (SD), were calculated for each variable, for each group (sound/lame) and for each condition (clockwise/counterclockwise direction). The four AIs calculated from the head and the withers were analyzed using the same methods as those described by Macaire et al. [15]. Normality was assessed using a graphical method [29]. Receiver Operating Characteristic (ROC) curves were plotted to discriminate, respectively, the right and left forelimb lame group (RF, LF) from the control group (sound horses) at lunge separately on the left and on the right rein. The AIs' discriminative power is indicated by the Area Under Curve (AUC) of the ROC curve. Given that AUC < 50% indicates discrimination no better than chance, higher AUC values (closer to 100%) indicate higher discriminative power. Finally, thresholds of indices with good discriminative power were calculated. In this study, indices were considered as having good discriminative power if the sum of sensitivity and specificity was strictly higher than 150% [30].

3. Results

3.1. Descriptive Results

The 158 horses included were 78 geldings, 72 females and 8 stallions; 94 Selle Français, 8 Zangersheide, 7 Hanoverian, 6 Koninklijk Warmbloed Paardenstamboek Nederland (KWPN), 6 French riding pony and 37 other breeds; 113 showjumpers, 12 dressage, 10 eventing and 23 other disciplines; and they were aged from 3 to 20 years (mean ± SD, 9 ± 3 years). Age, gender, breed and disciplines are detailed for each horse in the Supplementary Materials (Table S1). A mean ± SD of 20.4 ± 7.2 trot strides, 22.9 ± 5.8 on the right rein and 17.9 ± 7.6 on the left rein, were processed for each recording. The stride duration was 0.79 ± 0.05 s on both reins, respectively, and 0.80 ± 0.04 s for sound horses, 0.79 ± 0.04 s for RF lame horses and 0.78 ± 0.05 s for LF lame horses. The AIs of the head, the withers and the pelvis are detailed for each included horse in the Supplementary Materials: Table S2 shows AIs and ROM values measured on the left rein and Table S3 shows AIs and ROM values measured on the right rein.

The mean ± SD for each AI and for each horse group are summarized in Table 2 and boxplots are displayed in Figure 2. In sound horses, AIs calculated from the head (AI-min_H, AI-max_H and AI-up_H) were negative on the left rein and positive on the right rein, reflecting a reduced vertical range of motion of the head during the inside forelimb stance phase. AI-min of the withers also showed a reduced minimum (AI-min_W) during the inside forelimb stance phase. On the contrary, AI-max of the withers was positive on the left rein and negative on the right rein, reflecting a reduced maximum after the outside forelimb stance phase. Finally, in sound horses, the AI-Tmax of the head and of the withers, and AI-up of the withers were close to 0% of asymmetry on both reins.

Table 2. Mean ± SD of asymmetry indices (AIs) of the head and the withers in sound, left forelimb (LF) lame, right forelimb (RF) lame horses trotting on right rein and on left rein circles.

		Right Rein Circle			Left Rein Circle		
Location	AI	LF	Sound	RF	LF	Sound	RF
Head (_H)	AI-min_H (%)	−29 ± 39	7 ± 18	47 ± 32	−49 ± 26	−8 ± 20	28 ± 36
	AI-max_H (%)	−6 ± 34	16 ± 17	24 ± 23	−22 ± 28	−10 ± 14	9 ± 27
	AI-up_H (%)	−27 ± 48	22 ± 24	61 ± 32	−63 ± 28	−18 ± 25	31 ± 44
	AI-Tmax_H (%)	−15 ± 23	3 ± 9	28 ± 25	−26 ± 17	−2 ± 10	15 ± 21
Withers (_W)	AI-min_W (%)	0 ± 22	19 ± 10	36 ± 20	−28 ±24	−14 ± 11	4 ± 18
	AI-max_W (%)	−26 ± 16	−17 ± 12	−8 ± 16	15 ± 22	18 ± 8	26 ± 13
	AI-up_W (%)	−26 ± 25	2 ± 12	27 ± 22	−13 ± 21	4 ± 14	31 ± 19
	AI-Tmax_W (%)	−7 ± 9	0 ± 3	6 ± 9	−4 ± 9	0 ± 3	7 ± 6

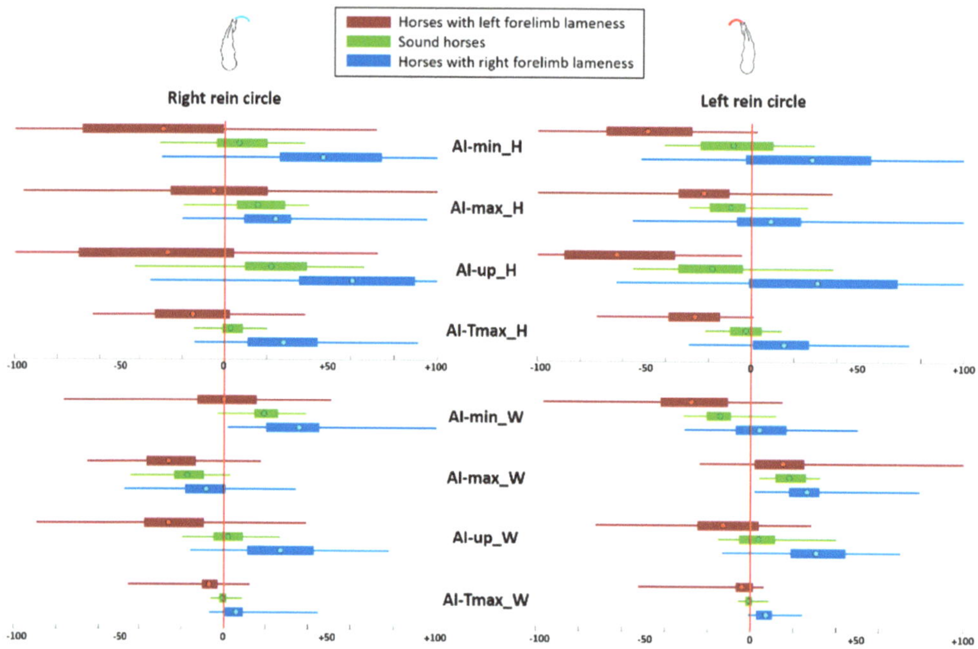

Figure 2. Boxplots of Asymmetry Indices (AIs) in percentage for sound horses and horses with a left forelimb lameness and right forelimb lameness. The dot represents the mean, the two extremities of the box are 25th and 75th percentiles, and extremities of the whiskers represent the minimum and maximum. A negative value reflects reduced movement or duration during the left limb stance, and positive value reflects reduced movement or duration during the right limb stance.

RF-lame horses showed higher mean values (sign of reduced movement on the right) than sound horses for all AIs of the head and withers. On the opposite hand, LF-lame horses showed lower mean values than sound horses for all AIs of the head and withers.

Horses with RF and LF lameness showed, respectively, positive and negative mean values (sign of reduced movement during the stance of the lame limb) for all AIs, except AI-max_W, when the lame limb was on the inside of the circle (RF at right rein and LF at left rein). When the lame limb was on the outside of the circle, AI-min_W was close to 0% of asymmetry.

3.2. Discrimination between Lame Horses with the Lame Forelimb on the Inside of the Circle and Sound Horses

ROC curves and associated results for the discrimination of forelimb lameness when the lame limb was on the inside of the circle (RF lameness on right rein and LF lameness on left rein) from sound horses are presented in Figure 3 and Table 3, respectively. The lowest AUC (lowest discrimination performance) value for the inside lameness detection was shown by the AI-max for the head (AUC $\leq$ 70%) and by the AI-max for the withers (AUC $\leq$ 67%). The indices with the highest AUC (AUC $\geq$ 83%) were in the following descending order: AI-min_H, AI-Tmax_H and AI-up_H for RF lameness on the right rein. For LF lameness on the left rein, the indices with the highest AUC (AUC $\geq$ 87%) were in the following descending order: AI-Tmax_H, AI-min_H and AI-up_H.

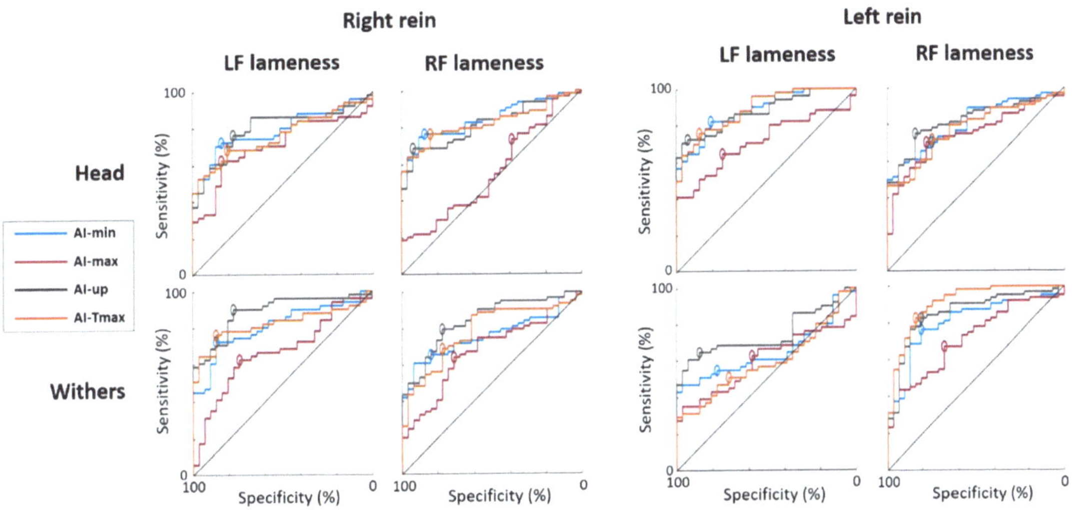

Figure 3. Receiver Operating Characteristic (ROC) curves discriminating horses with a constant Left Forelimb (LF) lameness from sound horses; and discriminating horses with a constant Right Forelimb (RF) lameness from sound horses, plotted for both reins on a circle. Tested Asymmetry Indices were AI-min (blue), AI-max (red), AI-up (grey) and AI-Tmax (orange). The highest specificity and sensitivity point of each curve is represented by a circle (top-left method). The black line is the hypothesized ROC curve with discriminative power only due to chance.

Table 3. Area Under the Curve (AUC) of the Receiver Operating Characteristic (ROC) curve discriminating forelimb lameness when the lame limb was on the inside of the circle from sound horses on circles, for each of the Asymmetry Indices (AIs). The highest sensitivity (Se), specificity (Sp) and associated threshold (Threshold) were calculated using the top-left method of ROC analysis. The 95% confidence intervals [;] were calculated by using a Bootstrap method, plotting ROC analysis on 400 population resamplings. Results for which the sum of sensitivity and specificity is over 150% for both circles (left and right reins) are in bold.

AI	Left Forelimb Lameness on the Left Rein (Inside Lameness on the Left Rein)				Right Forelimb Lameness on the Right Rein (Inside Lameness on the Right Rein)			
	AUC	Se	Sp	Threshold	AUC	Se	Sp	Threshold
AI-min_H (%)	**89 [83;94]**	**82 [72;94]**	**81 [65;90]**	**−25 [−30;−17]**	**86 [78;92]**	**79 [70;89]**	**87 [75;96]**	**23 [18;27]**
AI-max_H (%)	70 [60;80]	63 [47;76]	74 [57;89]	−17 [−25;−10]	57 [45;69]	74 [66;100]	39 [2;39]	9 [−11;12]
AI-up_H (%)	**87 [80;93]**	**72 [56;80]**	**94 [82;100]**	**−49 [−71;−37]**	**83 [74;90]**	**69 [54;78]**	**94 [84;100]**	**49 [41;65]**
AI-Tmax_H (%)	**90 [83;96]**	**79 [66;88]**	**87 [76;98]**	**−14 [−19;−11]**	**84 [76;91]**	**79 [70;90]**	**84 [71;95]**	**10 [6;12]**
AI-min_W (%)	66 [54;76]	53 [37;61]	87 [74;100]	−24 [−33;−19]	76 [67;86]	66 [52;77]	84 [69;97]	27 [24;32]
AI-max_W (%)	60 [49;73]	61 [46;83]	58 [23;71]	17 [11;25]	67 [56;77]	64 [48;74]	71 [56;88]	−11 [−15;−4]
AI-up_W (%)	76 [65;85]	67 [54;79]	81 [63;88]	−8 [−12;−3]	84 [76;91]	80 [69;92]	77 [62;88]	10 [4;14]
AI-Tmax_W (%)	61 [49;71]	60 [49;78]	61 [33;71]	−1 [−2;1]	79 [67;88]	67 [36;76]	77 [66;99]	2 [1;5]

3.3. Discrimination between Lame Horses with the Lame Forelimb on the Outside of the Circle and Sound Horses

The ROC curves and associated results for the discrimination of forelimb lameness when the lame limb was on the outside of the circle (LF lameness on right rein and RF lameness on left rein) from sound horses are presented in Figure 3 and in Table 4, respectively. The lowest AUC value for the outside lameness detection on the circle was shown by AI-max for the withers (AUC $\leq$ 71%) and by AI-max for the head (AUC $\leq$ 75%). The indices with the highest AUC (AUC $\geq$ 79%) were in the following descending order, AI-up_W, AI-Tmax_W, AI-up_H and AI-min_W, for LF lameness on the right rein. For RF lameness on the left rein, the indices with the highest AUC (AUC $\geq$ 81%) were in the following descending order: AI-Tmax_W, AI-up_W, AI-up_H and AI-min_W.

Table 4. Area Under the Curve (AUC) of the Receiver Operating Characteristic (ROC) curve discriminating forelimb lameness when the lame limb was on the outside of the circle from sound horses on circles, for each of the Asymmetry Indices (AIs). The highest sensitivity (Se), specificity (Sp) and associated threshold (Threshold) were calculated using the top-left method of ROC analysis. The 95% confidence intervals [;] were calculated by using a Bootstrap method, plotting ROC analysis on 400 population resamplings. Results for which the sum of sensitivity and specificity is over 150% for both circles (left and right reins) are in bold.

AI	Left Forelimb Lameness on the Right Rein (Outside Lameness on the Right Rein)				Right Forelimb Lameness on the Left Rein (Outside Lameness on the Left Rein)			
	AUC	Se	Sp	Threshold	AUC	Se	Sp	Threshold
AI-min_H (%)	79 [69;88]	70 [57;79]	84 [71;95]	−8 [−17;−1]	80 [73;88]	66 [45;75]	81 [63;98]	13 [0;34]
AI-max_H (%)	72 [60;82]	65 [50;75]	84 [73;99]	1 [−9;6]	75 [65;83]	70 [57;81]	77 [64;91]	−2 [−7;6]
AI-up_H (%)	**81 [71;90]**	**77 [62;89]**	**77 [61;89]**	**7 [−9;22]**	**82 [74;89]**	**74 [62;81]**	**84 [73;97]**	**0 [−9;11]**
AI-Tmax_H (%)	75 [65;85]	67 [55;79]	81 [65;91]	−3 [−7;4]	77 [68;85]	71 [57;82]	74 [59;88]	3 [−2;7]
AI-min_W (%)	**79 [71;89]**	**72 [60;82]**	**87 [75;99]**	**13 [11;15]**	**81 [72;89]**	**76 [63;86]**	**81 [66;94]**	**−7 [−12;−1]**
AI-max_W (%)	68 [57;79]	63 [49;75]	74 [59;88]	−23 [−28;−19]	71 [60;82]	66 [50;81]	68 [48;83]	22 [17;27]
AI-up_W (%)	**88 [81;95]**	**89 [81;100]**	**77 [60;85]**	**−5 [−9;1]**	**86 [78;93]**	**83 [73;94]**	**81 [65;89]**	**13 [5;17]**
AI-Tmax_W (%)	**81 [73;90]**	**74 [61;83]**	**87 [76;99]**	**−3 [−4;−3]**	**91 [86;97]**	**84 [72;93]**	**84 [71;94]**	**2 [1;3]**

3.4. Asymmetry Thresholds of Reliable Indices

For discriminating sound horses from lame horses with the lame limb on the inside of the circle, the indices with high sensitivity and specificity (sum of sensitivity and specificity greater than 150%) were three indices from the head (AI-up_H, AI-Tmax_H and AI-min_H). For discriminating forelimb lameness when the lame limb was on the outside of the circle, the indices with greater sensitivity and specificity were three indices from the withers (AI-up_W, AI-Tmax_W and AI-min_W) and one from the head (AI-up_H).

Figure 4 represents the thresholds and their 95% CI associated with a sum of sensitivity and specificity over 150% for inside (Figure 4a) and outside (Figure 4b) lameness discrimination on both reins.

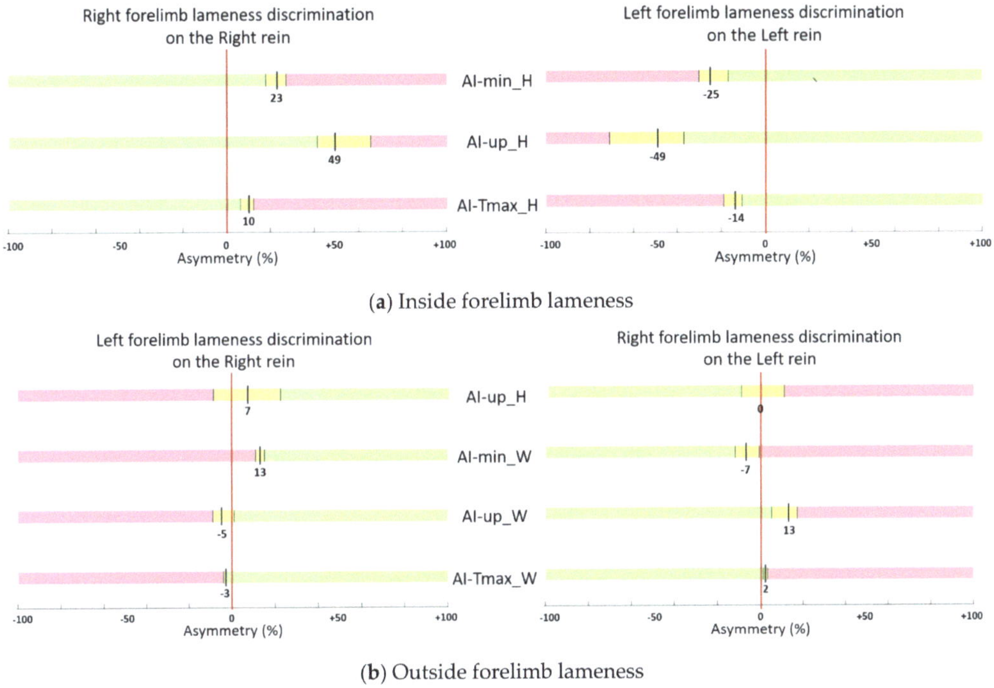

Figure 4. Thresholds (black line) of Asymmetry Indices (AIs) (in percentage of asymmetry) for lameness discrimination when the lame limb was on the inside of the circle (**a**) and when the lame limb was on the outside of the circle (**b**). Only the AIs with the sum of sensitivity and specificity over 150% for both right and left reins are plotted. Three ranges of values are represented: yellow for 95% confidence interval (95% CI) around the threshold, green for values below the 95% CI ("sound" horses) and red for values beyond the 95% CI ("lame" horses).

When comparing the absolute values of left rein and right rein thresholds for lameness discrimination when the lame limb was on the inside of the circle, the maximum difference between right and left rein was 4% of asymmetry for AI-Tmax_H (Figure 4a). When the lame limb was on the outside of the circle, the maximum difference between right and left was 8% of asymmetry for AI-up_W (Figure 4b).

4. Discussion

Asymmetry Indices (AIs) measured on sound horses showed a reduced head and withers movement during the inside forelimb stance phase, except for the AI-max of the withers. This goes with a larger downward movement of the trunk and head towards the outside forelimb, confirming the results of previous studies [12,22]. This physiological asymmetry observed on the circle means that we need to define the limit between a physiological asymmetry and an asymmetry that is amplified (or reduced) when a pathological phenomenon is superimposed.

Our study confirms the hypothesis that head and withers vertical displacements are indicators of forelimb lameness on the circle in a specific group of horses showing single-limb lameness on both reins, excluding a lameness grade of 1/10. In addition, the present study reveals that when the lame limb is inside the circle, head movements have the highest discriminative power. Conversely, when the lame limb is outside the circle, withers movements have the highest discriminative power. Practically, the AI-min and AI-Tmax of the head discriminated forelimb lameness when the lame limb was on the inside of the circle with the highest sensitivity (≥79%) and specificity (≥81%) on both reins. AI-up and AI-Tmax of the withers discriminated forelimb lameness when the lame limb was on the outside of the circle with the highest sensitivity (≥83% and ≥74%, respectively) and specificity (≥77% and ≥84%, respectively) on both reins.

Among the four indices (AI-min, AI-max, AI-up and AI-Tmax) used in this study, AI-max has systematically the lowest sensitivity and specificity for discriminating horses showing forelimb lameness on both reins from sound horses on a circle. In contrast, a previous study measured a reduced maximum altitude of the head after outside forelimb lameness induction [21]. There are several possible explanations for this discrepancy. On the one hand, the reference population for the two studies is not identical since we chose to concentrate on the lameness visible on both clockwise and counter clockwise circles. On the other hand, the type of lameness analyzed in the study by Rhodin et al. [21] was induced lameness (with a modified horseshoe) and not spontaneous lameness as in the present study.

Several studies describe variation in asymmetry but did not reach a consensus on the physiological asymmetry of sound horses induced by the circle [11,12,21,22]. Rhodin et al. [21] concluded a reduced head movement for the outside forelimb (HDmin). In 2016, Rhodin et al. [22] highlighted a non-uniform effect of the circle on the head. Other studies [11,12] showed results similar to those of the present study concerning physiological head asymmetry on a circle with a reduced head movement during the inside forelimb stance. The recorded asymmetries of the withers vertical displacements on sound horses trotting on a circle are consistent with a previous study [12] and showed a lowered minimum during and a reduced maximum after the stance phase of the outside forelimb. However, in the studies of Starke et al. [12] and Rhodin et al. [22], the inclusion criteria were based on the straight line and did not exclude visible lameness on the circle, meaning that some of the recorded asymmetries in their studies could be due to the apparition of a lameness on the circle that was not visible on the straight line.

Studies agree that forelimb lameness induces a reduced downward movement of the head (AI-min) during the stance phase of the lame limb [10,11,21,31], particularly for the inside lame limb when trotting on a circle [11,21,32]. The importance of the head movements for detecting the inside lameness and the withers for the outside lameness, as observed here, has been mentioned in the detailed results of a linear discriminant analysis discriminating positive and negative anesthesia realized by Pfau et al. [32]. They revealed that the minimum and upward movement asymmetry of the withers were the features with the most important weight to discriminate the anesthesia effect on the outside limb in circles on a hard surface, respectively, in each canonical discriminate function. Also, the minimum altitude of the head had the most important weight for the inside limb in the first canonical discriminate function. Marunova et al. [33], without the separation of outcomes from the inside and the outside limbs, measured significant differences in the head asymmetry indices and an upward withers asymmetry index before and after positive anesthesia.

No thresholds were previously determined for the locomotion on circles, allowing only comparisons with straight lines. For discriminating sound horses from lame horses with the lame limb on the inside of the circle, thresholds of head amplitude asymmetry (AI-up_H) showed higher values (−49% and +49% for respectively LF and RF lame limb) than thresholds for discriminating sound horses from lame horses established using similar methods on a straight line (−36% and +24% for respectively LF and RF lame limb) [15]. Conversely, thresholds of AI-up_H established for discriminating sound horses from lame horses with the lame limb on the outside of the circle showed lower values (+7%

and 0% for respectively LF and RF lame limb) than thresholds for discriminating sound horses from lame horses on a straight line (−36 and +24% for respectively LF and RF lame limb) [15]. This difference underlines the absolute need to take into account the physiological asymmetry induced by the circle on the head movements. In contrast, thresholds of withers amplitude asymmetry (AI-up_W) were less influenced by movement on the circle when the lame limb was on the outside (−5% and +13%, for respectively LF and RF lame limb, on the circle compared to −10% and +7%, for respectively LF and RF lame limb, on a straight line) [15].

The results obtained also demonstrate that, on the circle, the values of certain indices must be considered abnormal when they are equal to 0% (perfect symmetry between right and left). For example, when the index of the minimum withers height (AI-min_W) is equal to zero on a circle, this result indicates lameness on the limb outside the circle. An analysis of the symmetry indices on the circle must therefore take account of this shift in relation to what is expected on the straight line. This information is also useful for the clinician, who should consider that perfect symmetry on the circle could be interpreted as suspicious, as physiological asymmetry is to be expected.

In our study population, it appeared that the average grades attributed by the veterinary specialist to the inside forelimb lameness were slightly higher than the grade attributed to outside forelimb lameness. Means of lameness grade were indeed 3.5/10 for the inside forelimb and 3.1/10 for the outside forelimb. One hypothesis could be that injuries affecting the included horses were more painful for the inside limb than for the outside limb [1]. This could be a result of greater collateromotion and axial rotation movements in the inside limb than in the outside limb [1]. But, it should first and foremost be remembered that the main manifestation of an inside lameness is on the head, leading to a possible overestimation of lameness with an obvious head nod compared to a withers asymmetry [34].

In the present study, AIs were divided by the ROM to obtain relative indices expressed as a percentage. ROM values in centimeters are also provided in Table S2 for the locomotion on the right rein and in Table S3 for the locomotion on the left rein, meaning that the absolute value differences between the right and left limbs in centimeters can be easily recalculated using the formula AI(%) × ROM(cm)/100. However, normalizing values seems sensible in order to compare movements measured in a heterogeneous population, including individuals of different sizes (from pony to large horse) with varying vertical amplitudes of gaits. In addition, IMU systems differ in how they process accelerometric signals into displacement and this affects the threshold values that are used across systems [16]. Normalization can facilitate the comparison of asymmetry indices processed by different gait analysis systems, as suggested by Hardeman et al. [35].

In this study, an index based on temporal pattern asymmetry was used. AI-Tmax, reflecting a difference in duration of the down–up cycle between the right and left stance, showed a discriminative power as high as the amplitude asymmetry of the head and the withers. The results showed a reduction in the duration of the down–up cycle (time between two maxima) during the stance phase of the lame limb. Asymmetry indices based on Fourier transform have been shown to be indicators of lameness [17–19]. Also, Pfau et al. [36] found that the relative timing of the head movements compared to the withers or the pelvis was also an indicator of lameness. This underlines the importance of these temporal variables in the identification and analysis of lameness.

Horses were included in this study if they were lame on both reins. This selection criterion represents a unique subgroup of lameness cases, showing a specific manifestation. This choice has been made in order to guarantee unambiguous lameness under circle conditions, and in order to study the locomotion of the same horses whether they turn on the right rein or on the left rein. Otherwise, the locomotion of lame horses on the right rein would not be the locomotion of the lame horses, which were studied on the left rein. On the contrary, the group of sound horses would remain unchanged between the two reins, even though they are the reference group for comparison.

A well-known limitation of this study is the clinical reference used to distinguish lame horses from non-lame horses considering that visual clinical assessment is recognized by definition as being subjective [37,38]. This is a deliberate choice. Visual assessment is not considered here as a "gold standard" but only as a reference to what exists in the best possible conditions in order for clinicians to appropriate the tools for quantifying locomotor asymmetries compared to what they are used to seeing and concluding subjectively with the classical (even imperfect) methods. This is a key issue for "calibrating" these new quantitative tools and ensuring that the slightest asymmetry recorded by the machine is not wrongly considered to be an expression of lameness, particularly in the circle. However, in order to minimize the limits of subjective examination, the veterinarians chosen in this study were highly experienced and trained in the same clinic. These factors have been shown to improve agreement between vets [31,36]. Confounding specialists and unexperienced vets, a 69% agreement between veterinarians was reached on forelimb lameness detection on circles [31]. Moreover, the lowest grade of lameness (1/10) was excluded because of weaker agreement for very subtle asymmetries [38], and sound horses were included based on the agreement of three veterinary specialists in order to decrease uncertainty [34]. The strict selection criterion resulted in a sample that only represents a proportion of lameness cases. This choice was made in order to study unambiguous and simple lameness cases as a first step.

This study aims to investigate spontaneous cases of lameness of various origins. However, it is obvious that lameness can have different clinical expression depending on the type of injury [1,39]. Circles may further reveal lameness unseen on the straight line [1,2,26]. Some indices may be modified according to the type of injury. More horses with specific types of injuries should be included to go further in this direction.

Other limitations induced by circles were the radius, speed and body lean angle. The diameter of the circle was imposed with a standardized examination area. However, these factors are difficult to control precisely in practice. Yet, they have been shown to affect the symmetry [9,24], although the relationship between asymmetry and body lean angle has been considered unpredictable [40].

5. Conclusions

This study established preliminary thresholds for the clinical interpretation of asymmetry indices when the horses lunged at trot on short circles under clinical examination conditions for simple limb lameness shown on both reins with a grade over 1/10. For discriminating sound horses from lame horses with the lame forelimb on the inside of the circle, the asymmetry thresholds were approximatively (average between right and left absolute values) 24% and 49% for, respectively, the minimum and the amplitude of the elevation of the head, and 12% for the temporal phase shift of the head. For discriminating sound horses from lame horses with the lame forelimb on the outside of the circle, the asymmetry thresholds were approximately (average between right and left absolute values) 10% and 9% for, respectively, the minimum and amplitude of elevation of the withers, and 2.5% for the temporal phase shift of the withers.

The results confirmed that circles on a hard surface induce the asymmetry of movements in sound horses. This asymmetry should not be confused with lameness, making the notion of threshold particularly important in this circumstance of the locomotion. In this study, asymmetry of the head movements was shown to be more effective to discriminate forelimb lameness when the lame limb was on the inside of the circle (sensitivity $\geq$ 69% and specificity $\geq$ 81%), whereas asymmetry of the withers movements was shown to be more effective to discriminate lameness when the lame limb was on the outside of the circle (sensitivity $\geq$ 72% and specificity $\geq$ 77%). The temporal asymmetry between the left and right duration of the vertical displacement cycle of the head or of the withers showed a discriminative power as high as asymmetry indices calculated from the amplitude of the vertical displacements. These quantitative results are useful in objectively helping clinicians to establish an informed diagnosis. In the future, these thresholds will be refined by including more horses and will be specific to the anatomical location and to the type of lesion responsible for the lameness. Indeed, this study needs to be extended by adding horses with different lameness types and horses that show lameness on only one rein. Also, horses with subtle lameness (1/10 grade) have not been included here, considering that the level of agreement between clinicians for very subtle asymmetries is low [23]. However, further studies will be needed to refine thresholds for those more subtle and uncertain cases. In addition, the investigation should be extended to the detection of hindlimb lameness and to circles on a soft surface.

Supplementary Materials: The following supporting information can be downloaded at https://www.mdpi.com/article/10.3390/ani13213319/s1, Figure S1: Flowchart of the exclusion/inclusion criteria of the screened horses, which were visually considered lame at lunge on both reins on a hard surface by a veterinary specialist during his routine practice. Table S1: Table of detailed bread, age, discipline and gender of each included horse. "Other" is written for the rare mentions. Table S2: Table of detailed data measured on the head, the withers and the pelvis of each horse on the left rein. These include the horse identity; the group and the grade of lameness assigned by the veterinarian; the studied Asymmetric Indices (AI-up; AI-min; AI-max; AI-Tmax); the range of movement (maximum amplitude); and the stride duration averaged over all strides. Table S3: Table of detailed data measured on the head, the withers and the pelvis of each horse on the right rein. These include the horse identity; the group and the grade of lameness assigned by the veterinarian; the studied Asymmetric Indices (AI-up; AI-min; AI-max; AI-Tmax); the range of movement (maximum amplitude); and the stride duration averaged over all strides.

Author Contributions: Conceptualization, C.M., F.M., P.M. and H.C.; methodology, C.M., S.H.-P., F.M., P.M. and H.C.; software, C.M., S.H.-P., C.H. (Chloé Hatrisse) and C.H. (Camille Hébert); validation, C.M., S.H.-P., E.D.A. and C.H. (Camille Hébert); formal analysis, C.M. and S.H.-P.; investigation, E.D.A., J.-M.D., V.C., S.J., L.B. and A.T.; resources, E.D.A., J.-M.D., V.C., S.J., L.B., A.T., F.A., C.H. (Camille Hébert) and P.M.; data curation, C.M. and E.D.A.; writing—original draft preparation, C.M.; writing—review and editing, S.H.-P., F.A., F.M., P.M. and H.C.; visualization, C.M.; supervision, F.M., P.M. and H.C.; project administration, P.M. and H.C.; funding acquisition, P.M. All authors have read and agreed to the published version of the manuscript.

Funding: This research was funded by the Agence Nationale de la Recherche (LabCom "CWDVetlab", Contract ANR 16-LCV2-0002-01), the European Regional Development Fund (FEDER) and the Region Normandie (Project "EquiSym", Contract 20E01636).

Institutional Review Board Statement: The animal study protocol was approved by the Ethics Committee of COMITE D'ETHIQUE EN RECHERCHE CLINIQUE—ComERC (no2022-01-19).

Informed Consent Statement: Informed consent was obtained from the owner of all the subjects involved in the study.

Data Availability Statement: The data that support the findings of this study are available from the corresponding author upon reasonable request.

Acknowledgments: The authors thank the Centre d'Imagerie et de Recherche sur les Affections Locomotrices Equines (CIRALE). They also thank Alexandre Charles, Anne-Claire Idoux, Antoinette Terlinden and Alberto De la Rocha who actively contributed to data collection.

Conflicts of Interest: The project was supported by the Agence Nationale de la Recherche (ANR) which sponsors a collaborative project between a company (LIM France) and the Ecole Nationale Vétérinaire d'Alfort (ENVA).

References

1. Denoix, J.M. A Look at Lameness Through the Eyes of Functional Anatomy (and Biomechanics). *AAEP Proc.* **2021**, *67*, 106–133.
2. Chateau, H.; Camus, M.; Holden-Douilly, L.; Falala, S.; Ravary, B.; Vergari, C.; Lepley, J.; Denoix, J.-M.; Pourcelot, P.; Crevier-Denoix, N. Kinetics of the forelimb in horses circling on different ground surfaces at the trot. *Vet. J.* **2013**, *198*, e20–e26. [CrossRef] [PubMed]
3. Serra Bragança, F.M.; Rhodin, M.; van Weeren, P.R. On the brink of daily clinical application of objective gait analysis: What evidence do we have so far from studies using an induced lameness model? *Vet. J.* **2018**, *234*, 11–23. [CrossRef] [PubMed]

4. Weeren, P.R.; Pfau, T.; Rhodin, M.; Roepstorff, L.; Serra Bragança, F.; Weishaupt, M.A. Do we have to redefine lameness in the era of quantitative gait analysis? *Equine Vet. J.* **2017**, *49*, 567–569. [CrossRef]
5. Weeren, P.R.; Pfau, T.; Rhodin, M.; Roepstorff, L.; Serra Bragança, F.; Weishaupt, M.A. What is lameness and what (or who) is the gold standard to detect it? *Equine Vet. J.* **2018**, *50*, 549–551. [CrossRef] [PubMed]
6. Pfau, T.; Fiske-Jackson, A.; Rhodin, M. Quantitative assessment of gait parameters in horses: Useful for aiding clinical decision making? *Equine Vet. Educ.* **2016**, *28*, 209–215. [CrossRef]
7. Reed, S.K.; Kramer, J.; Thombs, L.; Pitts, J.B.; Wilson, D.A.; Keegan, K.G. Comparison of results for body-mounted inertial sensor assessment with final lameness determination in 1224 equids. *J. Am. Vet. Med. Assoc.* **2020**, *256*, 590–599. [CrossRef]
8. Kallerud, A.S.; Hernlund, E.; Byström, A.; Persson-Sjodin, E.; Rhodin, M.; Hendrickson, E.H.S.; Fjordbakk, C.T. Non-banked curved tracks influence movement symmetry in two-year-old Standardbred trotters. *Equine Vet. J.* **2021**, *53*, 1178–1187. [CrossRef]
9. Pfau, T.; Persson-Sjodin, E.; Gardner, H.; Orssten, O.; Hernlund, E.; Rhodin, M. Effect of Speed and Surface Type on Individual Rein and Combined Left–Right Circle Movement Asymmetry in Horses on the Lunge. *Front. Vet. Sci.* **2021**, *8*, 692031. [CrossRef]
10. Rhodin, M.; Egenvall, A.; Haubro Andersen, P.; Pfau, T. Head and pelvic movement asymmetries at trot in riding horses in training and perceived as free from lameness by the owner. *PLoS ONE* **2017**, *12*, e0176253. [CrossRef]
11. Pfau, T.; Jennings, C.; Mitchell, H.; Olsen, E.; Walker, A.; Egenvall, A.; Tröster, S.; Weller, R.; Rhodin, M. Lungeing on hard and soft surfaces: Movement symmetry of trotting horses considered sound by their owners: Movement symmetry on hard and soft surfaces on the lunge. *Equine Vet. J.* **2016**, *48*, 83–89. [CrossRef]
12. Starke, S.D.; Willems, E.; May, S.A.; Pfau, T. Vertical head and trunk movement adaptations of sound horses trotting in a circle on a hard surface. *Vet. J.* **2012**, *193*, 73–80. [CrossRef]
13. McCracken, M.J.; Kramer, J.; Keegan, K.G.; Lopes, M.; Wilson, D.A.; Reed, S.K.; LaCarrubba, A.; Rasch, M. Comparison of an inertial sensor system of lameness quantification with subjective lameness evaluation: Comparison of inertial system with subjective lameness evaluation. *Equine Vet. J.* **2012**, *44*, 652–656. [CrossRef]
14. Pfau, T.; Sepulveda Caviedes, M.F.; McCarthy, R.; Cheetham, L.; Forbes, B.; Rhodin, M. Comparison of Visual Lameness Scores to Gait Asymmetry in Racing Thoroughbreds during Trot In-hand. *Equine Vet. Educ.* **2020**, *32*, 191–198. [CrossRef]
15. Macaire, C.; Hanne-Poujade, S.; Azevedo, E.D.; Denoix, J.-M.; Coudry, V.; Jacquet, S.; Bertoni, L.; Tallaj, A.; Audigié, F.; Hatrisse, C.; et al. Investigation of Thresholds for Asymmetry Indices to Represent the Visual Assessment of Single Limb Lameness by Expert Veterinarians on Horses Trotting in a Straight Line. *Animals* **2022**, *12*, 3498. [CrossRef]
16. Pfau, T.; Boultbee, H.; Davis, H.; Walker, A.; Rhodin, M. Agreement between Two Inertial Sensor Gait Analysis Systems for Lameness Examinations in Horses. *Equine Vet. Educ.* **2016**, *28*, 203–208. [CrossRef]
17. Audigié, F.; Pourcelot, P.; Degueurce, C.; Geiger, D.; Denoix, J.M. Fourier analysis of trunk displacements: A method to identify the lame limb in trotting horses. *J. Biomech.* **2002**, *35*, 1173–1182. [CrossRef]
18. Kramer, J.; Keegan, K.G.; Kelmer, G.; Wilson, D.A. Objective determination of pelvic movement during hind limb lameness by use of a signal decomposition method and pelvic height differences. *Am. J. Vet. Res.* **2004**, *65*, 741–747. [CrossRef] [PubMed]
19. Keegan, K.G.; Arafat, S.; Skubic, M.; Wilson, D.A.; Kramer, J. Detection of lameness and determination of the affected forelimb in horses by use of continuous wavelet transformation and neural network classification of kinematic data. *Am. J. Vet. Res.* **2003**, *64*, 1376–1381. [CrossRef] [PubMed]
20. Hardeman, A.M.; Serra Bragança, F.M.; Swagemakers, J.H.; Weeren, P.R.; Roepstorff, L. Variation in gait parameters used for objective lameness assessment in sound horses at the trot on the straight line and the lunge. *Equine Vet. J.* **2019**, *51*, 831–839. [CrossRef] [PubMed]
21. Rhodin, M.; Pfau, T.; Roepstorff, L.; Egenvall, A. Effect of lungeing on head and pelvic movement asymmetry in horses with induced lameness. *Vet. J.* **2013**, *198*, e39–e45. [CrossRef]
22. Rhodin, M.; Roepstorff, L.; French, A.; Keegan, K.G.; Pfau, T.; Egenvall, A. Head and pelvic movement asymmetry during lungeing in horses with symmetrical movement on the straight. *Equine Vet. J.* **2016**, *48*, 315–320. [CrossRef] [PubMed]
23. Greve, L.; Pfau, T.; Dyson, S. Alterations in body lean angle in lame horses before and after diagnostic analgesia in straight lines in hand and on the lunge. *Vet. J.* **2018**, *239*, 1–6. [CrossRef] [PubMed]
24. Pfau, T.; Stubbs, N.C.; Kaiser, L.J.; Brown, L.E.A.; Clayton, H.M. Effect of trotting speed and circle radius on movement symmetry in horses during lunging on a soft surface. *Am. J. Vet. Res.* **2012**, *73*, 1890–1899. [CrossRef] [PubMed]
25. May, S.A.; Wyn-Jones, G. Identification of hindleg lameness. *Equine Vet. J.* **1987**, *19*, 185–188. [CrossRef]
26. Dyson, S. Can lameness be graded reliably? Can lameness be graded reliably? *Equine Vet. J.* **2011**, *43*, 379–382. [CrossRef] [PubMed]
27. Arkell, M.; Archer, R.M.; Guitian, F.J.; May, S.A. Evidence of bias affecting the interpretation of the results of local anaesthetic nerve blocks when assessing lameness in horses. *Vet. Rec.* **2006**, *159*, 346–348. [CrossRef]
28. Timmerman, I.; Macaire, C.; Hanne-Poujade, S.; Bertoni, L.; Martin, P.; Marin, F.; Chateau, H. A Pilot Study on the Inter-Operator Reproducibility of a Wireless Sensors-Based System for Quantifying Gait Asymmetries in Horses. *Sensors* **2022**, *22*, 9533. [CrossRef]
29. Oppong, F.B.; Agbedra, S.Y. Assessing Univariate and Multivariate Normality, A Guide For Non-Statisticians. *Math. Theory Model* **2016**, *6*, 26–33.
30. Power, M.; Fell, G.; Wright, M. Principles for high-quality, high-value testing. *Evid. Based Med.* **2013**, *18*, 5–10. [CrossRef]

31. Hammarberg, M.; Egenvall, A.; Pfau, T.; Rhodin, M. Rater agreement of visual lameness assessment in horses during lungeing. *Equine Vet. J.* **2016**, *48*, 78–82. [CrossRef]
32. Pfau, T.; Bolt, D.M.; Fiske-Jackson, A.; Gerdes, C.; Hoenecke, K.; Lynch, L.; Perrier, M.; Smith, R.K.W. Linear Discriminant Analysis for Investigating Differences in Upper Body Movement Symmetry in Horses before/after Diagnostic Analgesia in Relation to Expert Judgement. *Animals* **2022**, *12*, 762. [CrossRef] [PubMed]
33. Marunova, E.; Hoenecke, K.; Fiske-Jackson, A.; Smith, R.K.W.; Bolt, D.M.; Perrier, M.; Gerdes, C.; Hernlund, E.; Rhodin, M.; Pfau, T. Changes in Head, Withers, and Pelvis Movement Asymmetry in Lame Horses as a Function of Diagnostic Anesthesia Outcome, Surface and Direction. *J. Equine Vet. Sci.* **2022**, *118*, 104136. [CrossRef]
34. Starke, S.D.; May, S.A. Expert visual assessment strategies for equine lameness examinations in a straight line and circle: A mixed methods study using eye tracking. *Vet. Rec.* **2022**, *191*, e1684. [CrossRef] [PubMed]
35. Hardeman, A.M.; Egenvall, A.; Serra Bragança, F.M.; Koene, M.H.W.; Swagemakers, J.; Roepstorff, L.; Weeren, R.; Byström, A. Movement Asymmetries in Horses Presented for Prepurchase or Lameness Examination. *Equine Vet. J.* **2021**, *54*, 334–346. [CrossRef]
36. Pfau, T.; Noordwijk, K.; Sepulveda Caviedes, M.F.; Persson-Sjodin, E.; Barstow, A.; Forbes, B.; Rhodin, M. Head, withers and pelvic movement asymmetry and their relative timing in trot in racing Thoroughbreds in training. *Equine Vet. J.* **2018**, *50*, 117–124. [CrossRef] [PubMed]
37. Starke, S.D.; Oosterlinck, M. Reliability of equine visual lameness classification as a function of expertise, lameness severity and rater confidence. *Vet. Rec.* **2019**, *184*, 63. [CrossRef] [PubMed]
38. Keegan, K.G.; Dent, E.V.; Wilson, D.A.; Janicek, J.; Kramer, J.; Lacarrubba, A.; Walsh, D.M.; Cassells, M.W.; Esther, T.M.; Schiltz, P.; et al. Repeatability of subjective evaluation of lameness in horses: Repeatability of subjective evaluation of lameness in horses. *Equine Vet. J.* **2010**, *42*, 92–97. [CrossRef]
39. Ross, M.W.; Dyson, S.J. *Diagnosis and Management of Lameness in the Horse*, 2nd ed.; Elsevier: Amsterdam, The Netherlands, 2011.
40. Greve, L.; Dyson, S. Body lean angle in sound dressage horses in-hand, on the lunge and ridden. *Vet. J.* **2016**, *217*, 52–57. [CrossRef]

animals

MDPI

Article

Artificial Intelligence for Lameness Detection in Horses—A Preliminary Study

Ann-Kristin Feuser [1], Stefan Gesell-May [2], Tobias Müller [2] and Anna May [3,*]

1 Equine Hospital in Parsdorf, 85599 Vaterstetten, Germany
2 Anirec GmbH, Artificial Intelligence Solutions in Veterinary Medicine, 80539 Munich, Germany
3 Equine Hospital, Ludwig Maximilians University, 85764 Oberschleissheim, Germany
* Correspondence: anna.may@pferd.vetmed.uni-muenchen.de

Simple Summary: In the expanding field of artificial intelligence, deep learning and smart-device-technology, a diagnostic software tool was developed, which can help distinguish between lame and sound horses and locate the affected limb. As lameness influences the welfare of horses and is often difficult to detect, this tool can help owners and veterinarians in the process of evaluation. The technology is based on pose estimation, which is already used in human and veterinary science to study movement of limbs or bodies without the need to fix any devices onto the object of interest. In this study, 22 horses with unilateral fore- or hindlimb lameness and a control group of eight sound horses were analysed with the program. Based on the results of the program, it was possible to differentiate between horses with fore- and hindlimb lameness and sound horses. Difficult light settings, such as direct sunlight or darkness, or very even-coloured coats, complicate the precise placement of reference points. The analysis and detection with software-generated movement trajectories using pose estimation is very promising but requires further development.

Abstract: Lameness in horses is a long-known issue influencing the welfare, as well as the use, of a horse. Nevertheless, the detection and classification of lameness mainly occurs on a subjective basis by the owner and the veterinarian. The aim of this study was the development of a lameness detection system based on pose estimation, which permits non-invasive and easily applicable gait analysis. The use of 58 reference points on easily detectable anatomical landmarks offers various possibilities for gait evaluation using a simple setup. For this study, three groups of horses were used: one training group, one analysis group of fore and hindlimb lame horses and a control group of sound horses. The first group was used to train the network; afterwards, horses with and without lameness were evaluated. The results show that forelimb lameness can be detected by visualising the trajectories of the reference points on the head and both forelimbs. In hindlimb lameness, the stifle showed promising results as a reference point, whereas the tuber coxae were deemed unsuitable as a reference point. The study presents a feasible application of pose estimation for lameness detection, but further development using a larger dataset is essential.

Keywords: artificial intelligence; deep learning; pose estimation; lameness; equine

1. Introduction

Lameness is a term that describes a horse's change in gait, usually caused by pain or mechanical restriction. There are substantial economic losses attributed to lameness in the equine industry, due to interrupted or truncated sports careers, costs of veterinary services, drugs and additional treatment costs, as well as death [1]. Lameness is one of the most common medical issue in equine veterinary medicine [2], and it can affect any horse at any level of training [3,4].

As undetected lameness poses a significant welfare issue for the affected horse, owners and veterinarians need to be capable of recognising changes of gait as early as possible.

Studies have shown that owners are often unable to recognise lameness in their own horses [5] and that identifying whether the horse experiences musculoskeletal pain resulting in lameness can be very difficult, especially for inexperienced riders [6]. On the clinical side, veterinary experience influences subjective lameness evaluation. Veterinary students and recent graduates often exhibit difficulties in identifying the affected leg [7]. Even amongst experienced veterinarians, there is often a lack of agreement on the affected leg in horses with subtle lameness cases [8,9]. Further limitations to subjective lameness evaluation are the inaccuracy of the human eye and the influence of bias due to the assessment and interpretation of lameness after diagnostic anaesthesia [10,11].

Over the years, many technology-assisted methods have been developed to objectively evaluate gait, movement and lameness in horses. These systems can be divided into two major groups, depending on whether they are based on kinetic or kinematic measuring techniques. Kinetics describes the movement of a rigid body, depending only on the action of forces. In contrast, kinematic analysis characterises the spatio-temporal movement of a rigid body, using time and distance as measurable parameters, without considering the forces [12–14].

One of the first kinetic instruments for analysing lameness, which is still used in research and clinical cases [15,16], is the force plate [17]. By recording the ground reaction forces from a lame horse, asymmetrical distribution of body weight on the legs can be measured [18]. Though offering very precise data, lameness analysis with the force plate is expensive, time consuming and only applicable in institutions where this measuring platform is available [12,13,19]. Nevertheless, it is still seen as the gold standard in equine lameness evaluation [20,21]. Other options include a force-measuring horseshoe, which can record ground reaction forces. However, the additional weight and size of the shoe potentially influences the movement of the horse, which reduces its value in lameness evaluation [13,22]. The instrumented treadmill located at the University of Zurich, Switzerland [15,18], offers the possibility to measure the ground reaction forces from several consecutive strides and from all four limbs [21]. Still, horses need to be trained to walk on the treadmill, which is time-consuming. In addition, because of its custom-made, relatively expensive characteristics, the treadmill is not suitable for broad clinical use in the field [13,20,21].

Most of the kinematic lameness evaluation systems can be assigned to one of two groups: optical motion capture (OMC) and inertial measurement unit (IMU). OMC systems use infrared cameras with a recording speed between 100–300 Hz, allowing the collection of a large amount of three-dimensional (3D) coordinate data [21]. Most OMC systems capture data using retro-reflective, spherical markers that are attached to the skin over anatomical locations of interest [12,23,24]. In this setup, an OMC system enables precise recording of 3D movement. However, the cost-intensive nature of the equipment and the time-consuming setup largely limits the use of OMC systems to large clinics and universities [14]. In contrast, the functionality of IMUs is based on gyroscopes and accelerometers [14,20]. Usually both sensors work wirelessly and are attached to certain body segments of a horse, using straps or double-sided tape [25]. The number of sensors and the exact placement differ across IMU systems. While a gyroscope measures the angular velocity around an axis, accelerometers measure the velocity and acceleration along a single axis or multiple axes [13,22]. Even though IMUs are portable, they are still relatively cost-intensive and require a certain level of expertise for data collection, analysis and interpretation. Furthermore, the accumulation of drift errors, which are the sum of all minor measuring errors during one analysis, can influence the results and thereby the outcome of the examination [26].

In the last few years, there has been increasing development of these systems [27,28]. Considering the fact that they require markers or inertial sensors, which need to be fixed onto the object of interest, the studied body parts must be defined beforehand [29].

In this study, we attempt to combine pose estimation with lameness evaluation in horses. This offers a new approach that ameliorates some of the disadvantages of other objective lameness detection systems. The use of pose estimation offers a non-invasive way to track and record movements for further analysis. The development and use of pose estimation are based on deep learning. As part of the broad scientific field of artificial intelligence (AI), deep learning creates a neural network of multiple layers which relate to each other. By constantly incorporating new data into the network, it can be trained to recognise patterns in high-dimensional data. The significant difference in comparison to other computer programs is the fact that the filtering criteria of these layers are built autonomously from the algorithm itself, instead of by a software engineer [30].

The aim of this study was to evaluate the usability of pose estimation for detecting and marking specific anatomical reference points, using cell-phone videos of horses being lunged on a circle line. A secondary aim was to determine whether pose estimation can be used to differentiate between sound horses and horses with fore- and hindlimb lameness. We hypothesise that, using reference points on the head and forelimbs, it is possible to distinguish between a forelimb-lame and a non-lame horse. Furthermore, we hypothesize that a differentiation between hindlimb-lame horses and non-lame horses by using the stifle and the tuber coxae as reference points is feasible.

2. Materials and Methods

2.1. Technology

2.1.1. Deep Learning

In veterinary science, deep learning is already used in many areas. It offers the possibility to improve behavioural studies, for example of drosophila flies or mice [29], or to aid in developing a pain detection model for stabled horses [31]. Other fields of application are image recognition in radiology, such as the automatic classification of canine thoracic radiographs [32], or in equine ophthalmology, integrated in a diagnostic application with a focus on equine uveitis [33].

2.1.2. Pose Estimation

Pose estimation allows for the tracking and recording of the movement of humans, animals, or objects without the need to fix any markers or sensors directly onto the subject of interest [29]. For the study of human poses, several well-described programs such as ArtTrack (Saarbrücken, Germany) or Open-Pose already exist [34,35]. After showing promising results in prior studies with pose estimation on animals, the DeepLabCut (2.2rc3 and 2.2.0.6: https://github.com/DeepLabCut/DeepLabCut/tree/v2.2.0.6; accessed on 10 August 2022) program was used in this study [36]. DeepLabCut is a deep convolutional network based on DeeperCut, which is considered one of the best algorithms for pose estimation. In contrast to other pose estimation tools, such as the MPII Human Pose dataset, with approximately 25,000 datasets, DeepLabCut only requires a relatively small number of 200 training images to train a network [29,37]. The functioning of DeepLabCut is based on two main elements. On the one hand, it uses pre-trained residual neural networks (ResNets), which are trained beforehand on ImageNet (resnet_50: http://download.tensorflow.org/models/resnet_v1_50_2016_08_28.tar.gz; accessed on 10 August 2022), a database that provides images for large-scale object recognition models. On the other hand, it is based on deconvolutional layers, which help to increase the visual information inserted into the network and reach spatial probability densities. After being trained with only a small number of labelled images (~200), the algorithm can predict and mark body parts with accuracy comparable to humans [29].

2.1.3. Reference Point Selection

For the pose estimation, 58 reference points, as listed in Figure 1, were determined. Selection criteria were identifiable anatomical landmarks on the horse, with some of these already used and proven in other lameness detection systems [14,38]. There were four markers on the head, four markers on the neck and trunk, 11 on each forelimb from the shoulder down to the hoof and 14 on each hindlimb between the tubera sacrale and the hooves. Each reference point corresponded to one pixel in one picture.

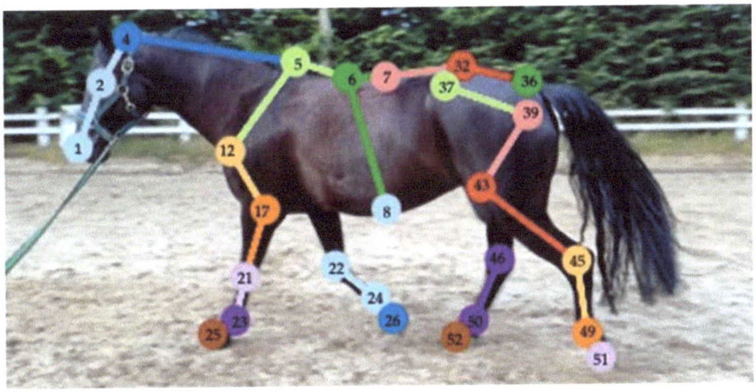

Head	Forelimb—proximal	Forelimb—distal	Hindlimb—proximal	Hindlimb—distal
1 Nostril	9 Spina scapulae left	19 Os carpi accessorium left	31 Croup middle	45 Tarsus left
2 Eye left	10 Spina scapulae right	20 Os carpi accessorium right	32 T. sacrale left	46 Tarsus right
3 Eye right	11 Tub. supraglenoidale left	21 Carpus left	33 T. sacrale right	47 Calcaneus left
4 Poll	12 Tub. supraglenoidale right	22 Carpus right	34 Kink left	48 Calcaneus right
Neck and trunk	13 Shoulder joint left	23 Fetlock left	35 Kink right	49 Fetlock left
5 Withers	14 Shoulder joint right	24 Fetlock right	36 Tail root	50 Fetlock right
6 Lowest back	15 Elbow hock left	25 Coronary band dorsal left	37 T. coxae left	51 Coronary band dorsal left
7 T18/L1	16 Elbow hock right	26 Coronary band dorsal right	38 T. coxae right	52 Coronary band dorsal right
8 Abdomen	17 Elbow joint left	27 Coronary band palmar left	39 Coxofemoral joint left	53 Coronary band plantar left
	18 Elbow joint right	28 Coronary band palmar right	40 Coxofemoral joint right	54 Coronary band plantar right
		29 Hoof tip left	41 T. ischiadicum left	55 Hoof pad left
		30 Hoof tip right	42 T. ischiadicum right	56 Hoof pad right
			43 Stifle joint left	57 Hoof tip left
			44 Stifle joint right	58 Hoof tip right

Figure 1. Reference points. Different combinations of reference points can be chosen in the program and offer multiple variations for gait analysis; the picture only shows a selection of the reference points which are enlarged in the image for better visibility. In the program, one reference point corresponds to one pixel. The accurate anatomical locations corresponding to the reference points of the program are listed in Table A1.

2.2. Collection of Data in Investigated Groups

All horses used in this study were assigned to one of three groups: one training group, one analysis group for lame horses and one analysis group for non-lame horses. Detailed information regarding all three groups is summarised in Table A2. Ethical approval for this study was obtained from the ethics committee of Ludwig Maximilians University, Munich, Germany.

Every horse of the three groups received a full orthopaedic lameness examination [39,40] by an orthopaedic specialist (German specialists for equine medicine), including flexion tests. All horses were examined on hard and soft ground in walk and trot on the straight line and on the circle. Horses with any sign of visible gait asymmetry, a positive flexion test or any pathological results in the lameness examination were excluded.

Lameness results were graded according to the AAEP lameness scale by the American Association of Equine Practitioners on a scale from 1 to 5.

All horses of the training group (n = 65) were filmed in various environmental surroundings, which included eight different indoor and 14 different outdoor riding arenas with varying sand and soil surfaces. In order to obtain high recognition probabilities on the labelled reference points, diversity in the coat colour of the horses and environmental backgrounds was necessary. Furthermore, care was taken to film in different weather conditions, such as under sunlight or clouded skies, and during different times of the day to obtain a broad spectrum of different video settings. Horses were recorded in walk and trot from the front, the back (11 s in walk and 7 s in trot, respectively), and from both sides on a straight line (12 s in walk and 7 s in trot, respectively). Horses were also recorded on a circle line with an approximate diameter of 12 m on soft ground (1 min in walk and trot) on both hands.

All horses included in the lame group were privately owned horses presented for lameness examination in the Equine Hospital in Parsdorf, Vaterstetten, Germany. In total, 22 horses were examined and included. Permission for the collection and use of data was obtained from the owners beforehand, and detailed information about the lameness history of the horses was documented. As part of the routine lameness examination in this clinic, the horses were first filmed in walk and trot on both hands for one minute on a 12 m diameter circle on soft ground. After performing flexion tests on concrete and examining gait on firm, as well as on soft, ground, horses were subjected to diagnostic anaesthesia. Depending on the results of the examination and the identified anatomical area, the horses underwent diagnostic imaging (radiographs, ultrasound, computed tomography) and treatment based on the diagnosis. The recorded lameness grades varied from 1 to 4 (AAEP). Horses with a lameness degree $\geq 4/5$ were excluded from the study, as well as horses that showed lameness on more than one leg.

The non-lame group represents the reference group and consisted of eight horses. All horses were privately owned by one owner/farm. The horses were filmed in walk and trot on a left (CL) and right (CR) circle line for one minute in each gait. Two additional horses were excluded due to positive flexion tests after lameness had been detected during lunging. All video-recordings were taken with an iPhone 11 (Apple), with the resolution set to 1080 p and 30 fps.

2.3. Training the Artificial Intelligence Tool Using Deep Learning

2.3.1. Data Processing and Training

For training the neural network, 454 still frames from 215 videos of the training group were extracted and the predetermined points of interest (reference points, as defined in Section 2.1.3) were labelled manually. To provide high diversity in the training data, attention was paid to select still frames with different limb positioning combined with varying overlay of limbs. Multiple intermediary trainings were conducted to find a suitable network configuration for the neural network. Additionally, frames with predicted poses that had a significant number of outliers were determined and labelled manually to improve the performance of the network. For the final training set of 454 labelled still frames, the ResNet50 network base architecture was utilised. Five percent of the images were reserved for evaluation during training. These images were used to survey the training status of the algorithm. As this application only had access to a limited amount of training data, the evaluation ratio was left at this default value. All hyperparameters related to the neural network and training process were set to the default values of DeepLabCut. This was to ensure that the neural network in this study was based on the stable results of DeepLabCut, using pre-trained and tested networks [29].

Initial tests were conducted using full resolution images (1920 × 1080 pixels) to preserve as much of the details as possible, but stable results could not be achieved. By reducing the resolution of the input images, a significant improvement in training was reached. In the end, a resolution of 768 × 432 pixels, which is 40% of the resolution of the original images, was chosen. This represents a balance of reduced image size without losing too much detail. The latest neural network was trained with 550,000 iterations with a resulting loss of 0.0013 of the training data. This low value indicates that the model fit the training data well. During training, the intention is to reach a preferably low value which must not become zero. This would reveal that the algorithm has learned the data by heart.

However, a comparison of training and evaluation data with respect to error probability showed that there was an average error of 2.6 pixels for training data, compared to as many as 8.22 pixels for evaluation data. Given the resolution of 432 pixels in the vertical axis, this error can make a difference of up to ~1.9% between training and evaluation data. Removing outliers with a likelihood below 60% in the predicted points led to an average error for training data of 2.59 pixels and 6.14 pixels for evaluation data. The small difference in error values for the training data shows its already-high certainty, combined with a distinctly lower certainty on unseen evaluation data. For the setup in this study, the threshold for the exclusion of data was set at a certainty of 60% to obtain high reliability for reference point detection, combined with a low error rate.

2.3.2. Data Analysis and Measurements and Mathematical Calculations in Trot Videos

For the following analysis, only the trot data were used. Each video included one minute of filming time with an average number of 74 strides per video for Warmbloods and 84 strides for German Riding Ponies. All horses of the second group were subdivided in two categories: A = forelimb-lame, B = hindlimb-lame.

Forelimb Lameness

The movement pattern of forelimb lame horses is marked by certain, distinguishable alterations. When trotting, a forelimb-lame horse demonstrates a typical, iterative head nod compared to a sound horse [39–41]. In an attempt to shift weight away from the painful leg, a left forelimb-lame horse lowers its head when stepping on the sound right leg and lifts the head up when loading onto the lame left leg [40,41]. Thus, to detect forelimb lameness in this study, the movement of the two forelimbs in comparison with the motion of the head was recorded. Reference points on the forelimbs and the neck were chosen. Reference points 17 (Elbow joint left) and 21 (Carpus left) were used for CL, and 18 (Elbow joint right) and 22 (Carpus right) were used for CR. Reference point 4 (poll) shows the movement of the head during trotting on both circles. To be able to distinguish between the left and right stance phase, points 19 (Os carpi accessorium left), 20 (Os carpi accessorium right), 45 (Tarsus left) and 46 (Tarsus right) were selected. For each horse, the recorded trajectory of the reference points from CL and CR were extracted from the program in csv-files and presented in charts. These data were analysed visually.

Hindlimb Lameness

Horses with hindlimb lameness show significant changes in their kinematic pattern [42,43]. In this study, two separate analysis parameters were investigated based on these known changes.

Stifle Reference Point

Horses with hindlimb lameness often present with a decreased protraction of the lame limb [39,42,43]. To compare the step length of both hindlimbs, the horizontal movement of points 43 (Stifle left) and 44 (Stifle right) on CL and CR was recorded and measured. It was estimated that horses with a hindlimb lameness show a shortened stride on the lame leg and, therefore, show a smaller difference between the measured minima and maxima of the stifle point on the lame side.

Tuber coxae reference point

As an approved reference point [41,44], the movement of the tuber coxae along the vertical axis was analysed. Studies have demonstrated that hindlimb-lame horses show an increased vertical displacement of the tuber coxae on the lame side [41,44,45]. Thus, it was estimated that horses with hindlimb lameness show a larger difference between the measured minima and maxima on the affected side.

For each horse, the recorded trajectory of the reference points from the CL and CR were extracted from the program in csv files and transferred into an Excel file (Microsoft Excel, Version 16.63.1). To avoid false results due to inaccurate placement of markers by the program, the maximum 5% (95–100%) and the minimum 5% (0–5%) of the recorded frames were excluded from the analysis. The maxima represent the highest measured values (90–95%) and the minima the lowest measured values (5–10%) of the stifle point and the tuber coxae points.

For the analysis of the stifle point, $\overline{Max}_{St}$ (mean value of the stifle maxima) and $\overline{Min}_{St}$ (mean value of the stifle minima) for every horse were calculated for the left and the right circle. The differences represent the length of the horizontal distance along which the stifle point is recorded during trotting on each circle:

$$DS_{St}(\text{CL}) = \left|\overline{Max}_{St}(\text{CL}) - \overline{Min}_{St}(\text{CL})\right|$$

$$DS_{St}(\text{CR}) = \left|\overline{Max}_{St}(\text{CR}) - \overline{Min}_{St}(\text{CR})\right|$$

For the analysis of the tuber coxae point, $\overline{Max}_{Tcox}$ (mean value of the tuber coxae maxima) and $\overline{Min}_{Tcox}$ (mean value of the tuber coxae minima) were calculated for both circles. The differences represent the length of the vertical distance between the highest and lowest tuber coxae values during movement on each circle:

$$DT_{Tcox}(\text{CL}) = \left|\overline{Max}_{Tcox}(\text{CL}) - \overline{Min}_{Tcox}(\text{CL})\right|$$

$$DT_{Tcox}(\text{CR}) = \left|\overline{Max}_{Tcox}(\text{CR}) - \overline{Min}_{Tcox}(\text{CR})\right|$$

In the next step the difference for the Stifle as a reference point was calculated to compare the CL and CR:

$$D_{St} = \left|DS_{St}(\text{CL}) - DS_{St}(\text{CR})\right|$$

The values for the tuber coxae measurements were calculated the same way for comparison of CL and CR:

$$D_{Tcox} = \left|DT_{Tcox}(\text{CL}) - DT_{Tcox}(\text{CR})\right|$$

Mean values $\overline{D}_{St}$ were calculated by summing up the DS_{St} of the individual horses, which should be compared, and dividing them by the number of included horses.

Mean values $\overline{D}_{Tcox}$ were calculated the same way with DS_{Tcox}.

2.3.3. Statistical Analysis

Diagnostic test properties based on the AI system in comparison to the clinical assessment (reference) were separately assessed for forelimb lameness, hindlimb lameness using the stifle reference point, and hindlimb lameness using the tuber coxae reference point, using 2 × 2 tables. Estimates for diagnostic sensitivity (SE) were calculated as the proportion of clinically lame horses that were correctly classified based on the AI results. Specificity (SP) was calculated as the proportion of clinically healthy horses that were correctly classified based on the AI results. Accuracy (ACC) was calculated as the proportion of correct (positive + negative) classifications based on the AI results. Positive predictive values (PPV), describing the probability that the AI positive result is correct, and negative predictive values (NPV), describing the probability that the AI negative result is correct, were evaluated. The agreement beyond chance (κappa), a statistical value for quantifying inter-rater reliability, was used in this study to measure agreement between clinical scoring of the horses and classification based on the AI. Kappa scores were calculated on the basis of a 3 × 3-table, including forelimb lameness, hindlimb lameness (only using stifle reference point data) and the non-lame control group. Finally, an overall accuracy (OA) was calculated as the percentage of all correctly classified horses based on the AI results [46].

3. Results

Of the 22 horses of the lame group, 13 horses were detected with forelimb lameness and nine horses with hindlimb lameness. The results of their analysis, together with the eight horses of the third group, are presented below.

3.1. Forelimb Lameness

In total, seven horses were diagnosed as left-forelimb-lame and six as right-forelimb-lame. The lameness degrees ranged from AAEP 1–2/5 in ten horses and AAEP 3–4/5 in three horses. As shown in Figure 2a), the upward and downward movement ("head nod") of the poll reference point was visually correlated with the loading of the lame and the non-lame limb, respectively. The non-lame horses did not show any signs of repetitive up-and-down motion of the head, as illustrated in Figure 2b).

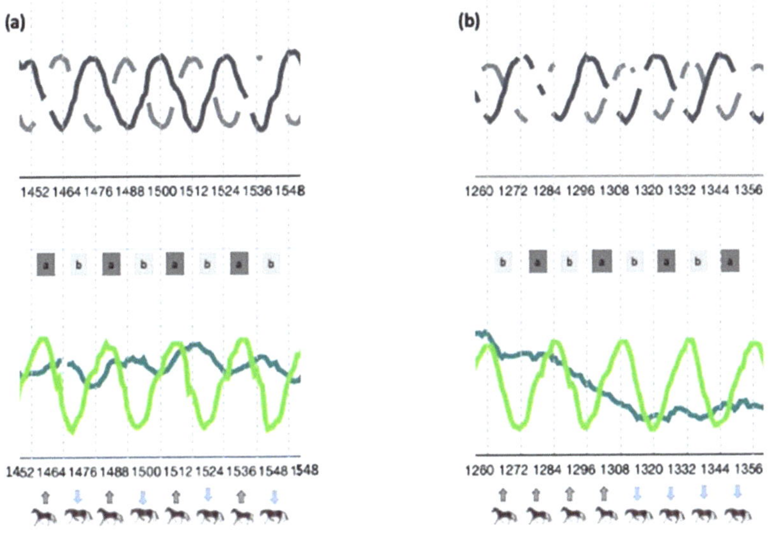

Figure 2. Graphical presentation of forelimb lameness in one representative horse (no. 11) (**a**) compared to a representative non-lame horse (no. 7), (**b**) on a left circle. a in the square = stance phase left forelimb, b in the square = stance phase right forelimb. Grey arrows indicate upward head movement, blue arrows indicate downward head movement. Upper graphs: grey lines show movements of left and right forelimb, with maximum values identifying the protracted foreleg = beginning of the stance phase (stride identification). Lower graphs: dark green line shows head movement, light green line shows movement of left forelimb; the numbers represent the frames of the video in the extracted sequence.

3.2. Hindlimb Lameness

The lameness degrees ranged from AAEP 1–2/5 in four horses and AAEP 3–4/5 in five horses. Five horses were lame on the left hindlimb, four horses were lame on the right hindlimb.

3.2.1. Stifle Reference Point

For every hindlimb-lame and every non-lame horse, the difference D_{St} was calculated. Results are presented in Tables 1 and 2. The median score of all D_{St} of the non-lame group was $\overline{D}_{St}(\text{non}-\text{lame}) = 0.55$ To verify detectability of hindlimb lameness with the stifle as reference point, a correlation between the lameness grade and the calculated D_{St} was constructed. After all videos were analysed, horses 2, 4, 7 and 9, were all classified with severe lameness and showed a clear difference in the calculated D_{St} compared to the median $\overline{D}_{St}$ of the sound group. For horses 3, 5 and 8, graded with subtle lameness, a smaller difference in the calculated D_{St} compared to the median $\overline{D}_{St}$ of the sound group could be illustrated. Therefore, a relation between the degree of lameness and the calculated D_{St} could be shown in all horses, except for horse 1.

Table 1. Stifle reference point—Hindlimb-lame horses.

Horse	Lameness	Degree of Lameness (1–5)		CL/CR	DS_{St}(CL) DS_{St}(CR)	Difference $D_{St} = \mid DS_{St}(CL) - DS_{St}(CR) \mid$	Classified Lame Based on AI
		1–2	3–4				
1	LH		X	CL CR	42.50 44.17	1.67	No
2	RH		X	CL CR	42.17 34.32	7.85	Yes
3	RH	X		CL CR	31.16 29.69	1.47	Yes
4	LH		X	CL CR	47.68 54.61	6.93	Yes
5	RH	X		CL CR	43.32 42.09	1.23	Yes
6	LH	X		CL CR	36.20 38.21	2.01	Yes
7	LH		X	CL CR	48.03 51.12	3.09	Yes
8	LH	X		CL CR	47.36 49.60	2.24	Yes
9	RH		X	CL CR	49.90 38.55	11.35	Yes

RH = Right hindlimb, LH = Left hindlimb, CL = Circle left, CR = Circle right.

Table 2. Stifle reference point—Non-lame horses.

Horse	CL/CR	DS_{St}(CL) DS_{St}(CR)	Difference $D_{St} = \mid DS_{St}(CL) - DS_{St}(CR) \mid$	Classified Sound Based on AI
1	CL CR	38.27 37.76	0.51	Yes
2	CL CR	35.82 34.95	0.87	Yes
3	CL CR	40.44 39.75	0.69	Yes
4	CL CR	46.58 46.51	0.07	Yes
5	CL CR	46.09 45.93	0.16	Yes
6	CL CR	42.35 41.53	0.82	Yes
7	CL CR	37.43 36.19	1.24	No
8	CL CR	40.18 40.18	0.	Yes

In the control group, with a calculated median $\overline{D}_{St} = 0.55$, all horses only showed small divergences in the comparison between CL and CR, except horse number 7.

3.2.2. Tuber Coxae Reference Point

For every hindlimb-lame and every non-lame horse, the difference D_{Tcox} was calculated. The results of the calculated D_{Tcox} for every hindlimb-lame horse are presented in Table 3, with the non-lame group in Table 4. The median score of all D_{Tcox} of the control group was $\overline{D}_{Tcox}$(non-lame) = 1.30. In three out of nine lame horses (horse 3, 5 and 9), the calculated D_{Tcox} corresponded with the lameness, as a larger difference between the measured minima and maxima on the lame side can be shown. In horses 1, 2, 4, 6, 7 and 8, D_{Tcox} indicated lameness on the contralateral non-lame limb. Comparing the median values of the detected lame, the non-detected lame and the non-lame horses, ($\overline{D}_{Tcox}$(lame) = 1.21, $\overline{D}_{Tcox}$(non-detected lame) = 3.08 and $\overline{D}_{Tcox}$(non-lame) = 1.30, respectively); therefore, no correlation between lameness, lameness grade and the absence of lameness could be drawn.

The mean values for SE, SP, ACC, PPV and NPV according to the analysis of the tuber coxae point of nine hindlimb-lame horses and eight non-lame horses are presented in Table 5. In comparison to the clinical assessment, the classification based on AI calculation was perfect (100% SE and SP) for forelimb lameness, close to 90% for hindlimb lameness when using the stifle reference point, but poor for hindlimb lameness when using the tuber coxae reference point (Table 5). The agreement beyond chance (κappa) was $\kappa = 0.92573$. Due to the unreliable results and the inapplicability of tuber coxae as a reference point, it was excluded in this setup. An overall accuracy (OA) of 95.3% could be reached (Table A1).

Table 3. Tuber coxae reference point—Hindlimb-lame horses.

Horse	Lameness	Degree of Lameness (1–5)		CL/CR	DS_{Tcox}(CL) DS_{Tcox}(CR)	Difference $D_{Tcox} = \mid DT_{Tcox}(CL) - DT_{Tcox}(CR) \mid$	Classified Lame Based on AI
		1–2	3–4				
1	LH		X	CL CR	11.29 19.21	7.92	No
2	RH		X	CL CR	13.18 12.17	1.01	No
3	RH	X		CL CR	11.81 14.62	2.81	Yes
4	LH		X	CL CR	15.68 20.89	5.21	No
5	RH	X		CL CR	9.22 9.95	0.73	Yes
6	LH	X		CL CR	11.53 12.13	0.60	No
7	LH		X	CL CR	13.69 15.02	1.33	No
8	LH	X		CL CR	7.98 10.36	2.38	No
9	RH		X	CL CR	11.18 11.27	0.09	Yes

Table 4. Tuber coxae reference point—Non-lame horses.

Horse	CL/CR	DS_{Tcox}(CL) DS_{Tcox}(CR)	Difference $D_{Tcox} = \mid DT_{Tcox}(CL) - DT_{Tcox}(CR) \mid$	Classified Sound Based on AI
1	CL CR	11.13 11.82	0.69	Yes
2	CL CR	12.06 11.55	0.51	Yes
3	CL CR	14.28 19.06	4.78	No
4	CL CR	13.99 14.49	0.50	Yes
5	CL CR	11.38 11.81	0.43	Yes
6	CL CR	9.96 10.64	0.68	Yes
7	CL CR	8.45 9.59	1.14	No
8	CL CR	8.15 9.79	1.64	No

Table 5. Diagnostic test characteristics SE, SP, ACC, PPV and NPV of forelimb and hindlimb classification based on AI calculations when compared to the full clinical assessment (reference) in a study of 22 horses with lameness and eight horses without lameness (calculations of table contents based on Tables A3–A6)).

Test	True Positive	False Positive	False Negative	True Negative	SE (%)	SP (%)	AC (%)	PPV (%)	NPV (%)
Forelimb AI	13	0	0	8	100	100	100	100	100
Hindlimb AI stifle	8	1	1	7	88.9	87.5	88.2	88.9	87.5
Hindlimb AI tuber coxae	3	3	6	5	33.3	62.5	47.1	50	45.4

4. Discussion

In this study, the usability of an AI-based program and its capacity, based on the implementation of pose estimation, to detect specific anatomical landmarks of horses was evaluated. Calculations were made based on these data to differentiate between non-lame and unilateral fore- and hindlimb lame horses. Furthermore, the assessments made based on the program were compared to clinical lameness examination.

We believe that the use of a smartphone application in a real-world, equestrian setting would provide a great advantage to the standard lameness examination. Video analysis is non-invasive, and videos can be obtained at any chosen location with no equipment needed, except for a cell phone camera [29]. The ground surface and training facilities can therefore be those to which the horse is accustomed. This is particularly relevant, as studies have shown adaptations in equine movement and gait when, for example, a treadmill is used [12,47]. Videos obtained using a smartphone are easy to transfer via the internet and can be exchanged with veterinary colleagues all over the globe. Deep learning software is a tool which can help to detect fore- and hindlimb lameness in horses. By applying pose estimation to videos of horses filmed on a circle line and further evaluating the generated data, it is possible to detect lameness without additional hardware.

4.1. Forelimb Lameness

With the application of the reference points on the forelimbs and the head, forelimb lameness was detectable in this study. The data revealed head nodding as a result of increased weightbearing on the non-lame limb during stance. By contrast, horses within the non-lame control group did not show any consistent head movement asymmetry in rhythm with the steps onto the right or left forelimbs. A sensitivity and specificity of 100% shows that, by viewing the graphical charts, it is possible to differentiate a forelimb lame from a non-lame horse with this application. The next step will be a further development of the program to classify the extracted parameters of head and limb movement in relation to the stride time. This will allow calculation of the measured values and the collection of more specific data.

4.2. Hindlimb Lameness

For analysing hindlimb lameness in this setup, different equine anatomical landmarks on the hindlimbs were considered as reference points. In the pre-evaluation, reference points on the tuber coxae and stifle proved to be the most promising in the detection of hindlimb lameness. The tuber coxae have been used as a reference point in various locomotion studies [41,44,45], while the stifle has not been evaluated previously with portable systems in the horse, as it is not feasible to fix an accelerometer onto this point. To the authors' knowledge, it has been used as a reference point only in studies with OMC [42,48].

4.2.1. Stifle

In this study, a correlation between the degree of lameness and the calculated D_{St} could be shown in eight out of nine horses. Horse 1 displayed a slight difference between CL and CR, which did not correspond to its lameness grade (3–4). This horse was a dark-brown Warmblood with a very even-coloured coat. As mentioned below, the colour of the horses, especially when showing little or no variance, influences the accuracy of the reference points and, consequently, the results. Horse 7 of the control group was filmed during sunset in an outdoor riding arena and part of the arena was still covered in sunshine. This can affect the quality of the video with the sunbeams causing a glare effect. As mentioned above, the error rate for data evaluation was higher compared to the training data when these effects were present. Given the resolution of 432 pixels in the vertical axis, this error can make a difference of up to ~1.9%. Consequently, the reference points cannot be detected correctly in a few frames per circle, which results in a higher percentage of inaccurate placement. A sensitivity and specificity of almost 90% when using the stifle reference point provides promising results in this first setup. Using more labelled data will help to improve and stabilise the placement of the markers despite disadvantageous light conditions and horses with less well-defined anatomical landmarks.

4.2.2. Tuber Coxae

On the other hand, the tuber coxae point was not suitable for use with videos of horses on a circle line. Comparing the median values between the horses detected as being lame, the horses not detected as being lame and the non-lame horses, no correlation between lameness, lameness grade and the absence of lameness could be drawn. Other studies have shown that left and right tuber coxae should be compared at the same time to detect asymmetry [42,44,49]. As videos of horses on a circle line only show one side of the horse, a direct comparison using this setup was not possible. Furthermore, the large divergence of the calculated values in the control group confirms the fact that the tuber coxae are not suitable as a reference point for this purpose in the given setup.

Depending on the choice of reference points, the AI-based classification showed high to perfect agreement with the clinical assessment. The use of pose estimation reduces some of the limitations that contemporary lameness analysis systems must cope with. The EquiMoves system® (www.equimoves.nl, accessed on 10 August 2022) uses four sensors on the trunk and one sensor on each limb. It detects upper-body movement asymmetries in horses. In comparison with other systems that employ fewer IMU sensors, it is possible to determine stride length and certain limb angles for pro- and retraction and for ad- and abduction [14]. Nonetheless, the sensors must be fixed onto the horse, and the number of reference points is limited compared to the program evaluated in this study. Another IMU system is the Equinosis Q Lameness Locator®, (Equinosis LLC, Columbia, MO, USA) which uses two accelerometers on the poll and tuber sacrale to measure the vertical maxima and minima of the head and pelvis during movement. A gyroscope attached to the right forelimb detects the stance phase to differentiate between movements of the left and right sides [25,50]. OMC systems such as QHorse from Qualisys Motion Capture Systems® (Qualysis AB, Motion Capture Systems, Göteborg, Sweden) allow marker fixation on different anatomical landmarks of the horse. With the need for a relatively large space to set up the cameras, evaluation and analysis of horses by this method are limited to large clinics and universities, reducing the flexibility and broad use of this system [18,51]. The use of pose estimation for equine gait analysis offers the possibility to record and analyse the movement of almost unlimited anatomical structures on a horse once the program has been adequately trained. Reference points can be selected before and after recording the horse and videos can be taken anywhere, with only a cellphone camera needed on site.

4.3. Limitations

There are some limitations in this study. Sample sizes were small, and larger studies on a broader range of patients are needed to derive robust estimates for SE and SP. To this point, a differentiation of the anatomical origin of lameness is not possible due to small study groups and a limited amount of data. With improvement and advanced training of the program, further studies on the comparison of different causes of lameness are planned.

Using this software on a smartphone device, filming must be standardised, as multiple factors can affect the quality of the videos. As mentioned before, bright sunlight and shade lower the quality of the videos. This problem has also been discussed in other studies [29]. Consequently, the DeepLabCut software has been trained to learn how to robustly extract body parts, even with a cluttered and varying background, inhomogeneous illumination, or camera distortion [36]. In our study, evening light or bright sunshine made filming more difficult, and the analysed data became more imprecise. To evaluate the performance of the tool with videos that were not taken under perfect conditions, different light settings were considered. The horses were filmed inside equestrian arenas with windows and other light sources in different locations, as well as in outside riding arenas with different backgrounds (trees, fields, grass, traffic). Nonetheless, the diversity of videos used to train the AI system needs to be increased.

To find the most suitable filming position, 215 videos were evaluated. It showed that filming the horse, trotting on a straight line, from in front, behind, or from the side, did not offer enough steps for evaluation. However, videos filmed from the inner circle provided good consistency and a sufficient number of strides for analysis. In a complete lameness examination, horses should be evaluated on a straight line and on a circle line [39]. There are differences in motion of the torso and the pelvic area when horses' motions on a straight line and on a circle line are compared [39,52]. With further development and improvement of the program, it should be possible to analyse shorter video sequences on a straight line.

Irregular movements (horses shaking their heads, vocalising or becoming distracted and showing horizontal or vertical head movements) or other horses in the vicinity decreased correct positioning of reference points by the program. This effect did not have much impact on the results, as the chosen videos of horses on a circle line provided sufficient data to evaluate the lameness, despite data outliers.

When the coat or hoof colour of the horse resembled the background, the sand or the ground, it was difficult to recognise the anatomical markers and their locations became imprecise, so they could not be used. The anatomical structures were less prominent in horses that were completely black or white, especially when they were filmed in direct sunlight, so that labelling became demanding or even impossible in some cases, and they had to be excluded from the study. Apart from these rare cases, coat colour did not cause any selection bias; there was variation of colour in all three categories and a large colour spectrum was covered in non-lame and lame horses. The error rate increased when horses were over-weight or had a long winter coat that made anatomical structures less visible. By excluding the maximum and minimum 5% of the measured values, these small errors could be removed from the data. While the reference points were difficult to evaluate under the above circumstances, markers on the "edge" of the horse, as well as on easily visible anatomical structures, such as the nostril, eye or coronary band, were reproducible.

Another limitation was the quality of footing. Deep sand was unstable, causing horses to stumble or show irregular movements that could resemble lameness. This complicates any lameness examination and is not unique to this study. This needs to be considered with regard to the future use of the tool when videos taken by owners or inexperienced veterinarians will be used. As the volume of labelled data grows, the reliability of the program is expected to increase.

Evaluation of error values for training data showed that excluding outliers with a certainty below 60% only reduced the average error from 2.6 pixels down to 2.59 pixels, indicating that it is unlikely to improve with more training on the current model with the same data. It also shows that the network has high uncertainty on unseen evaluation data, which could be solved by having a greater variety of labelled images in the dataset. With additional augmentation through modification of the images, for example, by adding noise or changing colours or brightness, stability in difficult situations could be improved.

Additionally, with more data and different hyperparameters this error can be reduced in future iterations of the neural network.

4.4. Outlook for the Future

Pose estimation has the potential to improve gait analysis and lameness diagnostics in equine medicine and veterinary science. It can be applied to various gait or training assessments and can be used in various species such as horses, dogs, cats and dairy cattle. Studies have shown that dairy farmers do not recognise lameness in their cattle, even though it has a large impact on animal welfare, milk yield and, therefore, emerging costs [53,54]. With the help of this new, easily applicable pose estimation program, objective lameness evaluation can be efficiently executed, offering various possibilities for veterinary students and veterinarians to improve their abilities to assess horses' movements and, therefore, improve welfare for the affected animals [31,55].

Studies have shown that the quality of lameness examination improves with years of work experience, as veterinarians expand their skills and become better in detecting lameness [7]. In addition to these years of training, this tool may serve as a valuable system to improve learning quality and to refine and improve the veterinarian's ability to evaluate equine gait. Experienced veterinarians can use it for confirmation during daily clinical work and to keep records for retrospective evaluation of treatment. With increasingly more data being assessed and used to train the pose estimation tool, it may be possible to detect subtle gait changes, such as mild lameness or ataxia. Another possible use for the tool could be to compare different trainers or training methods. For example, gait analysis using all reference points to show swinging back movements or different swing-phase trajectories could be quantified to assess training efficacy.

5. Conclusions

This study demonstrated the feasibility of obtaining accurate measurements and data that match the clinical presentation in moderately lame horses (grade 3–4/5 AAEP). For horses that were only slightly lame (grade 1–2/5 AAEP), the smartphone app provided less distinct measurements, a sign that the program needs more labelled data and training to become more accurate and reliable. Furthermore, extended studies on the feasibility of the different reference points must be obtained, but these preliminary results are regarded as promising with regard to proof of concept.

Author Contributions: Conceptualization, A.-K.F., S.G.-M., A.M. and T.M.; methodology, S.G.-M. and T.M.; software, T.M.; validation, A.M., A.-K.F. and S.G.-M.; formal analysis, T.M.; investigation, A.-K.F.; resources, A.M., S.G.-M. and A.-K.F.; data curation, T.M. and A.-K.F.; writing—original draft preparation, A.-K.F. and A.M.; writing—review and editing, A.M.; visualization, A.-K.F., A.M. and T.M.; supervision, A.M.; project administration, A.M. and S.G.-M. All authors have read and agreed to the published version of the manuscript.

Funding: This research received no external funding.

Institutional Review Board Statement: The animal study protocol was approved by the Ethics Committee of Ludwig Maximilians University, Munich, Germany. (approval AZ 322-18-08-2022, August 2022).

Informed Consent Statement: Informed consent was obtained from the owners of the horses.

Data Availability Statement: The data presented in this study are available on request from the corresponding author.

Acknowledgments: The authors would like to thank Marcus Doherr and Mathias Raths for valuable comments and help with statistics.

Conflicts of Interest: The authors declare no conflict of interest.

Appendix A

Table A1. Reference points of the program with the correct anatomical location.

Reference Point in the Program	Anatomical Location	Reference Point in the Program	Anatomical Location
1. Nostril	nostril	30. Hoof tip right	hoof tip right forelimb
2. Eye left	left eye	31. Croup middle	midpoint between left and right tuber sacrale
3. Eye right	right eye	32. T. sacrale left	left tuber sacrale
4. Poll	poll	33. T. sacrale right	right tuber sacrale
5. Withers	withers	34. Kink left	midpoint between left tuber coxae and left tuber sacrale (view from behind)
6. Lowest back	lowest part of the dorsal line	35. Kink right	midpoint between right tuber coxae and right tuber sacrale (view from behind)
7. T18/L1	position of the 18th thoracic vertebra/first lumbar vertebra	36. Tail root	tail root
8. Abdomen	deepest part of the abdomen	37. T. coxae left	left tuber coxae
9. Spina scapulae left	scapular spine left	38. T. coxae right	right tuber coxae
10. Spina scapulae right	scapular spine right	39. Coxofemoral joint left	left coxofemoral joint
11 Tub. supraglenoidale left	supraglenoid tubercle left	40. Coxofemoral joint right	right coxofemoral joint
12. Tub. supraglenoidale right	supraglenoid tubercle right	41. T. ischiadicum left	left ischial tuberosity
13. Shoulder joint left	left shoulder joint	42. T. ischiadicum right	right ischial tuberosity
14. Shoulder joint right	right shoulder joint	43. Stifle joint left	left stifle joint
15. Elbow hock left	left elbow hock	44. Stifle joint right	right stifle joint
16. Elbow hock right	right elbow hock	45. Tarsus left	left tarsus
17. Elbow joint left	left elbow joint	46. Tarsus right	right tarsus
18. Elbow joint right	right elbow joint	47. Calcaneus left	left calcaneus
19. Os carpi accessorium left	left accessory carpal bone	48. Calcaneus right	right calcaneus
20. Os carpi accessorium right	right accessory carpal bone	49. Fetlock left	fetlock left hindlimb
21. Carpus left	left carpus	50. Fetlock right	fetlock right hindlimb
22. Carpus right	right carpus	51. Coronary band dorsal left	dorsal part of the coronet band left hindlimb
23. Fetlock left	fetlock left forelimb	52. Coronary band dorsal right	dorsal part of the coronet band right hindlimb
24. Fetlock right	fetlock right forelimb	53. Coronary band plantar left	plantar part of the coronet band left hindlimb
25. Coronary band dorsal left	dorsal part of the coronet band left forelimb	54. Coronary band plantar right	plantar part of the coronet band right hindlimb
26. Coronary band dorsal right	dorsal part of the coronet band right forelimb	55. Hoof pad left	heel bulb left hindlimb
27. Coronary band palmar left	palmar part of the coronet band left forelimb	56. Hoof pad right	heel bulb right hindlimb
28. Coronary band palmar right	palmar part of the coronet band left forelimb	57. Hoof tip left	hoof tip left hindlimb
29. Hoof tip left	hoof tip left forelimb	58. Hoof tip right	hoof tip right hindlimb

Table A2. Horses of Groups 1–3 (classified into sex, median age, median height, breed and colour).

		Group 1	Group 2	Group 3
Total Number		**65**	**22**	**8**
Sex	Mare	24	13	3
	Gelding	41	9	5
Median Age (in years)		13.8	11.6	12.4
Median Height (in meter)		1.60	1.61	1.62
Breeds	Warmblood	31	16	6
	Quarter Horse	7		
	PRE	5		
	Lusitano	3		
	Friese	1		
	Pinto	2		
	Knabstrupper	1		
	Arabian	1	1	
	Lewitzer	1		
	Haflinger	1		
	German Riding Pony	12	5	2
Colours	Black	8	1	
	Dark Bay	10	7	3
	Bay	11	6	3
	Chestnut	15	5	2
	Flaxen Chestnut	3		
	Buckskin	1		
	Palomino	3		
	Grey	4		
	White	4	2	
	Tobiano	5		
	Leopard	1	1	

Table A3. 3 × 3-Table and statistical evaluation of κ (without reference point tuber coxae).

	Classified by AI Non-Lame	Classified by AI Forelimb-Lame	Classified by AI Hindlimb-Lame Stifle	Total
Clinically non-lame	20	0	1	**21**
Clinically forelimb-lame	0	13	0	**13**
Clinically hindlimb-lame stifle	1	0	8	**9**
Total	**21**	**13**	**9**	43

Appendix B

Table A4. Statistical classification of horses with and without forelimb lameness.

Forelimb Lameness	Clinically Forelimb-Lame	Clinically Non-Lame	Total	
AI classified as forelimb-lame	13	0	**13**	Positive predictive value **1**
AI classified as non-lame	0	8	**8**	Negative predictive value **1**
Total	**13**	**8**	21	
AI diagnostic test evaluation	Sensitivity of AI **1**	Specificity of AI **1**	Accuracy of AI **1**	

Table A5. Stifle reference point—Statistical classification of horses with and without hindlimb lameness.

Hindlimb Lameness Stifle	Clinically Hindlimb-Lame	Clinically Non-Lame	Total	
AI classified as hindlimb-lame	8	1	**9**	Positive predictive value **0.888888889**
AI classified as non-lame	1	7	**8**	Negative predictive value **0.875**
Total	**9**	**8**	17	
AI diagnostic test evaluation	Sensitivity of AI **0.888888889**	Specificity of AI **0.875**	Accuracy of AI **0.882352941**	

Table A6. Tuber coxae reference point—Statistical classification of horses with and without hindlimb lameness.

Hindlimb Lameness Tuber Coxae	Clinically Hindlimb-Lame	Clinically Non-Lame	Total	
AI classified as hindlimb-lame	3	3	**6**	Positive predictive value **0.5**
AI classified as non-lame	6	5	**11**	Negative predictive value **0.454545455**
Total	9	**8**	17	
AI diagnostic test evaluation	Sensitivity of AI **0.333333333**	Specificity of AI **0.625**	Accuracy of AI **0.470588235**	

References

1. Seitzinger, A.H. A comparison of the economic costs of equine lameness, colic, and equine protozoal myeloencephalitis (EPM). In Proceedings of the 9th International Symposium on Veterinary Epidemiology and Economics, Breckenridge, CO, USA, 6–11 August 2000; pp. 1–4.
2. Nielsen, T.D.; Dean, R.S.; Robinson, N.J.; Massey, A.; Brennan, M.L. Survey of the UK veterinary profession: Common species and conditions nominated by veterinarians in practice. *Vet. Rec.* **2014**, *174*, 324. [CrossRef] [PubMed]
3. USDA. *Part I: Baseline Reference of 1998 Equine Health and Management*; USDA: Washington, DC, USA, 1998; p. N280.898.

4. Slater, J. *National Equine Health Survey (NEHS) 2016*; Blue Cross for Pets: Burford, UK, 2016.
5. Muller-Quirin, J.; Dittmann, M.T.; Roepstorff, C.; Arpagaus, S.; Latif, S.N.; Weishaupt, M.A. Riding Soundness-Comparison of Subjective With Objective Lameness Assessments of Owner-Sound Horses at Trot on a Treadmill. *J. Equine Vet. Sci.* **2020**, *95*, 103314. [CrossRef] [PubMed]
6. Dyson, S.; Pollard, D. Application of a Ridden Horse Pain Ethogram and Its Relationship with Gait in a Convenience Sample of 60 Riding Horses. *Animals* **2020**, *10*, 1044. [CrossRef] [PubMed]
7. Starke, S.D.; May, S.A. Veterinary student competence in equine lameness recognition and assessment: A mixed methods study. *Vet. Rec.* **2017**, *181*, 168. [CrossRef]
8. Keegan, K.G.; Dent, E.V.; Wilson, D.A.; Janicek, J.; Kramer, J.; Lacarrubba, A.; Walsh, D.M.; Cassells, M.W.; Esther, T.M.; Schiltz, P.; et al. Repeatability of subjective evaluation of lameness in horses. *Equine Vet. J.* **2010**, *42*, 92–97. [CrossRef]
9. Fuller, C.J.; Bladon, B.M.; Driver, A.J.; Barr, A.R. The intra- and inter-assessor reliability of measurement of functional outcome by lameness scoring in horses. *Vet. J.* **2006**, *171*, 281–286. [CrossRef]
10. Parkes, R.S.; Weller, R.; Groth, A.M.; May, S.; Pfau, T. Evidence of the development of 'domain-restricted' expertise in the recognition of asymmetric motion characteristics of hindlimb lameness in the horse. *Equine Vet. J.* **2009**, *41*, 112–117. [CrossRef]
11. Arkell, M.; Archer, R.M.; Guitian, F.J.; May, S.A. Evidence of bias affecting the interpretation of the results of local anaesthetic nerve blocks when assessing lameness in horses. *Vet. Rec.* **2006**, *159*, 346–349. [CrossRef]
12. Back, W.; Clayton, H.M. 1. History. In *Equine Locomotion*, 2nd ed.; van Weeren, P.R., Ed.; Saunders Elsevier: Edinburgh, UK; New York, NY, USA, 2013; pp. 1–30.
13. Keegan, K.G. Evidence-based lameness detection and quantification. *Vet. Clin. North Am. Equine Pract.* **2007**, *23*, 403–423. [CrossRef]
14. Bosch, S.; Serra Bragança, F.; Marin-Perianu, M.; Marin-Perianu, R.; van der Zwaag, B.J.; Voskamp, J.; Back, W.; van Weeren, R.; Havinga, P. EquiMoves: A Wireless Networked Inertial Measurement System for Objective Examination of Horse Gait. *Sensors* **2018**, *18*, 850. [CrossRef]
15. Weishaupt, M.A.; Hogg, H.P.; Wiestner, T.; Denoth, J.; Stussi, E.; Auer, J.A. Instrumented treadmill for measuring vertical ground reaction forces in horses. *Am. J. Vet. Res.* **2002**, *63*, 520–527. [CrossRef] [PubMed]
16. Back, W.; Clayton, H.M. 9. Gait Adaption in Lameness. In *Equine Locomotion*; Buchner, H.H., Ed.; Saunders Elsevier: Edinburgh, UK; New York, NY, USA, 2013; pp. 175–197.
17. Morris, E.; Seeherman, H. Redistribution of ground reaction forces in experimentally induced equine carpal lameness. In *Equine Exercise Physiology*; Wiley: Hoboken, NJ, USA, 1987; pp. 553–563.
18. Byström, A.; Egenvall, A.; Roepstorff, L.; Rhodin, M.; Bragança, F.S.; Hernlund, E.; van Weeren, R.; Weishaupt, M.A.; Clayton, H.M. Biomechanical findings in horses showing asymmetrical vertical excursions of the withers at walk. *PLoS ONE* **2018**, *13*, e0204548. [CrossRef] [PubMed]
19. Oosterlinck, M.; Pille, F.; Huppes, T.; Gasthuys, F.; Back, W. Comparison of pressure plate and force plate gait kinetics in sound Warmbloods at walk and trot. *Vet. J.* **2010**, *186*, 347–351. [CrossRef] [PubMed]
20. Keegan, K.G. Objective measures of lameness evaluation. In Proceedings of the American College of Veterinary Surgeons Symposium, National Harbor, MD, USA, 1–3 November 2012; pp. 127–131.
21. Serra Bragança, F.M.; Rhodin, M.; van Weeren, P.R. On the brink of daily clinical application of objective gait analysis: What evidence do we have so far from studies using an induced lameness model? *Vet. J.* **2018**, *234*, 11–23. [CrossRef]
22. Keegan, K.G.; Yonezawa, Y.; Pai, P.F.; Wilson, D.A.; Kramer, J. Evaluation of a sensor-based system of motion analysis for detection and quantification of forelimb and hind limb lameness in horses. *Am. J. Vet. Res.* **2004**, *65*, 665–670. [CrossRef] [PubMed]
23. Barrey, E. Methods, applications and limitations of gait analysis in horses. *Vet. J.* **1999**, *157*, 7–22. [CrossRef]
24. Rhodin, M.; Persson-Sjodin, E.; Egenvall, A.; Serra Bragança, F.M.; Pfau, T.; Roepstorff, L.; Weishaupt, M.A.; Thomsen, M.H.; van Weeren, P.R.; Hernlund, E. Vertical movement symmetry of the withers in horses with induced forelimb and hindlimb lameness at trot. *Equine Vet. J.* **2018**, *50*, 818–824. [CrossRef]
25. Keegan, K.G.; Kramer, J.; Yonezawa, Y.; Maki, H.; Pai, P.F.; Dent, E.V.; Kellerman, T.E.; Wilson, D.A.; Reed, S.K. Assessment of repeatability of a wireless, inertial sensor-based lameness evaluation system for horses. *Am. J. Vet. Res.* **2011**, *72*, 1156–1163. [CrossRef]
26. Titterton, D.; Weston, J. 4 Gyroscope Technology 1. In *Strapdown Inertial Navigation Technology*; Institution of Engineering and Technology: London, UK, 2004; pp. 59–112.
27. van Weeren, P.R.; Pfau, T.; Rhodin, M.; Roepstorff, L.; Serra Bragança, F.; Weishaupt, M.A. Do we have to redefine lameness in the era of quantitative gait analysis? *Equine Vet. J.* **2017**, *49*, 567–569. [CrossRef]
28. van Weeren, P.R.; Pfau, T.; Rhodin, M.; Roepstorff, L.; Serra Bragança, F.; Weishaupt, M.A. What is lameness and what (or who) is the gold standard to detect it? *Equine Vet. J.* **2018**, *50*, 549–551. [CrossRef]
29. Mathis, A.; Mamidanna, P.; Cury, K.M.; Abe, T.; Murthy, V.N.; Mathis, M.W.; Bethge, M. DeepLabCut: Markerless pose estimation of user-defined body parts with deep learning. *Nat. Neurosci.* **2018**, *21*, 1281–1289. [CrossRef] [PubMed]
30. LeCun, Y.; Bengio, Y.; Hinton, G. Deep learning. *Nature* **2015**, *521*, 436–444. [CrossRef] [PubMed]
31. Kil, N.; Ertelt, K.; Auer, U. Development and Validation of an Automated Video Tracking Model for Stabled Horses. *Animals* **2020**, *10*, 2258. [CrossRef] [PubMed]

32. Banzato, T.; Wodzinski, M.; Burti, S.; Osti, V.L.; Rossoni, V.; Atzori, M.; Zotti, A. Automatic classification of canine thoracic radiographs using deep learning. *Sci. Rep.* **2021**, *11*, 3964. [CrossRef] [PubMed]
33. May, A.; Gesell-May, S.; Muller, T.; Ertel, W. Artificial intelligence as a tool to aid in the differentiation of equine ophthalmic diseases with an emphasis on equine uveitis. *Equine Vet. J.* **2022**, *54*, 847–855. [CrossRef]
34. Insafutdinov, E.; Andriluka, M.; Pishchulin, L. ArtTrack: Articulated Multi-Person Tracking in the Wild. In Proceedings of the IEEE Conference on Computer Vision and Pattern Recognition, Honolulu, HI, USA, 21–26 July 2017; pp. 6457–6465. [CrossRef]
35. Cao, Z.; Simon, T.; Wei, S.-E. Realtime Multi-person 2D Pose Estimation Using Part Affinity Fields. In Proceedings of the IEEE Conference on Computer Vision and Pattern Recognition, Honolulu, HI, USA, 21–26 July 2017.
36. Nath, T.; Mathis, A.; Chen, A.C.; Patel, A.; Bethge, M.; Mathis, M.W. Using DeepLabCut for 3D markerless pose estimation across species and behaviors. *Nat. Protoc.* **2019**, *14*, 2152–2176. [CrossRef]
37. Andriluka, M.; Pishchulin, L.; Gehler, P. 2D Human Pose Estimation: New Benchmark and State of the Art Analysis. In Proceedings of the IEEE Conference on computer Vision and Pattern Recognition, Columbus, OH, USA, 23–28 June 2014.
38. Keegan, K.G.; Wilson, D.A.; Kramer, J.; Reed, S.K.; Yonezawa, Y.; Maki, H.; Pai, P.F.; Lopes, M.A. Comparison of a body-mounted inertial sensor system-based method with subjective evaluation for detection of lameness in horses. *Am. J. Vet. Res.* **2013**, *74*, 17–24. [CrossRef]
39. Baxter, G.M.; Adams, O.R.; Stashak, T.S. *Adams and Stashak's Lameness in Horses*, 6th ed.; Wiley-Blackwell: Chichester, UK; Ames, IA, USA, 2011; p. xxviii. 1242p.
40. Ross, M.W.; Dyson, S.J. *Diagnosis and Management of Lameness in the Horse*, 2nd ed.; Saunders: St. Louis, MO, USA, 2011.
41. Buchner, H.H.; Savelberg, H.H.; Schamhardt, H.C.; Barneveld, A. Head and trunk movement adaptations in horses with experimentally induced fore- or hindlimb lameness. *Equine Vet. J.* **1996**, *28*, 71–76. [CrossRef]
42. Kramer, J.; Keegan, K.G.; Wilson, D.A.; Smith, B.K.; Wilson, D.J. Kinematics of the hind limb in trotting horses after induced lameness of the distal intertarsal and tarsometatarsal joints and intra-articular administration of anesthetic. *Am. J. Vet. Res.* **2000**, *61*, 1031–1036. [CrossRef]
43. Buchner, H.H.; Savelberg, H.H.; Schamhardt, H.C.; Barneveld, A. Limb movement adaptations in horses with experimentally induced fore- or hindlimb lameness. *Equine Vet. J.* **1996**, *28*, 63–70. [CrossRef]
44. May, S.A.; Wyn-Jones, G. Identification of hindleg lameness. *Equine Vet. J.* **1987**, *19*, 185–188. [CrossRef] [PubMed]
45. Church, E.E.; Walker, A.M.; Wilson, A.M.; Pfau, T. Evaluation of discriminant analysis based on dorsoventral symmetry indices to quantify hindlimb lameness during over ground locomotion in the horse. *Equine Vet. J.* **2009**, *41*, 304–308. [CrossRef] [PubMed]
46. Altman, D.G. *Practical Statistics for Medical Research*; Chapman & Hall/CRC: London, UK, 1999; p. XII. 611p.
47. Buchner, H.H.; Savelberg, H.H.; Schamhardt, H.C.; Merkens, H.W.; Barneveld, A. Kinematics of treadmill versus overground locomotion in horses. *Vet. Q.* **1994**, *16* (Suppl. 2), S87–S90. [CrossRef]
48. Audigié, F.; Pourcelot, P.; Degueurce, C.; Geiger, D.; Denoix, J.M. Kinematic analysis of the symmetry of limb movements in lame trotting horses. *Equine Vet. J. Suppl.* **2001**, *33*, 128–134. [CrossRef]
49. Kramer, J.; Keegan, K.G.; Kelmer, G.; Wilson, D.A. Objective determination of pelvic movement during hind limb lameness by use of a signal decomposition method and pelvic height differences. *Am. J. Vet. Res.* **2004**, *65*, 741–747. [CrossRef] [PubMed]
50. Leelamankong, P.; Estrada, R.; Mählmann, K.; Rungsri, P.; Lischer, C. Agreement among equine veterinarians and between equine veterinarians and inertial sensor system during clinical examination of hindlimb lameness in horses. *Equine Vet. J.* **2020**, *52*, 326–331. [CrossRef]
51. Hardeman, A.M.; Serra Bragança, F.M.; Swagemakers, J.H.; van Weeren, P.R.; Roepstorff, L. Variation in gait parameters used for objective lameness assessment in sound horses at the trot on the straight line and the lunge. *Equine Vet. J.* **2019**, *51*, 831–839. [CrossRef] [PubMed]
52. Rhodin, M.; Pfau, T.; Roepstorff, L.; Egenvall, A. Effect of lungeing on head and pelvic movement asymmetry in horses with induced lameness. *Vet. J.* **2013**, *198* (Suppl. 1), e39–e45. [CrossRef]
53. Whay, H.R.; Main, D.C.; Green, L.E.; Webster, A.J. Assessment of the welfare of dairy cattle using animal-based measurements: Direct observations and investigation of farm records. *Vet. Rec.* **2003**, *153*, 197–202. [CrossRef]
54. Whay, H.R.; Shearer, J.K. The Impact of Lameness on Welfare of the Dairy Cow. *Vet. Clin. N. Am. Food Anim. Pract.* **2017**, *33*, 153–164. [CrossRef]
55. Haubro Andersen, P.; Bech Gleerup, K.; Wathan, J. Can a Machine Learn to See Horse Pain?: An Interdisciplinary Approach Towards Automated Decoding of Facial Expressions of Pain in the Horse. *Animals* **2018**, *11*, 1643. [CrossRef]

MDPI AG
Grosspeteranlage 5
4052 Basel
Switzerland
Tel.: +41 61 683 77 34

Animals Editorial Office
E-mail: animals@mdpi.com
www.mdpi.com/journal/animals

www.ingramcontent.com/pod-product-compliance
Lightning Source LLC
Chambersburg PA
CBHW041403210926
51850CB00013B/3160
* 9 7 8 3 7 2 5 8 4 1 3 1 8 *